The Academic Health Center

Leadership and Performance

The leadership and management of academic health centers present challenges as complex as any in the corporate environment. A consensus is emerging about their integrated mission of education, research, and service, and this book, focusing on value-driven management, is the most up-to-date and comprehensive review of these issues available.

Based on reports produced by the Blue Ridge Academic Health Group, which has developed a framework for meeting the challenges of improving health in the twenty-first century, it also contains invited commentaries and case studies from leading authorities in and beyond the United States. It identifies the public policies and organizational practices required to maximize the health status of individuals and the population, and highlights innovative practices.

It is essential reading for managers and leaders of clinical and basic science departments in academic health centers, and for all those involved in health systems management studies.

Don E. Detmer is Professor of Medical Education at the University of Virginia, Senior Scholar at the Judge Institute of Management Studies, University of Cambridge, and President and Chief Executive Officer of the American Medical Informatics Association. He founded the Blue Ridge Academic Health Group in 1997, and has served as the CEO of the Health Sciences Centers of the Universities of Utah and Virginia.

Elaine B. Steen is a health policy analyst affiliated with the University of Virginia, and served as project manager and editor of the Blue Ridge Academic Health Group.

The
Academic Health Center

Leadership and Performance

Edited by

Don E. Detmer

University of Virginia, Cambridge University

Elaine B. Steen

University of Virginia

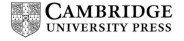

CAMBRIDGE UNIVERSITY PRESS
Cambridge, New York, Melbourne, Madrid, Cape Town, Singapore, São Paulo

Cambridge University Press
The Edinburgh Building, Cambridge, CB2 2RU, UK

Published in the United States of America by Cambridge University Press, New York

www.cambridge.org
Information on this title: www.cambridge.org/9780521827188

First published 2005

Printed in the United Kingdom at the University Press, Cambridge

Typefaces Minion 11/14 pt. and Helvetica   *System* LaTeX 2_ε [TB]

A catalog record for this book is available from the British Library

Library of Congress Cataloging in Publication data
The Academic Health Center: Leadership and Performance
edited by Don E. Detmer, Elaine B. Steen.
    p.   cm.
Includes bibliographical references and index.
ISBN 0 521 82718 3 (alk. paper)
1. Academic medical centers – United States – Administration.   I. Detmer, Don E. II.
Steen, Elaine B.
RA966.O68   2005
362.12′068 – dc22   2004054620

ISBN 0 521 82718 3 hardback
ISBN 978-0-521-82718-8 hardback

Contents

Figures

Tables

Foreword

Roger J. Bulger, M.D. and Jordan J. Cohen, M.D.

The leadership and management of academic health centers are increasingly in the spotlight during these uncertain times at the dawn of the 21st century. Many business leaders and management experts have openly recognized the more complex array of challenges that face chief executive officers of academic health centers (AHCs) compared with those faced by the average corporate leader. It has been repeatedly shown to be exceedingly difficult to implement standard business management strategies within the environment that has evolved from the deeply rooted culture of American university-based AHCs.

Great leaders are often depicted as shepherds, but great shepherds lead flocks of sheep or cows, accustomed to work together in going where the shepherd leads. Great shepherds do not shepherd cats, but herding cats is in fact one over-simplified way of describing the leadership and management challenge facing AHCs. We need leaders and management tools that can get cats to work as a team for institutional goals. AHC leaders need to create an organizational culture with incentives sufficient to sustain required integration. The culture must foster coordination and collaboration not only among individual cats, but also among the several species of cats composing the various silos typical of our academic centers. How to herd academic health center cats is one of the themes this book addresses.

Clearly, many changes have occurred and much progress has been made over the past decade in re-shaping our academic organizations to meet their challenges. We must not lose sight of that. However, the past decade also has witnessed both an escalation of new threats and challenges and an unprecedented expansion of our scientific horizons and technological achievements. Indeed, some of our greatest successes have sown the seeds of much of our current fiscal fragility. This book addresses that theme as well.

Roger J. Bulger is President and Chief Executive Officer of the Association of Academic Health Centers. Jordan J. Cohen is President and Chief Executive Officer of the Association of American Medical Colleges.

A consensus is emerging about the leadership and management issues with which academic health centers of the future must be prepared to deal. These issues include, but are not limited to the following challenges.

- AHCs must manage to the individual missions of education, research, and service (both health care and community service). These separate missions require individual business plans, but also need a strategy for integration across the missions to serve the overall purposes of the center.
- Fiscal and outcomes data must be transparent in a "learning" organization.
- The evolving focus on patient-centered care and improving population health is the central starting point for service, for discovery, and for workforce development. This new focus leads to new or modified action agendas and organizational functions and structures.
- Finding and deploying the resources, fiscal and otherwise, to fuel the cultural modifications required for the desired changes will be perhaps the greatest challenge.

This book represents the most up-to-date and comprehensive review of these issues to be found in one place. It underscores a new leadership slogan, "Value-Driven Management," and produces a credible vision about the growing potential of information technologies to help construct an effective herd out of the wonderfully productive and creative individual cats who energize our academic health centers. The editors deserve our gratitude for pulling together so many vital issues.

Acknowledgments

We would like to thank the individuals and organizations that participated in the remarkable collaborative process that created this book. We begin by recognizing and thanking the members of the Blue Ridge Academic Health Group who generously shared their time and expertise during the preparation of the reports on which this volume is based. These individuals brought a critical view and sense of urgency to their deliberations that enabled them to challenge the status quo. We thank the invited participants who enlightened and broadened the dialogue with their expertise and perspectives. We also thank the current members of the Blue Ridge Academic Health Group who continue to work to help academic health centers create greater value for society. These individuals are listed below.

We greatly appreciate the willingness of the authors of the new chapters, case studies, and commentaries to help us expand upon the original work of the Blue Ridge Group. We would also like to recognize the contributions of Jon Saxton who drafted and edited the original reports on organizational culture and e-health on behalf of the Blue Ridge Group.

We gratefully acknowledge the support of Cap Gemini Ernst & Young US, LLC, the University of Virginia, and Emory University in providing financial and in-kind support for the Blue Ridge Group. The support of Cambridge University Press has been crucial and a special thanks goes to Richard Barling, Joseph Bottrill and Sarah Price for their help.

Charlotte Ott deserves particular recognition for all of her administrative support for the Blue Ridge Group and for holding down the fort in Charlottesville while we worked on this manuscript from Cambridge University and North Carolina. Finally, we thank our spouses, Mary Helen and Bruce, for the patience and support they have shown to us over the years as we have collaborated on this work and on related health policy studies, especially with respect to health information technology.

As the co-editors of this volume, we have sought to capture the sense of the Blue Ridge Reports and add additional content to advance its themes. Any failure in this regard is solely our responsibility and not that of the Blue Ridge Group or its members.

BLUE RIDGE ACADEMIC HEALTH GROUP MEMBERS, 1997–2001

David Blumenthal, M.D., M.P.P., Samuel, O. Thier Professor of Medicine and Health Policy, Harvard Medical School; Director, Institute for Health Policy, Massachusetts General Hospital/Partners Health Care System

Enriqueta C. Bond, Ph.D., President, The Burroughs Wellcome Fund

Roger J. Bulger, M.D., President and Chief Executive Officer, Association of Academic Health Centers (rotating member)

Robert W. Cantrell, M.D., Director, Virginia Health Policy Center, University of Virginia Health System (retired)

Jordan J. Cohen, M.D., President and Chief Executive Officer, Association of American Medical Colleges (rotating member)

*Don E. Detmer, M.D., Professor of Medical Education, University of Virginia; Senior Associate, Judge Institute of Management Studies, University of Cambridge; President and Chief Executive Officer, American Medical Informatics Association

Michael A. Geheb, M.D., Professor of Medicine, and Vice President for Institutional Advancement, Oregon Health & Science University

Jeff C. Goldsmith, Ph.D., President Health Futures, Inc.

Michael M. E. Johns, M.D., Executive Vice President of Health Affairs, Emory University; Chief Executive Officer, Robert W. Woodruff Health Sciences Center

Peter O. Kohler, M.D., President, Oregon Health & Sciences University

Edward D. Miller, Jr., M.D., Chief Executive Officer, Johns Hopkins Medicine; Dean, Medical Faculty, The Johns Hopkins University

John G. Nackel, Ph.D., Executive Vice President, US Technology Resources

Jeff Otten, Chief Executive Officer, Brigham & Women's Hospital

Mark L. Penkhus, M.H.A., M.B.A., Senior Vice President and Chief Development Officer, Sheridan Healthcorp

Paul L. Ruflin, Vice President, Health Managed Care, Cap Gemini Ernst & Young US, LLC

George F. Sheldon, M.D., Professor of Surgery and Social Medicine, Chair of Surgery (1984–2001), University of North Carolina Chapel Hill

Katherine W. Vestal, Ph.D., Cap Gemini Ernst & Young US, LLC

INVITED PARTICIPANTS 1997–2001

(Affiliations listed are those at time of Blue Ridge Group meetings)

Ron J. Anderson, M.D., President and Chief Executive Officer, Parkland Health and Hospital System

*Chair

Gerard N. Burrow, M.D., Special Advisor to the President, David Paige Smith Professor of Medicine, Yale University

David J. Campbell, Chief Executive Officer and President, Detroit Medical Center

Richard Couto, Ph.D., Chair, Leadership Studies, Jepson School, University of Richmond

Haile Debas, M.D., Executive Director, Global Health Sciences, Chancellor and Dean Emeritus, University of California San Francisco

Tipton Ford, Senior Partner, Cap Gemini Ernst & Young US, LLC

Mark Frisse, M.D., M.S., M.B.A., Associate Dean for Academic Information Management, Associate Professor of Medicine, Adjunct Professor of Health Management and Information Systems, Washington University School of Medicine

Arthur (Tim) Garson, Jr., M.D., M.P.H., Senior Vice President and Dean for Academic Operations, Professor of Cardiology, Baylor College of Medicine; Vice President, Texas Children's Hospital

John P. Glaser, Ph.D., Vice President and Chief Information Officer, Partners HealthCare System

Dennis Gillings, Ph.D., Chairman and Chief Executive Officer, Quintiles Transnational Corporation

Michael J. Goran, M.D., Partner, Cap Gemini Ernst & Young US, LLC

Mary Jane Kagarise, R. N., M.S.P.H., Associate Chair of Surgery, School of Medicine, University of North Carolina

John Lynch, Vice President, Human Resource, Medical Systems, General Electric Corporation

Gabriele McLaughlin, M.B.A., Senior Advisor, Xerox Corporation

John G. Peetz, Jr., Partner, Chief Knowledge Officer, Cap Gemini Ernst & Young US, LLC

Stephanie Reel, Vice President Information Services, Johns Hopkins Medicine

Jay E. Toole, Partner, Health Care Consulting, Cap Gemini Ernst & Young US, LLC

Andrew Vaz, Partner, Cap Gemini Ernst & Young US, LLC

CURRENT BLUE RIDGE ACADEMIC HEALTH GROUP MEMBERS

David Blumenthal, M.D., M.P.P., Samuel O. Thier Professor of Medicine and Health Policy, Harvard Medical School; Director, Institute for Health Policy, Massachusetts General Hospital/Partners Health Care System

Enriqueta C. Bond, Ph.D., President, The Burroughs Wellcome Fund

Roger J. Bulger, M.D., President and Chief Executive Officer, Association of Academic Health Centers (rotating member)

Jordan J. Cohen, M.D., President and Chief Executive Officer, Association of American Medical Colleges (rotating member)

Catherine DeAngelis, M.D., M.P.H., Editor, *Journal of the American Medical Association*

Haile Debas, M.D., Executive Director, Global Health Sciences, Chancellor and Dean Emeritus, University of California San Francisco

*Don E. Detmer, M.D., Professor of Medical Education, University of Virginia; Senior Associate, Judge Institute of Management Studies, University of Cambridge; President and Chief Executive Officer, American Medical Informatics Association

Michael A. Geheb, M.D., Professor of Medicine and Vice President for Institutional Advancement, Oregon Health & Science University

Steven Lipstein, President and Chief Executive Officer, BJC HealthCare

*Michael M. E. Johns, M.D., Executive Vice President of Health Affairs, Emory University; Chief Executive Officer, Robert W. Woodruff Health Sciences Center

Peter O. Kohler, M.D., President, Oregon Health & Sciences University

Jeffrey P. Koplan, M.D., M.P.H., Vice President for Academic Health Affairs, Emory University

Lawrence Lewin, Executive Consultant

Arthur Rubenstein, M.B.B.Ch., Dean, Executive Vice President, University of Pennsylvania School of Medicine

George F. Sheldon, M.D., Professor of Surgery and Social Medicine, Chair of Surgery (1984–2001), University of North Carolina Chapel Hill

*Co-chairs

Contributors

Ron J. Anderson, M.D.
President and Chief Executive Officer
Parkland Health and Hospital System

Cynthia L. Bero, M.P.H.
Chief Information Officer
Partners Community Healthcare, Inc.

David Blumenthal, M.D.
Samuel O. Thier Professor of Medicine
    and Health Policy
Harvard Medical School
Director, Institute for Health Policy
Massachusetts General
    Hospital/Partners Health Care System

Enriqueta C. Bond, Ph.D.
President
The Burroughs Wellcome Fund

Jim Brophy
PatientSite Project Leader
CareGroup Healthcare System

Roger J. Bulger, M.D.
President and CEO
Association of Academic Health Centers

Jordan J. Cohen, M.D.
President and CEO
Association of American Medical
    Colleges

Haile Debas, M.D.
Executive Director
Global Health Sciences
Chancellor and Dean Emeritus
University of California
    San Francisco

David Delaney, M.D.
Technical Director, Web Applications
CareGroup Healthcare System

Don E. Detmer, M.D.
Professor of Medical Education
University of Virginia
Senior Associate
Judge Institute of Management Studies
University of Cambridge
President and Chief Executive Officer
American Medical Informatics
    Association

Sherrilynne Fuller, Ph.D.
Professor
Biomedical and Health Informatics
School of Medicine
Director
Health Sciences Libraries
University of Washington

Robert Galvin, M.D.
Director, Global Healthcare
General Electric

Arthur (Tim) Garson, Jr., M.D., M.P.H.
Vice President and Dean
School of Medicine
University of Virginia

Michael A. Geheb, M.D.
Professor of Medicine
Senior Vice President for Clinical
    Programs
Oregon Health & Science University

John P. Glaser, Ph.D.
Vice President and Chief Information
    Officer
Partners HealthCare System

R. Edward Howell
Vice President and Chief Executive
    Officer
University of Virginia Medical Center

Michael M.E. Johns, M.D.
Executive Vice President of Health
    Affairs
Emory University

Robert P. Kelch, M.D.
Executive Vice President for Medical
    Affairs
University of Michigan

Michael G. Kienzle, M.D.
Special Assistant to the Dean
Director, Office of Economic and
    Business Development
Roy J. and Lucille A. Carver College of
    Medicine
University of Iowa

Peter O. Kohler, M.D.
President
Oregon Health & Science University

Alice Lee
Vice President of Clinical
    Systems
CareGroup Healthcare System

Steven Lipstein
President and Chief Executive
    Officer
BJC HealthCare

Edward D. Miller, Jr., M.D.
Chief Executive Officer
Johns Hopkins Medicine
Dean, Medical Faculty
The Johns Hopkins University

J. Michael McCoy, M.D.
Chief Information Officer, UCLA
    Healthcare
Associate Professor of Medicine
David Geffen School of Medicine at
    UCLA

John G. Nackel, Ph.D.
Executive Vice President
US Technology Resources

Mark L. Penkhus, M.H.A., M.B.A.
Senior Vice President and Development
    Officer
Sheridan Healthcorp

Sue Pickens, M.Ed.
Director of Strategic Planning and
    Population Medicine
Parkland Health and Hospital
    System

Jonathan F. Saxton, J.D.
Health Policy Analyst
Emory University

Steven Shea, M.D., M.S.
Professor of Medicine and Epidemiology
   (in Biomedical Informatics)
Chief, Division of General Medicine
Columbia University

George F. Sheldon, M.D., FACS,
FRCS(Edin), FRCS(Eng)Hon
Professor of Surgery and Social
   Medicine
Chair of Surgery (1984–2001)
   School of Medicine
University of North Carolina Chapel
   Hill

Tom Smith
Senior Policy Analsyst
Health Policy and Economic Research
   Unit
British Medical Association

Justin Starren, M.D., Ph.D.
Assistant Professor of
   Biomedical Informatics
   and Radiology
Columbia University, College
   of Physicians and Surgeons

Douglas S. Wakefield, Ph.D.
Professor and Head
Department of Health Management
   and Policy
College of Public Health
University of Iowa

Linda Watson
Associate Dean and Director
Claude Moore Health Sciences
   Library
University of Virginia

Ruth S. Weinstock, M.D., Ph.D.
Professor of Medicine
Chief, Endocrinology, Diabetes, and
   Metabolism
SUNY Upstate Medical Center and
Department of Veterans Affairs
   Medical Center at Syracuse

LuAnn Wilkerson, Ed.D.
Sr. Associate Dean for Medical
   Education
David Geffen School of Medicine at
   UCLA

Introduction

This book began with a set of questions. What are society's health needs in the twenty-first century? What kind of health system will be able to meet those needs? How can academic health centers (AHCs)[1] and other health sector leaders help create a health system and health organizations that meet the health challenges of the twenty-first century? What capabilities should AHCs and other health care organizations develop for short- and long-term success in such a health system?

This book is based on a series of reports produced by the Blue Ridge Academic Health Group (Blue Ridge Group). The Blue Ridge Group seeks to help academic health centers better meet the needs of society. Towards that end, the Group has explored a set of pivotal health policy, leadership, and management issues and identified ways that AHCs can strengthen their viability while striving to improve the health of individuals as well as the general population. Through the course of its work, the Blue Ridge Group has developed a framework for how the health system and health care organizations should evolve to meet the challenges of improving health in the twenty-first century.

The Blue Ridge Group began its work in 1997 with three basic premises. First, demographic changes, technology, economic forces, and societal developments demand new approaches in health care delivery systems, education, and research. Second, the reforms that created upheavals in the health care delivery system during the 1980s and 1990s were primarily structured to achieve financial objectives. Yet, the potential exists for fundamental changes in the health sector to improve health *and* better manage costs. Third, AHCs

---

[1] As described in Chapter 1, an academic health center (AHC) is a health education, research, and service center that encompasses a school of allopathic or osteopathic medicine, a teaching hospital with associated primary and secondary care sites, and at least one additional health sciences professional school such as a school of nursing, dentistry, or pharmacy. There are over 100 such centers in North America and they typically are major institutions in their own regions and perform much of North America's biomedical research, education, and health care service delivery including a disproportionate share of care for the society's lower socio-economic groups.

play a unique role in the US health care system as they develop, apply, and disseminate knowledge to improve health and educate many if not most health workers. In so doing, they assume responsibilities and encounter challenges other health care provider institutions typically do not bear. Thus, AHCs face additional risks as they grapple with the evolving health care environment. And, at the same time, they hold within their talented workforce the opportunity to be the fulcrum for constructive change.

The Blue Ridge Group's first report focused fairly narrowly on how AHCs could use business practices to strengthen their financial viability and protect their tradition of public service. Despite the brevity of this report, it introduced themes that would be revisited and expanded upon in later reports (e.g., performance measures, broadening AHC mission). The second report's scope was significantly broader as the Blue Ridge Group studied the issue of the uninsured and concluded that this complex challenge can only be addressed fully in the context of a *value-driven health system* for the United States. The concept of a value-driven health system became a cornerstone for all subsequent work of the Blue Ridge Group and continued to evolve as the Group explored organizational issues such as leadership, culture, knowledge management, and e-health.

This volume updates and restructures the content of the first six Blue Ridge Group reports (Blue Ridge Group, 1998a, 1998b, 2000a, 2000b, 2001a, 2001b).[2] Two invited chapters, six invited case studies, and nine invited commentaries provide additional depth and breadth for the themes originally addressed by the Blue Ridge Group. David Blumenthal's description of the challenges facing twenty-first century health care organizations and the status of AHCs in the United States sets the stage for this volume by pointing to the need for dramatic changes in AHCs and the health system as a whole. Chapter 2 explores what those changes should be and presents the framework of a value-driven health system. Chapters 3 through 6 address specific issues – leadership, culture, knowledge management, and e-health – that require attention and action by twenty-first century health care organizations. Tom Smith's discussion of the challenges facing European AHCs highlights the similar issues facing US and European AHCs and the potential for international collaboration on organizational and health system development.

This book has two goals. First, we seek to advance understanding of and the need for a value-driven health system in the United States. Second, we seek

---

[2] The Group's seventh report, *Reforming Medical Education: Urgent Priority for the Academic Health Center in the New Century*, was published in 2003 and its eighth report, *Converging on Consensus? Planning the Future of Health and Health Care*, was published in 2004.

to provide AHC leaders, senior administrators, faculty, policy-makers, and interested scholars with a guide to the essential tasks for fostering a value-driven culture for their organizations and building a value-driven health system anywhere in the world where biomedical research, teaching, and services coexist.

Although the Blue Ridge Group focuses its attention on AHCs, the Group addresses issues faced by all health care organizations grappling with increasingly powerful market forces, growing societal expectations, growing consumerism, diffusion of new technology, a constantly expanding base of medical knowledge, reimbursement mechanisms that do not reinforce desired behaviors, and inadequate national health policy on the uninsured. This book explores how health care organizations may improve their performance in terms of quality and efficiency and how they can help to influence changes in the broader health system. It highlights innovative practices consistent with value-driven care and identifies where additional practical action is needed. Thus, this text may be of interest to all individuals in the health sector committed to creating health care organizations capable of meeting the health challenges of the twenty-first century.

REFERENCES

Blue Ridge Academic Health Group (1998a). *Academic Health Centers: Getting Down to Business*. Washington, DC: Cap Gemini Ernst & Young US, LLC.

(1998b). *Promoting Value and Expanded Coverage: Good Health is Good Business*. Washington, DC: Cap Gemini Ernst & Young US, LLC.

(2000a). *Into the 21st Century: Academic Health Centers as Knowledge Leaders*. Washington, DC: Cap Gemini Ernst & Young US, LLC.

(2000b). *In Pursuit of Greater Value: Stronger Leadership in and by Academic Health Centers*. Washington, DC: Cap Gemini Ernst & Young US, LLC.

(2001a). *e-Health and the Academic Health Center in a Value-driven Health Care System*. Washington, DC: Cap Gemini Ernst & Young US, LLC.

(2001b). *Creating a Value-driven Culture and Organization in the Academic Health Center*. Washington, DC: Cap Gemini Ernst & Young US, LLC.

1 Academic health centers: current status, future challenges

David Blumenthal, M.D., M.P.P.

Introduction

The decade of the 1990s was unprecedented in the history of the modern academic health centers (AHCs) in the United States, as it was for health care institutions generally. The nation's 125 AHCs had for the previous 40 years grown steadily larger, more powerful, and more lustrous. They had built or acquired hospitals, outpatient buildings, and research facilities. Their faculties had captured an enviable share of Nobel prizes in their fields and pioneered life-saving treatments for cardiovascular disease, cancer, and other illnesses. Despite occasional storms associated with the introduction of new Medicare payment policies (i.e., diagnosis-related groups or DRGs and the resource-based relative value system or RBRVS), AHCs' clinical facilities had mostly sailed to higher volumes of patient care, higher clinical income, and increasing fiscal reserves. If few administrators or board members from parent universities understood the intricacies of these complex medical institutions – their peculiar organizational structures, accounting practices, promotion rituals, and cultures – well, there were other parts of the university that were both more comprehensible and more problematic. Academic health centers did not appear broken, or to need fixing.

All that changed dramatically for many AHCs and their parent universities in the middle and late 1990s. Out of a seemingly clear horizon, a tidal wave of red ink crashed across the balance sheets of some of the nation's most eminent and heretofore invulnerable AHCs. In anticipation or response, many AHCs embarked on unprecedented internal reforms: buying up primary care practices, selling teaching hospitals, creating new internal

David Blumenthal is Samuel O. Thier Professor of Medicine and Health Policy, Harvard Medical School; Director, Institute for Health Policy, Massachusetts General Hospital Partners Health Care System.

organizational arrangements such as physician–hospital organizations and integrated faculty group practices, and merging with teaching hospitals and schools from other universities. In many cases, these radical course changes seemed only to make matters worse – and infinitely more confusing to those leading, working in, or developing policy for these huge, apparently floundering health care institutions.

This chapter reviews the current status of and future challenges for AHCs. It begins by defining what an AHC is and what confers distinctive identity to AHCs in the modern US health care system.

Defining and describing the AHC

Academic health centers consist of medical schools and their closely affiliated or owned clinical facilities and professional schools. There are roughly 125 such complexes in the United States. Parent institutions wholly own some of these institutions (e.g., University of Pennsylvania Health System; Johns Hopkins University Health System; University of California San Diego; University of Virginia). Other AHCs consist of close affiliations between medical and other health professional schools and independent nonprofit and for-profit clinical entities (e.g., Harvard Medical School and its clinical affiliates; Washington University and the BJC Health System; Columbia and Cornell Medical Schools and the NewYork–Presbyterian Health System).

Diversity, commonality, and complexity

Recently, the clinical component of the AHC has become increasingly diverse. For much of the twentieth century, AHCs' clinical facilities typically included hospitals and faculty group practice plans. In the 1990s, as part of their response to external financial threats, a number of AHCs sought to compete more effectively in clinical markets by creating integrated health care systems. Thus, the AHC of the early twenty-first century frequently includes networks of primary care physicians, community hospitals, community health centers, nursing homes, health plans, and home health care services. At the same time, some AHCs decided to shield themselves from market forces by withdrawing from formal ownership of any clinical facilities, selling off hospitals and even faculty group practices (Blumenthal and Weissman, 2000). The AHC sector thus constitutes a varied and evolving set of institutions.

This variety should not, however, obscure their commonality. Regardless of their precise organizational and ownership arrangements, AHCs share certain common purposes and missions. They exist to improve the health of their communities and the larger society in which they reside (Blue Ridge Academic Health Group, 2000; Commonwealth Fund Task Force on Academic Health Centers, 2003). In this endeavor, they have capabilities and roles that set them apart to some extent from other institutions in our health care system. These distinctive capabilities lie in the areas of biomedical research, education of health professionals, provision of rare and high technology medical services, and continuous innovation in patient care. In addition, many AHCs play a major role in caring for poor and uninsured patients in their communities. The distinctive roles and capabilities of AHCs are often referred to as their "social missions."

A common characteristic of these social missions is that they are unlikely to be optimally produced and distributed in freely competitive private markets. Several missions have attributes that economists associate with public goods (Garber, 1995). Basic biomedical research is a classic public good. Other missions of AHCs do not meet the classic definition of public goods but, nevertheless, have characteristics which make it unlikely that they will be handled well by private markets. Some of these mission-related activities produce so-called merit goods (Allan, 1971). Private markets for merit goods exist because these goods benefit the individuals who purchase them. Consumption of merit goods also benefits other members of society; that is, the use of these goods has positive externalities. Medical education is an example of a merit good. By paying tuition, medical students are prepared for a career that benefits them financially. At the same time, society clearly benefits from having a well-educated medical profession with certain characteristics. Left to their own devices, medical students paying the full cost of their education may choose to enter specialties that maximize their own future income, and neglect areas of work (such as geriatrics, primary care, and care for poor and uninsured patients) whose full social benefits may not be rewarded in current health care markets.

Academic health centers play a prominent role in the following social missions that have characteristics of either public or merit goods:

1. AHCs perform nearly 30 percent of all the health care research and development in the United States and more than 50 percent of research supported by the National Institutes of Health (NIH).

2. AHCs train the great majority of the nation's allopathic medical students and nearly half its residents and interns.

3. AHCs provide large amounts of specialized, costly services (such as burn, transplant, and trauma care).
4. AHCs play major roles as safety net institutions caring for poor and uninsured patients in their communities.
5. AHCs are uniquely suited to conduct clinical research that enables the innovation of clinical care.

The effort to serve these multiple and complex missions makes AHCs extraordinarily complex institutions. From the special standpoint of their parent universities, AHCs are rendered more confusing by having one foot solidly rooted in the university, and the other planted just as firmly in the turbulent health care market place. Some elements of AHC faculty, such as their basic investigators and heavily committed teachers, occupy themselves with work that is absolutely typical of the university faculty in the arts and sciences and other professional schools. In contrast, many clinical faculty seem to be providing what look like routine health care services, and to have earned faculty status (including tenure) by virtue of the quantity and quality of services provided. The law or business school analogy would be to grant tenure to law professors if they achieved partnership in university-owned or affiliated law firms, or to business professors if they became chief executive officers (CEOs) of university-owned or affiliated businesses.

Nevertheless, clinical faculty contribute to core academic activities. They provide supervision to medical students and residents in patient care settings, thus assuring the competence of graduates. They participate in clinical innovation, using protected time afforded by faculty status to conduct funded and unfunded clinical research that translates basic knowledge into applied technologies (Weissman *et al.*, 1999). The revenues from their clinical activities support research and teaching. In one study, 30 percent of clinical revenues of faculty group practices were diverted to fund academic activities within those practices and at affiliated medical schools (Jones and Sanderson, 1996).

Financing

Uniform, integrated financial data on the diverse components of AHCs as we have defined them are virtually nonexistent. To understand their finances, Figure 1.1 shows trends in the contribution of various sources to the income of medical schools for which data are available. As these data make clear, medical schools have become increasingly dependent on clinical revenues, and grants and contracts supporting research. The latter component has

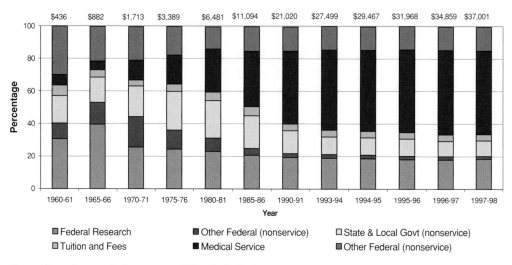

Figure 1.1   Revenues for the programs of US medical schools

grown dramatically over the last five years as Congress has doubled the budget of the National Institutes of Health. This may partly explain why medical schools seem to have suffered less than hospitals over the last five years, despite the vulnerability of clinical incomes to market forces. Schools were able to continue to raise faculty salaries throughout the late 1990s at or above the rate of inflation (Studer-Ellis, Gold, and Jones, 2000). In contrast to medical schools, AHC clinical facilities (with a handful of exceptions) realize virtually all their revenues from clinical sources, which makes them much more vulnerable than medical schools and other health professional schools to perturbations in health care markets.

Current status

The extent of the financial difficulties plaguing AHCs is surprisingly hard to pinpoint because of time lags in available data, variable accounting practices, and anomalies in the way universities and their affiliated institutions keep their books. Nevertheless, it seems clear that 1999–2000 constituted a period of unprecedented financial stress for these institutions. Figure 1.2 shows trends in total and operating margins for AHC hospitals during the 1990s and into the year 2000.

As these figures make clear, total margins for AHC hospitals averaged one to two percent nationally in 1999–2000, compared to five to six percent in the

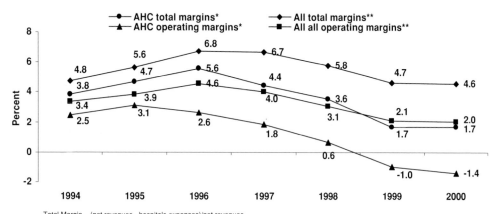

Figure 1.2   Trends in the aggregate total margins and operating margins for AHCs, 1994–2000

mid 1990s. Operating margins were negative by the end of the decade. AHCs performed considerably less well throughout the decade than did nonAHC facilities. In 1999, the major clinical affiliates of 14 of the 18 medical schools that received the largest amounts of NIH research funding suffered operating losses, received a negative outlook from bond-rating agencies, or had their bond ratings downgraded. Incomplete, unaudited quarterly reports nevertheless suggest that after several years of decline, average teaching hospital operating margins stabilized and even increased for private AHC hospitals, though declines continued for public-owned facilities.

Skeptics correctly point out that the majority of the nation's AHC hospitals and medical schools continue in the black (at least judged by total margins), that a few bad years may not constitute a crisis, and that AHCs have often cried wolf about their finances in the past. Yet, it seems clear that, never since the Great Depression, have so many eminent university teaching facilities been in such distress simultaneously. Their extreme reactions seem to support their claims. AHCs do not lightly sell their teaching hospitals, especially to for-profit corporations, nor do they casually lay off 10 to 20 percent of their workforce, as have the University of Pennsylvania, Beth Israel Deaconness Medical Center, San Diego, San Francisco, and Stanford.

Since AHCs are such large, complex institutions, it should come as no surprise that the sources of their distress are similarly intricate and multifaceted. The advent of economic competition in health care during the 1990s took most AHCs (like most other health care institutions) by surprise. The prices

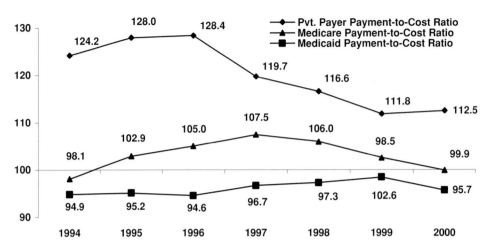

Figure 1.3   Trends in payment-to-cost ratios by payer for AHCs, 1994–2000

they could charge for patient care fell dramatically as a result of pressure from managed care companies, which were doing the bidding of cost-conscious employers. Traditionally, fees from private patients had been AHCs' most lucrative source of income. Over the last half of the 1990s, however, payment-to-cost ratios (Figure 1.3) for private payers declined precipitously. Then, in 1997, the federal government piled on the pressure by reducing Medicare payments for all hospitals (including AHCs) under provisions of the Balanced Budget Act (BBA) of 1997. AHCs, however, took a special hit that is not reflected in their simple payment numbers. This was because the Medicare program began reducing graduate medical education (GME) payments that provided extra payments to teaching hospitals to reflect the higher costs of care provided in these institutions. Even though some Medicare payments were restored through BBA revisions in 1999 and 2000, payments to AHCs did not regain pre-BBA levels, and further cuts in Medicare GME payments became effective in 2003 because of Congress' decision not to address Medicare payment issues in its 2002 lame duck session. Another factor affecting AHCs more severely than other hospitals was a rise in uncompensated care payments. As the Lewin Group has documented, public AHC facilities in particular have experienced disproportionate increases in uncompensated care, especially in markets of high managed care penetration (Dobson *et al.*, 2002).

The responses of AHCs to these developments in some cases helped, but in other cases exacerbated, their problems. A first response was to cut costs through reducing lengths of hospital stays and re-engineering clinical processes. Virtually every AHC hospital undertook cost reduction programs during the late 1990s. The result was that, during the latter part of the decade, real hospital costs per admission at AHCs fell by several percent annually. These cost reductions have provided teaching hospitals critical breathing room as their revenues have fallen.

AHCs also re-organized to improve their positions in health care markets, with somewhat problematic results. Fearful that managed care companies would channel patients to less expensive facilities (AHCs' costs average nearly 30 percent more than their community competition) some AHCs began buying up primary care practices and community hospitals in their markets, hoping that they could thereby assure themselves referrals from these institutions (Commonwealth Fund Task Force on Academic Health Centers, 1997). AHCs also theorized that the acquisitions would make them such large players in local markets that they could negotiate better prices from managed care companies.

Unfortunately, these acquisitions were costly, sometimes excessively so. In retrospect, AHCs often overpaid for primary care practices. Furthermore, primary care is a marginal business at best, and newly acquired networks proved financial drains for many AHCs. The infrastructures required to manage far flung clinical enterprises were also costly, and anticipated economies of scale through consolidation of departments and backroom functions sometimes fell victim to internal politics as some powerful department chairs, faculty members, and administrators resisted efforts to merge and downsize their units and services.

Another organizational maneuver pursued by AHCs during the 1990s produced mixed results. Several major nationally prominent teaching hospitals merged with local rivals in an effort to cut costs and improve bargaining power with local managed care organizations. Harvard institutions pioneered this trend with the 1994 merger of the Brigham and Women's Hospital (BWH) and the Massachusetts General Hospital (MGH) to form the Partners Health-Care System (PHCS). Boston's Beth Israel Hospital and Deaconness Medical Center followed to form the BIDMC, which became the core of the larger Caregroup system. In New York City, Columbia Presbyterian Hospital merged with New York-Cornell, and Mt. Sinai with New York University Hospital. In the San Francisco Bay Area, the University of California, San Francisco (UCSF) and Stanford merged their teaching facilities. Penn State University's Medical Center merged with the nearby Geisinger Clinic, and Dartmouth's Mary Hitchcock Clinic and Hospital affiliated with the Lahey Clinic.

Among these mergers, only the BWH–MGH union has proved a clear success. The UCSF–Stanford merger was abandoned after only a year, and the NYU–Mt. Sinai merger has been largely abandoned. Also dissolved were unions between Dartmouth and Lahey Clinic and the Penn State Medical Center and the Geisinger. The final word is out on the other major combinations, but there is no question that such mergers have major financial costs in the short term. Their benefits in terms of cost reduction and improved market position are realized later, if at all. Cultural differences, even those among teaching hospitals affiliated with the same medical schools, have proved major impediments to effective governance. Furthermore, consolidations of hospitals nationally are now prompting antitrust reviews by the Federal Trade Commission that will undoubtedly sweep up some AHC combinations in their nets (Abelson, 2002). The North Shore Medical Center (resulting from a merger of Long Island Jewish and North Shore Hospitals) recently emerged unscathed from lengthy federal antitrust litigation, and other affected AHCs may beat back such assaults. However, the legal and public relations costs of such defenses are considerable.

In responding to the shock of health care's market transformation, AHCs have often taken cues from the playbooks of large corporations in other economic sectors and the consultants who peddle those solutions. Given the suddenness and surprise of events, AHCs' reactions were logical and predictable. Yet, they may not have been well suited to their own unique circumstances. A critical component of AHCs' workforce is professors and professorial aspirants. Faculty cannot be ordered willy-nilly out of the lab and classroom and into the clinical breech when a threat arises on the perimeter of an AHC market. Nor is it clear that a major reallocation of faculty time, even among clinical faculty, to provision of health care services would be socially desirable in the long term. The lighter clinical loads that some faculty sustain are clearly important in liberating time for their teaching and research activities. For this and other reasons, AHCs social missions add to their costs and are likely to frustrate their ability to reduce expenses and reorganize quickly (Commonwealth Fund Task Force on Academic Health Centers, 2002). The unique situation of AHCs makes it questionable that they will find adequate solutions to their economic problems using classic competitive strategies.

Another consideration that AHCs and other interested stakeholders must bear in mind is that, despite their financial problems, these institutions have enjoyed notable successes in the service of their social missions, and are shouldering greater burdens now in certain ways than ever before.

In biomedical research, AHCs have been at the forefront of the most exciting developments in the biological revolution – including the mapping of the human genome – that have led to the development, testing and clinical application of new therapeutic modalities (e.g., solid organ transplant, treatment of cardiovascular disease using both medications and invasive procedures, the progress in treating childhood cancers). The vitality of local AHCs has played a pivotal role in the economies of major high technology areas, such as Boston's Route 128 (now a mecca for pharmaceutical research institutes), the San Francisco Bay Area and San Diego. In the area of medical education, AHCs are in the midst of profound changes designed to measure the outcomes of the educational process, and are increasingly putting curricula on-line (Commonwealth Fund Task Force on Academic Health Centers, 2002). Both high technology care and indigent care are more concentrated in AHCs now than they were at the beginning of the 1990s. Especially in markets with large amounts of managed care, AHCs now take care of larger proportions of those regions' poor and uninsured patients than they did before managed care began to spread (Weissman, Gaskin, and Reuer, 2003).

Ownership of clinical facilities

A fundamental question facing AHCs and their parent institutions is whether they should continue to own and manage clinical facilities. This issue has major implications for all AHCs' missions. Given the diversity of AHCs and universities, no single correct answer is likely to emerge but a few salient considerations bear importantly on this decision in the short run. First, the financial pressures on AHCs' clinical programs are likely to ease in the short term as managed care retreats, health care prices rise, and internal cost cutting in university health systems takes effect. Even AHCs under the greatest financial pressure, such as University of Pennsylvania and the BIDMC, experienced marked improvements in their bottom lines in 2001 and 2002. This provides universities and their governing boards some breathing space in which to contemplate whether to fundamentally change traditional relationships with clinical affiliates.

Second, universities cannot sustain world-class medical schools without intimate partnerships with world-class clinical facilities. To provide excellent clinical education to medical schools, medical schools depend on partnerships with inpatient and outpatient settings with a diverse patient mix and with a clinical faculty that provide lifetime role models for excellence in clinical care and commitment to continuous learning. To conduct clinical research, medical schools must also have access to patient populations of sufficient size and diversity, and must attract clinical faculty with the drive and intellect to ask the key questions and attract the necessary funding. These faculty will demand access to excellent clinical institutions.

Examples of successful partnerships between medical schools and superb, independent clinical facilities exist, and provide hope that universities can achieve excellence in their social missions without incurring the burdens and risks of owning a health system. For example, neither Harvard University nor Washington University in St. Louis owns any hospitals or clinics. In the case of Harvard University, long-standing tradition, mutual dependency, and interlocking faculties assure that the medical school secures the teaching resources it needs from a range of affiliated clinical entities. In the case of Washington University, these informal connections are complemented by a formal agreement through which the Barnes-Jewish Hospital provides financial support each year to the medical school.

There are also several examples of universities selling teaching hospitals and group practices to nonprofit and for-profit chains (e.g., Tulane, University of Minnesota, Georgetown) without obvious catastrophes. However, it should be pointed out that in cases like Harvard and Washington University, the relationships have evolved over a century or more. It is not clear that the same relatively seamless interdependence will emerge in the case of recent sales, especially where for-profit entities are involved, or if it does, how long this will take (Blumenthal and Weissman, 2000). Experience with these sales suggests that, when universities sell clinical facilities, important cultural differences do emerge between universities and their new partners, and that the details of contracts are critical to maintaining commitment to academic mission. Furthermore, none of the universities selling their teaching hospitals has been among the nation's most research intensive. Given the breathing space afforded by easing markets, universities have some time to learn what the experience will be over the long term with recent sales and to see how much managers can improve economic performance under current ownership.

Public policy

Academic health centers exert an influence on the health care system that extends well beyond their walls, and affects the average citizen in the United

States and beyond. They play a pivotal role in applying the fruits of the biological revolution, much of it funded by NIH dollars, to relieving human suffering. They maintain the quality of our health care workforce. And they are providers of last resort both for highly specialized and high technology services, and for patients who lack the means to pay for their care. The extent to which the fiscal pressures are affecting AHCs' ability to serve these missions is not precisely known at this time. However, these institutions have definitely come to rely on excess revenues from their clinical arms to subsidize their academic and charitable work. The financial problems of AHCs, therefore, constitute legitimate concerns for community leaders and policy-makers at all levels of government and within AHCs' communities.

Legitimate concerns, of course, need not translate into action. AHCs are far from perfect. As suggested above, some of their current problems are self-inflicted, the results of unwise responses to competitive pressures. Those problems cannot be remedied without tough, internal reforms at AHCs themselves, including continued cost cutting and improvements in management. The wider community could decide that forcing AHCs to undertake these painful changes requires external fiscal pressure, and is worth short-term disruptions in their social missions.

If policy-makers do wish to protect AHCs from the full brunt of market forces and the consequences of their own missteps, a variety of options are available. One of these, already underway, is to continue to restore recent cuts in Medicare payments to hospitals. The Congress has enacted two measures adding back funds that were removed under provisions of the Balanced Budget Act of 1997, including monies targeted at teaching hospitals.

Cuts in the Medicare program were not solely responsible for the difficulties facing AHCs, however, and Medicare add-backs are unlikely, therefore, to make them whole. The competitive transformation of health care markets and reductions in payments by private insurance companies and managed care have also been major factors. Academic health center advocates believe that their involvement in research, teaching, care of indigent, and health care innovation render them incapable of competing on a level playing field with nonacademic providers of care, and that AHCs should receive additional, direct governmental support for these social missions (Commonwealth Fund Task Force on Academic Health Centers, 1997). The goal in this regard should be to create a mechanism that is administratively simple, transparent, accountable, and predictable, so that taxpayers and legislators can understand where the money is going and how well it is being used, and AHCs can plan their investments in mission-related activities. One possible approach would be to create a federal Academic Health Center Trust Fund that would funnel such support to AHCs that demonstrate substantial involvement in teaching, research, indigent care, and innovation. The Commonwealth Fund Task Force on Academic Health Centers studied the problems of AHCs from 1996 to 2003 and endorsed this approach (Commonwealth Fund Task Force on Academic Health Centers, 1997). Congress passed a version of such a fund as part of Medicare legislation in 1995, but President Clinton vetoed the bill over unrelated matters.

The federal cavalry seems unlikely to rescue AHCs anytime soon. Federal intervention was a long-shot even before the election of George W. Bush, and prospects have declined further with the retirement and death of Daniel Patrick Moynihan who was ranking minority on the influential Senate Finance Committee, and the Congress' most tireless advocate of AHCs. However, through the convoluted pathways of our national political process, the enactment of prescription drug coverage may prompt debate about the role of AHCs in society. This is because the Bush Administration and its congressional allies linked Medicare drug benefits to major reforms in the Medicare program. Such reforms will inevitably raise questions about how Medicare's current special payment to AHCs will be organized and funded. Once opened, this debate could easily be extended to consider the merits of the generic Trust Fund.

Long-term challenges

As the universities and their AHCs look to the future, immediate issues actually pale in importance compared to long-term trends in the economic, social, and health care environment that will confront AHCs. Private and public policy-makers concerned about the missions of AHCs and about the institutions that serve those missions must take these trends into account when formulating short- and long-term plans.

Demographic developments

At least three demographic trends in the US population could have significant implications for AHCs in the future. These include: the aging of the population, its increasing diversity, and its changing geographic distribution. The numbers of older Americans will increase dramatically over the next 20 years as the baby boom generation reaches maturity. Immigration and varying rates of reproduction within different population subgroups will produce a US population that, in 20 years, will display much greater racial and ethnic diversity than it has in the past (US Census Bureau, 2000). The most rapidly growing group is Hispanic Americans, which will comprise 18 percent of the population by 2025, compared with 12 percent now. Interestingly, levels of diversity will vary considerably in different parts of the United States, with the West and Southwest showing the greatest levels, and the Northern and Central areas the least. Profound shifts are also occurring in the geographic distribution of the American population, with dramatic growth in the South and West.

Taken together, these demographic developments suggest that, in the future, AHCs will have to be prepared to educate a more diverse, culturally competent, health professional work force, and will also have to be prepared to offer services that take into account the needs of populations that are older, more chronically ill and more racially, ethnically, and linguistically varied than has ever been true in the past. Educationally, this will mean that medical schools, schools of public health, nursing schools, and other health professional training programs will have to reform their curricula to include programs with more social and cultural content, more emphasis on proficiency in relevant foreign languages (especially Spanish), and exposure to role models who deliver care that is appropriate for patients of diverse ethnic and cultural backgrounds. Clinical curricula will have to provide more systematic exposure to chronic illness, the care of elderly populations at home and in long-term care facilities, and the skills necessary to care for patients in teams, which is required for effective chronic care. These changes will require investments of necessary resources, recruitment and training of new and more diverse faculty, and development of relationships with a more diverse set of clinical facilities.

Demographic trends further suggest that AHCs in the South and West are likely to face greater pressures to make these changes, and increased demand for their services generally. Over time, this will likely lead to the addition of new AHCs in these geographic locales. In contrast, AHCs in the North and Northeast are less likely to grow in number.

Increasing importance of public health problems

Several recent events have increased awareness of the need for the US health care system to improve its public health infrastructure. The anthrax scare of

2001 dramatically increased attention on the potential effects of infectious diseases on the health of populations both in the United States and abroad. This has revived interest in neglected areas of research, medical education, and health care practice related to the microbiology and epidemiology of infectious illnesses, both common and uncommon; their recognition and treatment in daily practice; and the development of population-based strategies for preventing them and limiting their spread.

Behavioral trends within the US population also remain a vital public health concern. Among the most important behavioral influences on health are obesity, smoking, and alcoholism (Sturm, 2002). In 1998, 23 percent of the population was obese, 24 percent smoked, and 17 percent engaged in binge drinking. These behaviors have been associated with heart disease, cancer, emphysema, asthma, diabetes, and other afflictions that represent the most frequent causes of death in the United States.

These trends have implications for education, research, and clinical care at AHCs. Schools of public health, where they exist within AHCs, will undoubtedly face increased burdens of service and education. Traditionally, these institutions have been woefully under-resourced. Correcting this imbalance will be a challenge for university development offices, and will put additional strains on endowments. Where AHCs lack access to the talents and skills of public health schools, existing faculty will have to assume burdens for which they are not currently prepared. Universities should be prepared to manage these increasing demands on the public health resources of their schools, including requirements to invest more resources in schools of public health. Those institutions that lack such schools may also find that they face proposals to start them. In some cases, pressures to invest in public health infrastructure may be difficult to resist because they arise in the context of local efforts to manage bioterrorism and the emergence of new types of infectious illnesses, such as West Nile virus, dengue fever, and even malaria, which may re-emerge in the United States with global warming and the decline in mosquito control programs.

National and international economic trends

Several powerful and persistent economic trends seem likely to profoundly affect the environment in which AHCs function over the next several decades. The first is globalization which is taking shape in the spread of market forces around the world with most countries engaging in freer trade and widespread deregulation. For the United States, open markets and international competition mean that international trade and investment will play a much greater role in our economic life than before. The second trend is the revolution in information technology. The digitalization of our homes and our workplaces has vastly improved communications and increased the pace at which we compete in global markets. The third trend is the emergence of a knowledge-based economy (Blue Ridge Academic Health Group, 2000). This economy is dominated by intangible assets and resources such as the unique knowledge held by individual firms, a focus on services, and marketing of valuable patents. These three trends are creating a world in which innovation is often more important than industrial production, ideas are more profitable than tangible products, and change is accelerating.

These macroeconomic shifts have implications for health and health care nationally and worldwide. To begin with, there is new concern in the developed world with so-called diseases of globalization (Epstein and Chen, 2002). In the early to mid twentieth century, US public health officials were concerned with diseases of poverty, including infectious diseases, childhood illnesses, and infant and maternal mortality. In the latter part of last century, more attention was given to diseases of affluence and older populations, including cardiovascular diseases, diabetes, and cancers. To these familiar concerns have been added new public health challenges symbolized by the diseases of globalization. Examples include acquired immune deficiency syndrome (AIDS), new infectious agents such as a variant of Creutzfeldt–Jakob disease, West Nile virus, and multi-drug-resistant tuberculosis. These concerns have the potential to threaten the entire globe and can only be addressed through coordinated, cross-national efforts. At the same time, globalization has led to economic inequality and social dislocation, which are associated with the spread of unsafe sex, violence, and terrorism, including bioterrorism.

Whereas many ideas and services are readily traded in global markets, until recently health services delivery has been almost exclusively a local activity. However, advances in telecommunication and robotics are permitting the delivery of health services over long distances (Sable *et al.*, 2002). This raises the prospect that health care services may be susceptible to export in new, unanticipated ways. If so, it is possible to imagine a highly competitive international trade in a variety of health care services that could create new opportunities and challenges for AHCs and other US health care institutions.

The explosion of Internet usage has likewise led to multiple new applications for health care with potentially profound implications for all providers and consumers of services in the United States and abroad. The Robert Wood Johnson Foundation defines the new phenomenon of *eHealth* as the

use of emerging information and communication technology, especially the Internet, to improve or enable health and health care. This term bridges both the clinical and nonclinical sectors and includes both individual and population health-oriented tools. (Eng, 2001)

As of this date, about 60 million Americans have used the World Wide Web to seek out information on their health or the medical care system (Rainie and Packel, 2001). Yahoo lists over 19 000 web sites dealing with health care, but this may represent only a minority of the available sites (Eng, 2001). The availability of new electronic sources of health information can empower both patients and physicians to improve the health care services they receive and provide, and may create unpredictable changes in the optimal organization of services.

These issues have implications for a number of the social missions conducted by AHCs. As do so many of these long-term trends, these developments suggest that the content of undergraduate and post-graduate medical education will have to include training in illnesses that were once rare in the United States, but now may appear unpredictably and with greater frequency. From a clinical standpoint, AHCs may face new types of opportunities and challenges related to competing in global, on-line markets for the provision of health care services. Local monopolies of specialized services may no longer be secure in the future. AHCs in California and Massachusetts may find themselves competing not only with Hopkins and Mayo, but with Cambridge, Oxford, and the University of Tokyo. Finally, AHCs as a class of institutions may no longer have the monopoly they once had as authoritative dispensers of the most advanced information – the places where patients with the most difficult, complex, and apparently insoluble health problems seek help when all else has failed. Instead, new eHealth resources may emerge as the equivalent of virtual AHCs, providing expert advice and direction in cyberspace.

How AHCs should respond to these challenges remains to be seen. However, it seems clear that investments in new infrastructure and increased organizational nimbleness will be critical. New faculty and research in the area of infectious disease will be required, and greatly increased bioinformatics and information technology capabilities will also be needed. If AHCs wish to remain the sites where young health professionals learn the skills they will need to be competitive in the fast-changing, global health care market, they will have to be exposed to the diagnostic and therapeutic potential of new information technology and robotics. They will have to be prepared to use these resources to serve their patients, and young faculty members will have to be prepared to build their research and teaching around these new modalities for care and communication. One can begin to imagine the new educational buildings that will dot AHC campuses, the new high technology research and clinical laboratories, the international exchange programs that will be required to acquaint physicians and researchers in training with international health care problems and resources, and the accelerating pace of change in all dimensions.

Rising health expenditures

Health care expenditures in the United States have resumed their apparently relentless upward surge. In retrospect, the mid 1990s provided only brief relief from a trend that persisted with temporary interruptions throughout most of the last century. After a brief period of relative calm, private health insurance premiums are again outpacing other economic indicators. The *New York Times* reported that Health Maintenance Organizations (HMOs) in 2001 asked for increases in premiums more than 18 percent over the prior year, with some companies charging as much as 60 percent more (Freudenheim, 2001). The likely persistent increases in health care expenditures will be an important environmental factor affecting the future of AHCs. In particular, it seems likely that purchasers of care will find new approaches to constraining health care expenditures that will in some way or other reduce revenues of AHCs in the future. This will place inevitable, renewed pressure on their ability to cross-subsidize mission-related activities. Cost containment will be a continual, evolving challenge for AHCs, requiring continuing reorganization of their clinical facilities, and tough continuing negotiations between medical schools and their faculty on the one hand, and stressed clinical partners on the other. These developments emphasize the difficulty of continuing to rely on clinical cross-subsidies to fund AHC missions. Such clinical funds will remain an unstable and unpredictable source of support for public and merit goods of widely acknowledged national importance. AHCs and their parent universities will need to provide leadership in examining alternative, more reliable, and accountable mechanisms to fund their social missions.

The biological revolution

References to the biological revolution in the late twentieth and early twenty-first centuries are so common as to be almost cliched. But the reality of this development remains undeniable. The mapping of the human genome has come to symbolize this phenomenon, but other comparable accomplishments, perhaps less heralded, undoubtedly lie ahead as the knowledge gained is exploited in other basic and clinical applications. The sciences of genomics and proteomics, genetic epidemiology, immunology, cancer biology, and many others are poised to take advantage of and spur on the work of the Human Genome Project.

Academic Health Centers have enjoyed an important public trust as recipients of enormous amounts of public funding for biomedical research. As a result, they have played and have the opportunity to continue to play a pivotal role in the biological revolution. However, as the pace of change continues to accelerate, and opportunities to apply new knowledge grow, AHCs will likely face new challenges. They will likely be called upon to demonstrate that they are efficient producers of new knowledge, can apply that knowledge effectively, can partner with nonacademic institutions, and can do so in ways that meet public expectations for disinterestedness, objectivity, and protection of human participants in research.

Persistent and increasing barriers to care

Given their prominent role in caring for disadvantaged populations, AHCs' missions will be importantly affected by trends in the numbers and characteristics of such populations. Two developments have important implications in this regard. One is the growing diversity in the population, documented above, and the increasing information that, even when insured, patients from underrepresented minorities receive care that is inferior to that provided to white Americans (Institute of Medicine, 2002). A recent report from the Institute of Medicine found substantial evidence that racial and ethnic disparities in health care exist, and that they result in unacceptable consequences for health outcomes. As they educate young health professionals, conduct research, and care for vulnerable patients groups, AHCs must confront the implications of these cultural, racial, and ethnic differentials in access to health care services.

A second important trend concerns the number of uninsured in the United States. Though insurance may not be sufficient to guarantee access to services, it is clearly necessary. Some analysts fear that recent economic trends have unleashed a "perfect storm" that could increase dramatically the number of uninsured people in the United States (Miller, 2001). Changes in the unemployment rate are particularly troubling. A new analysis from Massachusetts Institute for Technology, the National Bureau of Economic Research, and Kaiser Family Foundation shows that for every 100 people who lose their jobs, 85 will also lose their insurance (Kaiser Family Foundation, 2002). Rapidly rising health insurance premiums also will increase the number of uninsured, all else equal, because of the difficulty some people will have in maintaining their coverage. Rising premiums combined with even a mild recession could increase the percentage of uninsured Americans to as high as 23 percent nationally in the next six to seven years, with the number reaching 60 million or more. For AHCs, which provide disproportionate amounts of care to racial minorities and uninsured patients, these trends are ominous. They are almost certain to increase financial pressures on institutions struggling to remain international innovators in education, research, and clinical care. Solving the problem of uninsurance in the United States could be vital to the continued preeminence of US AHCs in the nation and the world. This gives the parent universities of these facilities a vital interest in the resolution of what would otherwise seem a vexing, but somewhat tangential, public policy issue.

The future

Responding to the challenges posed by environmental forces and past missteps will require changes in the ways that both AHCs and public policy-makers do business. An enduring question facing AHCs, their university parents, and policy-makers is how to improve the efficiency and resilience of these organizations without causing unintended reductions in the quality or quantity of their social missions. The remainder of this volume seeks to provide guidance on how to achieve these pivotal objectives. In so doing, it explores reforms that are applicable to the entire AHC enterprise, reforms that are specific to the individual AHC missions, and reforms that are needed in the entire health system.

To paraphrase Yogi Berra, prediction is hard, especially when it's about the future. To contribute as effectively as possible to the health and health care of the American people, the future AHC will have to be prepared for change and uncertainty. Academic Health Centers, collectively and individually, must be able to learn quickly and act expeditiously. They must learn about the evolving needs of the American people and new ways to serve those needs and then implement rapidly and effectively the changes necessary to respond to those needs and opportunities. There will be no shortage of challenges for the leaders of these institutions, their faculties, or their parent universities. While this may be said of all the functions of modern universities to some extent, the dual role of AHCs as academic institutions and as vital providers of an essential societal service magnifies the uncertainties many fold. In both the short and long term, the future is destined to be interesting for those individuals who choose to play a role in shaping the nation's health care future.

REFERENCES

Abelson, R. (2002). Merged hospitals gain both power and critics. *New York Times*, 26 September, Late Edition, Final: C1.

Allan, C. M. (1971). *The Theory of Taxation, Microeconomics, Penguin Modern Economics Texts*. Harmondsworth, UK: Penguin.

Blue Ridge Academic Health Group (2000). *Into the 21st Century: Academic Health Centers as Knowledge Leaders*. Washington, DC: Cap Gemini Ernst & Young US, LLC.

Blumenthal, D. and Weissman, J. S. (2000). Selling teaching hospitals to investor-owned hospital chains: three case studies. *Health Affairs*, **19**(2), 158–66.

Commonwealth Fund Task Force on Academic Health Centers (1997). *Leveling the Playing Field: Financing the Missions of Academic Health Centers*. New York: Commonwealth Fund.

(2002). *Training Tomorrow's Doctors: the Medical Education Mission of Academic Health Centers*. New York: Commonwealth Fund.

(2003). *A Vision of the Future Academic Health Center*. New York: Commonwealth Fund.

Dobson, A., Koenig, L., Sen, N., Ho, S. and Gilani, J. (2002). *Financial Performance of Academic Health Center Hospitals, 1994–2002*. New York: Commonwealth Fund.

Eng, T. R. (2001). *The Ehealth Landscape: a Terrain Map of Emerging Information and Communication Technologies in Health and Health Care*. Princeton, NJ: Robert Wood Johnson Foundation.

Epstein, H. and Chen, L. (2002). Can AIDS be stopped? *The New York Review of Books*, March 14.

Freudenheim, M. (2001). Medical costs surge as hospitals force insurers to raise payments. *New York Times*, May 25.

Garber, A. (1995). *Evaluating the Federal Role in Financing Health Related Research*. Presentation to the Roundtable on Economics at the National Institutes of Health. Bethesda, MD: National Institutes of Health.

Institute of Medicine (2002). *Unequal Treatment: Confronting Racial and Ethnic Disparities in Health Care*. Washington, DC: National Academy Press.

Jones, R. F. and Sanderson, S. C. (1996). Clinical revenues used to support the academic mission of medical schools, 1992–93. *Academic Medicine*, **71**(3), 299–307.

Kaiser Family Foundation (2002). *Rising Unemployment and the Uninsured*. Washington, DC: Kaiser Family Foundation. Online at www.kff.org.

Miller, J. E. (2001). *A Perfect Storm: the Confluence of Forces Affecting Health Care Coverage*. Washington, DC: National Coalition on Health Care.

Rainie, L. and Packel, D. (2001). *More Online, Doing More: 16 Million Newcomers Gain Internet Access in the Last Half of 2000 as Women, Minorities, and Families with Modest Incomes Continue to Surge Online*. Washington, DC: Pew Internet Project. Online at http://www.pewinternet.org/.

Sable, C. A., Cummings, S. D., Pearson, G. D., Schratz, L. M., Cross, R. C., Quivers, E. S., Rudra, H. and Martin, G. R. (2002). Impact of telemedicine on the practice of pediatric cardiology in community hospitals. *Pediatrics*, **109**(1), e3. Online at http://pediatrics.aappublications.org/cgi/content/full/109/e3.

Studer-Ellis, E., Gold, J. S. and Jones, R. F. (2000). Trends in US medical school faculty salaries, 1988–1989 to 1998–1999. *Journal of the American Medical Association*, **284**(9), 1130–5.

Sturm, R. (2002). The effects of obesity, smoking, and drinking on medical problems and costs. Obesity outranks both smoking and drinking in its deleterious effects on health and health costs. *Health Affairs*, **21**(2), 245–53.

US Census Bureau (2000). *Statistical Abstract of the US*. Washington, DC: US Census Bureau.

Weissman, J. S., Gaskin, D. J. and Reuer, J. (2003). Hospitals' care of uninsured persons during the 1990s: the relation of teaching status and managed care to changes in market share and market concentration. *Inquiry*, **40**(1), 84–93.

Weissman, J. S., Saglam, D., Campbell, E. G., Causino, N. and Blumenthal, D. (1999). Market forces and unsponsored research in academic health centers. *Journal of the American Medical Association*, **281**(12), 1093–8.

2 A health system for the twenty-first century

Introduction

Health care spending in the United States is massive and on the rise. We do not, however, spend our health care dollars wisely. Despite the importance of health and health care to individual, community, and national productivity, we have not designed a health system that assiduously leverages its resources to maximize health. Rather, we continue to support a health care system that does not provide access to basic care for all citizens and does not fully exploit either established knowledge or technologies proven to improve health.

Our health care spending and policy is heavily skewed towards treating rather than preventing illness (leading to higher treatment costs). We overemphasize the care of individuals to the detriment of the health of populations. We do not organize our practice systems to manage chronic illnesses as well as we could. Quality and safety of care are highly variable; both over-treatment and under-treatment are commonplace. Such practices waste dollars and patient time and expose patients to unnecessary risk. Typically, incentives are not aligned with desired behaviors of patients and health professionals. Further, administrative costs are high and regulations are often beside the mark. In short, we must make substantial reforms.

The Blue Ridge Academic Health Group (Blue Ridge Group) believes that it is both possible and essential for the United States to spend its health care dollars much more rationally and effectively. We can build a true *health system* that is capable of maximizing the health of individuals and populations. To do so, the United States must conceive of its health care expenditures as an investment in the health of both populations and individuals and see the entire population of the nation as the appropriate target for system planning. By basing our spending decisions on the expected value or return on health investment (as measured in terms of health improvement), both the nature of care and the deployment of resources will shift.

The Blue Ridge Group calls this approach a *value-driven health system*. This chapter reviews the need for and presents the emerging vision for a value-driven health system. It also outlines first steps that academic health centers (AHCs), other health organizations, policy-makers, and business leaders should take to help create such a system. We begin by addressing the "elephant in the corner" of the US health care system – the lack of universal health insurance.

Intertwined challenges

Despite being a nation of wealth, over 43 million people in this country lack health insurance and 47 million are underinsured (Kaiser Commission on Medicaid and the Uninsured, 2002; Pear, 2003). These individuals often go without needed health care services (Institute of Medicine (IOM) 2001a, 2002a). When the uninsured receive care it is often less organized, later than optimal, at greater cost, and with poorer outcomes than the insured population experiences (IOM, 2002a; Weissman, Gatsonis, and Epstein, 1992). Studies have found that uninsured populations experience higher hospitalization rates for problems that generally do not require inpatient care, receive different care than the insured population, and have poorer survival rates for some conditions (e.g., breast cancer) (Ayanian *et al.*, 1993; Weissman, Gatsonis, and Epstein, 1992; Weissman *et al.*, 1991). Uninsured adults have been found to have lower health status and to be at a higher risk of premature death than insured adults (IOM, 2002a).

Having even one uninsured person in a family can jeopardize the entire family's financial stability (IOM, 2002b). The United States is one of only three developed countries in which a working family can experience economic hardship because of bad health (Anderson, 1997; Reinhardt, 1998). Uninsured individuals typically pay 35 percent of the overall cost of their medical services; this sometimes requires that they deplete their savings, borrow from friends or a bank, or, in the most severe cases, declare bankruptcy (IOM, 2002b).

A sizable uninsured population increases strain on a community by forcing health care providers and public health agencies to divert resources towards services for the uninsured and away from other investments that would benefit the community (IOM, 2003a, 2003b). It can also increase a community's burden of disease and disability. This increased burden is due to poorer health of uninsured individuals and a spillover effect on the health of other residents due to "the spread of communicable diseases from unvaccinated or ill individuals, shortages of health care providers and loss of local capacity to deliver health care services" (IOM, 2003b).

Further, the poorer health and shorter lifespan that can be attributed to lack of health insurance coverage result in lost productivity and reduced educational achievement. These costs are estimated to reach $65–130 million each year (IOM, 2003a). Uninsured adults have a 25 percent greater mortality risk than adults with health insurance. Each year, lack of health insurance can be linked to an estimated 18 000 deaths among people younger than 65 (IOM, 2002a).

The uninsured problem has grown substantially during the last 15 years; there are 9 million more uninsured Americans today than in 1987. Even with the robust economy of the late 1990s, the number of uninsured individuals only dipped slightly before increasing again in 2001 (Holahan and Pohl, 2002; Pear, 2003). Predictions for the future are even more dire – ranging from 48 to 61 million uninsured individuals by 2009 (Custer and Ketsche, 2000).

Meanwhile, declining subsidies and growth in Medicaid managed care have adversely affected safety net providers that deliver health care and related services to uninsured, Medicaid, and other vulnerable patients (IOM, 2000). Hospitals once relied on cross-subsidies from insured patients to pay for care to uninsured individuals. Employers and insurers no longer tolerate this practice as they are urgently seeking to manage their own health care costs. Moreover, cost shifting as a strategy for providing care to the uninsured results in an implicit and irrational rationing of health care resources.

Many proposals for addressing the uninsured issue represent incremental expansions of existing programs (e.g., expansion of Medicaid and implementation of the State Children's Health Insurance Program) rather than an overhaul of the voluntary employer-based approach to health insurance in the United States. This strategy is politically prudent in light of past experience and the current political climate. Phased implementation of programs aimed at expanding coverage is reasonable and likely necessary. Incremental approaches that simply extend coverage to more people and perpetuate current behaviors and resource allocation patterns are, however, inherently incomplete and will not produce desired results (Oberlander, 2003). As long as the United States has a patchwork of health insurance coverage that relies predominately on fee-for-service reimbursement, it will be impossible to align incentives with desired stakeholder behavior across the entire system.

The uninsured issue is juxtaposed against a health care system that consumed $1.6 trillion dollars in 2002 and is projected to consume twice as much within the next decade (Heffler *et al.*, 2004; Levit *et al.*, 2004). Not surprisingly, the nation is resistant to additional increases in health care spending for expanded health insurance coverage without commensurate benefits. Indeed, the nation may not support additional investment to expand health insurance coverage even for increases in health status or productivity. As a result, improving our health care system is intertwined with eliminating the uninsured problem.

Only if we improve the effectiveness and efficiency of the health care system, can we afford to extend coverage to all residents. And, at the same time, only with universal coverage will we be able to create a health care system devoted to the health management of both individuals and the entire population. Since health status is influenced by a variety of determinants, universal coverage alone will not assure the health of those insured today and those who are currently uninsured. Multiple strategies must be pursued. Thus, the issue of the uninsured ultimately must be addressed in the context of what the US health care system should become in the twenty-first century.

The need to enhance value

The United States spends more on health care than any other industrialized nation (Anderson, 1997). Spending $1.6 trillion dollars a year on health care produces many positive results. For those who can access the sophisticated technology of American medicine, our system of care can be uniquely lifesaving. Its curative successes attract patients from around the globe. Our medical research infrastructure continually generates discoveries that help to expand the treatment arsenal in America and throughout the world. For example, today it is possible to customize treatment for some diseases (such as some breast cancers) to match an individual's genes and improve the likelihood of successful outcomes.

The US health care system is, however, too far from its full potential (American Public Health Association, 2003; IOM, 2001b, 2003b). In addition to the uninsured issue, our health care spending does not provide a safe environment, strong public health capabilities, or a healthy populace. The mortality rate from gunfire in the United States is 28 times that of Japan, and, despite a recent decline, is the highest among all Western industrialized nations (Thompson, 1998). The US public health system is in "disarray" and facing "increasingly diverse threats and challenges" – including but not limited to bioterrorism (IOM, 2003c). The health of US citizens, as measured by variables such as life expectancy and infant mortality, lags behind that of most industrialized countries. Further, within the United States, disparities in health status persist between racial and ethnic groups, men and women, and populations with lower and higher levels of income and education. And while some progress has been made with regard to tobacco addiction, over the past decade millions of the nation's adults and children have become overweight or clinically obese.

Most of our health care spending is allocated to health care services, yet even here we are far from providing uniform quality and safety. Poll data indicate that four in ten Americans personally have had a "bad experience" with medical care (Miller, 1998). In 1999 the IOM reported that medical errors are a leading cause of death in the United States and called for a 50 percent reduction in medical errors over five years (IOM, 1999). In a broader survey of health care quality issues, the IOM found a "chasm" between the promise and the realities of the health care system (IOM, 2001b). The IOM concluded that our existing systems of care are inadequate given the complexity of modern health care and the growth in the health sciences' knowledge base. Health professionals are hampered in their efforts to provide high quality care by a delivery system with deficient processes, inadequate information systems, and misaligned incentives.

After a brief respite in the 1990s, health care costs and insurance premiums are climbing again and creating budgetary stresses for individuals, businesses, states, and the federal government. Generally, the increased expenditures purchase the same level and kinds of service; the increases do not consistently offer improvement in health status. The techniques used over the past decade to control rising health care costs have taken a toll on public confidence in the health care system and on the morale and motivation of health care professionals. Trust in large institutions and organizations throughout society has eroded in recent years and health care has not been excluded. Public opinion surveys repeatedly report concerns about quality and safety and the erosion of trust in the system, particularly in managed care organizations. A substantial percentage of the public attributes the high costs of health care to the greed of insurers and for-profit health care delivery organizations and believes that profits are put before quality (Miller, 1998). Within the health care community, there are concerns about professionalism and the incentives created by managed care organizations for physicians (Blumenthal, 1994; Iglehart, 1998; Kassirer, 1995).

As the twenty-first century progresses and until substantial corrections are applied, several trends will exacerbate the deficiencies of our health care system's performance and create even greater cost pressures. The aging population sharpens the need for more effective chronic disease management and greater continuity of care across time and organizations. Our health care facilities and processes have been designed to support centralized, acute care rather than at-home chronic care. Their sheer size and scale create an underlying drive to maintain the infrastructure of bricks and mortar while emerging and more important priorities do not receive adequate investment. The sedentary and increasingly overweight population will create additional disease burden on the system. The changing ethnic composition of the population will require multi-cultural capabilities within health care organizations.

Substantial investments in information technology and the national health information infrastructure (NHII) need to be made by individual organizations and the federal government if we are to strengthen the health sector's decision-support and knowledge-management capabilities. (See discussion in Chapter 5.) Pharmacogenomics will be coming progressively onto the scene over the next decade. Our expanding set of treatment capabilities and an increasingly informed public will create greater demand for new services and higher expectations for outcomes. Many patients are assuming greater responsibility for managing and coordinating their medical care and these people would benefit from both education and tools that support personal health management. Bioterrorism preparedness represents a significant and expensive new challenge for the public health community. The roles of health professionals are evolving and complicating the already difficult challenge of attracting qualified individuals to the health sector and adequately preparing them to do their jobs, including enhanced expertise in communications.

Given the enormous level of resources allocated to health care in this country (USA) and the lack of uniformly desirable results, it is clear that simply adding more money to the current system will not secure the gains needed by the nation. Managing the costs and improving the quality, safety, and availability of health care services are necessary, but not sufficient to meet the health care needs of the United States. Thus, the US health sector stands at a turning point. Will we build on our achievements in improving health and fulfill the promise offered by our ever-expanding knowledge on human health? Or, will we allow the deficiencies of our current approach to health to persist and muddle through the next quarter century without sufficiently realigning our health system? Are we willing to change our thinking, our behaviors, and our financial allocations to create a system that maximizes the health of individuals and the population?

Tools for building the future

A series of developments provides us with the tools that can make improved health a reality in an environment of constrained resources. These tools include:

- A broader understanding of the determinants of health – ranging from environmental to behavioral to genomic factors.
- Growing expectations for accountability of health care organizations and professionals with associated transparency with respect to health status, patient satisfaction, and the costs, quality, and safety of services.
- Increasing capabilities in the assessment of satisfaction and measurement of health status and outcomes.
- The maturing of information technology applications in health care service delivery and emergence of a national health information infrastructure.
- The increasing effectiveness of pharmaceuticals and medical technology.
- Lessons learned from the evolution of managed care, especially population health management.
- An ever-expanding base of knowledge that supports the practice of medicine and tools to help clinicians manage that knowledge, especially computer-based adaptive decision support systems.
- Growing interest in and research to improve the safety and quality of health care services.
- Examples of successful collaborations and partnerships within communities and regions to promote health.
- A growing trend of individuals assuming greater responsibility for maintaining their health and managing their care or at least their being more aware of their need to do so.
- Greater understanding of complex adaptive systems and how to introduce successful change within such systems.

    Further, the Institute of Medicine developed an explicit set of aims for improvement in the US health care system to guide health care organizations (IOM, 2001b). These aims prescribe that health care services should be:

- **Safe** – Avoid injuries to patients from the care that is intended to help them.
- **Effective** – Provide services based on scientific knowledge to all who could benefit and refrain from providing services to those not likely to benefit (avoiding underuse and overuse, respectively).

- **Patient-centered** – Provide care that is respectful and responsive to individual patient preferences and needs and ensure that patient values guide clinical decisions.
- **Timely** – Reduce waits and potentially harmful delays for both those who receive and those who give care.
- **Efficient** – Avoid waste, including waste of equipment, supplies, ideas, and energy.
- **Equitable** – Provide care that does not vary in accessibility and quality because of personal characteristics such as gender, ethnicity, geographic location, and socio-economic status.

By drawing upon these varied assets and innovations, health care leaders and policy-makers can stimulate the development of a system in the United States that is focused on health, driven by value, and offers far more than today's system.

A value-driven health system

There are three ways in which an individual, organization, or system can be driven by value. The individual or entity can base decisions and actions on principles deemed to be *desirable*, act to *create worth*, or seek a *fair price* on goods and services. A value-driven health system encompasses each of these dimensions of value. It is driven by the belief that health is both a social and an economic good and that there should be equity of access and quality of essential evidence-based care services in our health system. It is driven to maximize the health of the nation. And it is driven to achieve good health as efficiently as possible.

A value-driven health system promotes and improves the health of the nation while maximizing the effectiveness of health care spending for individuals and populations. It minimizes risk of disease and injury through individual, community, and national initiatives that enable more healthy work, home, and community environments, encourage wellness and prevention practices, and support health education and health maintenance programs. A value-driven health system also enables health care professionals and organizations to consistently provide evidence-based, high quality, patient-centered health care services when disease or injury does occur. It accomplishes these objectives by applying sound health professional and business practices – maximizing return on investment, managing risk, and aligning incentives with desired outcomes – within the framework established by its guiding principles.

Guiding principles

A value-driven health system begins with a basic premise. The health of the population is a pivotal factor in determining equity for our citizens and the wealth of our nation. Whether viewed from an ethical or economic perspective, we are all impacted by the health status of our communities. Thus, a healthy population is a paramount social and economic good, health care spending is an investment in our nation, and we all bear a level of collective responsibility for managing our health.

Articulating the full value of health to our society is a fundamental step in the transformation of the US health care system. A healthy nation is a strong nation. Healthy citizens can work productively, take advantage of educational opportunities, participate in democratic processes, and support community organizations. Health contributes to personal success, sustainable economic growth, and social stability. In turn, "disease and ill-health interfere with our happiness and undermine our self-confidence" (Green, 1976). Poor health is expensive for the individual, the family, the community, the employer, and the nation as a whole (Knowles and Owen, 1997; Ram and Schultz, 1979; Smart, Mann and Adrian, 1993; Vinni, 1983).

The United States has focused its health care delivery system and health policy primarily on the value of health to individuals. In contrast, Europeans view health care predominantly as a social or collective good in which all citizens benefit when an individual receives needed care (World Health Organization, 1996). Most European countries provide universal coverage for their residents, spend less than the United States on health care services, and in so doing have achieved better health status for their citizens (Anderson, 1997). If we view health as a determinant of the nation's wealth, then universal health insurance (as a primary means of improving health status for over 40 million Americans) is also a means of strengthening the nation. Thus, the benefits of universal coverage accrue to all citizens, not just those who previously lacked health insurance.

Individual choice is a fundamental value for Americans, but some individual behaviors adversely impact others. As a result, some federal, state, and local policies limit individual choices to protect citizens' health (e.g., mandated childhood immunizations, seat belt and air bag requirements, gun control legislation, and restrictions on smoking). Not all health promotion activities can, however, be legislated and individuals must assume responsibility for choices that affect their health.

The obesity epidemic illustrates this point. Obesity is caused by a complex set of factors including genetics, nutrition, environment, and individual behaviors, but in most cases it is preventable. The human and financial costs of obesity are staggering. Each year an estimated 300 000 adults die from causes that can be attributed to obesity; many others experience chronic disease and lower quality of life (Allison *et al.*, 1999; Mokdad *et al.*, 2000). In economic terms, annual direct and indirect costs of obesity are $100 billion (Wolf and Colditz, 1998). The Medicare and Medicaid programs bear a significant portion of these costs. Employers do as well. So ultimately individual taxpayers and consumers are funding the costs of individual behaviors or choices. Viewed in another way, we are treating the avoidable condition of obesity instead of funding other critical social and/or medical needs of our society.

Maximizing return on investment

If health spending is an investment in our nation's social and human capital, then it follows that decisions about health spending should be framed in terms of how to maximize the return on that investment or how to maximize the health achieved for the dollars spent. At present, health care spending decisions can be vastly improved to obtain greater value. A study by the Dartmouth Center for Evaluative Clinical Services found that Medicare spending per person varies more than twofold among regions of the country (Wennberg, Fischer, and Skinner, 2002). These variations in expenditure are not reflected in differences in health status and have not resulted in more effective care or better health outcomes. Use of treatments that are supported by clinical evidence varies extensively among hospital referral regions. For example, the percentage of patients who met criteria for receiving beta-blockers and actually received them ranged from 5 to 92 percent across the regions. Eliminating regional disparities would yield an estimated $40 billion that could be reallocated elsewhere in the system.

In contrast, scientifically valid evidence drives decisions in a value-driven health system. Each decision point is evaluated in terms of how a finite set of resources can be optimized for the particular population or subset of the population. A basic question must be asked repeatedly by all decision-makers – federal, state, and local policy-makers, health care provider organization managers, public health officials, health care professionals, insurers, and in some cases, patients:

With the available level of resources, what action(s) will yield the highest benefit toward our objective for this population and/or individual patient?

The actions under consideration will span preventive, clinical, and social interventions. The objectives likely will include: keep people healthy, return them to health and to their gainful labors, maximize their ability to function independently, manage their chronic pain or ease their terminal pain. The populations in question will include the nation, state, region, community, insured group, or patients in a physician's practice.

In essence, a value-driven health system expands the concept of evidence-based medicine from an overwhelming focus on the care of individual patients to include the proper care of populations of patients (Sackett *et al.*, 1996). Evidence-based decision-making for individuals and populations requires access to sound evidence applicable to the question at hand (Gray, 1997). Thus, a value-driven health system depends on ongoing generation, evaluation, refinement, and dissemination of evidence on the quality, efficiency, and effectiveness of all health system activities (e.g., health care services, health promotion programs). It also depends on the presence of a robust information technology infrastructure that enables accurate and timely data collection and analysis and facilitates access to existing evidence on a need-to-know and right-to-know basis. (See Chapter 5.)

A value-driven health system requires that health professionals and organizations, nonhealth organizations, communities, and regions shift investment to what makes a difference in the health status of the population. Stakeholders at all levels – from policy-makers to health professionals to patients – must be evidence-driven and be willing to act on timely, accurate knowledge to eliminate treatments and interventions that have been shown to be ineffective. Following this path will not be easy. It requires a reallocation of resources not only within the medical infrastructure (e.g., away from treatments shown to be ineffective or provider organizations with poor performance), but also to other domains that are known to contribute to improved health status (e.g., literacy). For instance, approximately 50 percent of deaths can be attributed to behavioral and environmental factors, yet only 5 percent of the US health care budget is allocated to prevention activities (McGinnis and Foege, 1993). Courageous and sound leadership is needed to realign incentives and structures toward the appropriate performance-based rewards.

In addition, the health care community, policy-makers, and citizens must accept that explicit rationing of resources is a likely and equitable step toward achieving universal coverage and maximizing the effectiveness of health care spending in the United States. As a first step, the health community and general public should acknowledge that our current approach rations health resources away from millions of uninsured citizens. Further, patients, citizens and health professionals need to be educated about the benefits and wisdom of redirecting resources to effective interventions and of withholding funding for ineffective and marginally beneficial treatments. The difficulty associated with allocating resources in terms of greatest benefit reinforces the need for a solid, objective, and more refined base of knowledge on which to make those decisions and an ongoing dialogue about the ethics of health care spending decisions.

Maximizing health or value achieved for resources expended is also a function of the safety, quality, and efficiency of health care services. Once the decision about the most appropriate treatment is made, we must have confidence that it will be implemented properly (i.e., meet the six aims for health care services outlined by the IOM, as described earlier). Further, although cost reduction is not the primary objective of a value-driven health system, the health care delivery system can and should optimize available resources and provide services as efficiently as possible.

Managing risk

An estimated 75 percent of current health care spending in the United States can be attributed to treating the 125 million Americans with one or more chronic diseases (Snyderman, 2002). Irreversible damage (e.g., amputation, blindness or renal failure due to diabetes) and expensive treatment can often be avoided by early diagnosis or prevention of chronic disease. Yet, typically the health system directs it resources to treating rather than preventing disease. Moreover, the health system is inconsistent in its application of and results achieved from treatment. New technologies and knowledge allow both earlier diagnosis of, and identification of risk for, many diseases. Emerging information and communication technologies support organizational structures that can assure much more effective management of chronic conditions when disease cannot be prevented. (See Chapter 6.)

Thus, managing risk for populations and individuals is at the heart of the value-driven health system. It involves identifying health risks, communicating those risks, and managing the health risks collaboratively before the onset of disease and associated treatment costs. It also requires mechanisms for assessing risk and motivating individuals to respond to that risk. Finally, it is organized to manage the care of those who still face advancing morbidity over time.

Populations

Population health management primarily focuses on modifying risk for an entire population but also includes selective preventive measures for members of subgroups at above-average risk. Population health management activities range from immunization programs to public education campaigns to legislation (e.g., seatbelt laws or minimum wage increases) to systematic population-based application of effective treatment for common diseases. Population health management offers a viable mechanism for improving health while reducing costs of health care services. Health education programs designed to reduce health risks have been shown to "improve population health and at the same time reduce medical costs by 20 percent or more" (Fries *et al.*, 1998).

Two conditions must be met for population health management to be effective at the health system level. First, it must be possible to collect and analyze data on the population. These data are used to determine health risk, to track interventions or preventive strategies used, to monitor health resources consumed, and to assess the resulting outcomes for members of a given population. These data become the basis for new knowledge about improving the health of the population.

Second, it must be possible to establish incentives that affect all members of the population so that a free-rider problem does not emerge. Individuals who choose to pursue less healthy behaviors or more expensive care approaches should know and bear these costs. The entire population must be part of the health system for these two conditions to be met. Universal coverage provides the best mechanism for bringing as many citizens as possible into the system.

Individuals

A new truly "patient-centered" model for managing risk to individuals' health is emerging. Prospective heath care or personalized health planning begins with a risk analysis based on an individual's genetic, environmental, and lifestyle factors. This risk analysis is used to develop a plan that identifies "the best countermeasures for each individual to minimize the probabilities for development or progression of major chronic disease" (Snyderman and Williams, 2003). Individuals are stratified according to their risk, linked to the appropriate programs (e.g., education, behavior modification, or disease management), and monitored by health coaches to assure that individuals are following their health plan. To date, prospective health care has been shown to be effective for patients with congestive heart failure, diabetes, and asthma. For this approach to become widely applied, advanced information systems that integrate multiple streams of information about a patient to generate both a personalized risk profile and a set of recommendations aimed at reducing that risk must be implemented.

Aligning incentives

One of the greatest challenges in creating a value-driven health system will be to establish incentives that motivate individual patients, health professionals, and health care organizations to choose behaviors and actions that will lead to the desired outcomes of health and efficiency. In contrast to current practice, it is essential that the system distributes responsibility and financial risks and rewards appropriately. A value-driven system needs to reward:

- Individuals for healthy lifestyle choices and being prudent purchasers of health services.
- Health care professionals and organizations for promoting and improving the health of populations and individuals, managing risk, and providing high quality and efficient services.
- Researchers for pursuing research areas that support value-driven health.

It also needs to recognize and support employers, communities, and federal and state policy-makers for creating health-promoting environments. In short, a value-driven system rewards (i.e., pays for) performance that is consistent with system objectives.

The prevalent, fee-for-service reimbursement system rewards the treatment of acute disease and tends as well to favor expensive interventionist technologies. It pays for the costs of professional time spent with a patient, facility costs, and supplies associated with treating episodic services for acute care provided in a physician's office or hospital. It does not recognize the costs nor reward the benefits of health promotion, coordination for chronic care services or disease management, time spent weighing available evidence, development of robust information systems, population health management or community health improvement. It does not recognize the possibility that health care services can be consumed from home (e.g., telemedicine or email communication between doctor and patient). It does not encourage individuals to make decisions to promote health or to be prudent consumers of health services. Nor does it encourage communities to address the social determinants of health.

In theory, managed care provides incentives for health care professionals and organizations to focus on health promotion and disease management. In practice, one approach to managed care (i.e., health maintenance organizations), where physicians' incentives are closely aligned with organizational objectives and a stable population of patients is present, has led to some value-driven practices (e.g., health promotion, disease management, investment in information systems) (Dixon *et al.*, 2004; Feachem, Sekhri, and White, 2002). But in general, managed care programs have focused on controlling utilization and thereby limiting choices rather than offering sufficient incentives or additional value to consumers.

Underpinning the emerging consumer-driven health plans is the belief that "individual consumers of health care should assume greater financial responsibility for the decisions they make when selecting insurance and seeking medical treatment" (Iglehart, 2002). Consumers are given a bigger role in choosing their health insurance coverage and are provided with more information about health service quality and cost to aid in their selection of providers and treatments. This approach shows early promise. By providing consumers with data on price and quality, the Minnesota's Buyer Health Care Action Group has increased enrollment in provider groups with lower prices and higher ratings for quality (Christianson *et al.*, 1999). (See Chapter 6.)

Consumer-driven health plans may well constitute an important breakthrough in managing the cost and improving the quality of health care services, but a value-driven health system encompasses more than the health care delivery system. Thus, additional incentives that stimulate population health management, community health improvement, and personal responsibility for behaviors that impact health will be critical.

Towards a value-driven health system

The success of a value-driven system will depend on: innovation in designing and delivering services; investment of short-term savings into a long-range strategy that promotes health, lowers disability, and reduces morbidity and mortality; and streamlined administration at the organizational and system level. Elements of a value-driven health system are already in place or under development (e.g., increasing sophistication and use of outcome measures, implementation of clinical information systems that offer decision support to clinicians), but these components are too fragmented today. Both the integration and acceleration of development and implementation are needed. This will require both public and private sectors – particularly those who purchase health services, award grants, and allocate resources to localities – to establish incentives that reward individuals and organizations for value-driven practices.

In addition, three inter-related steps are needed to make real progress toward universal coverage and a value-driven health system. First, Congress must declare that universal coverage is a national priority and set a date for its enactment. Second, health care organizations, public health agencies, and local communities and regions must strengthen their focus on population health management and community health improvement through education, research, and demonstration projects. Third, each health care organization should assure that its mission is focused on improving individual and population health and that its resources and capabilities are aligned accordingly.

The Blue Ridge Academic Health Group developed the following set of recommendations for moving toward a value-driven health system. Each of these is discussed in the sections that follow. In addition, Chapters 3 through 6 address challenges associated with becoming value-driven organizations.

Universal coverage recommendations

- Congress should begin to address the uninsured problem by passing legislation that mandates health insurance coverage, whether privately or publicly funded, for all residents as a national objective. Subsequently, Congress should pass legislation that creates the framework and authorizes funding for insurance to be extended to all residents. This insurance should provide access to a minimum set of effective health services, including preventive, health maintenance, and acute and chronic illness care.
- Federal and state governments should assure that existing, expanded, or new publicly funded health insurance programs promote value-driven practices through appropriate incentives and support the information infrastructure needed for a value-driven health system (i.e., national, local, and organizational health information infrastructures).

Population health recommendation

- The Department of Health and Human Services, state and local health departments, health care provider organizations, schools of public health, private foundations, and other public and private health-related organizations should make population health the primary objective of public health.

Community health improvement recommendations

- Each community or region should assume responsibility for improving the health of the residents in its area.
- Each health care delivery organization (public or private) within the community or region should help to initiate (if necessary), actively participate in, and support through their clinical and service programs, efforts to advance the health of residents of the community or region.
- Federal and state legislators and agencies should support community and regional efforts by developing policies (including distribution of resources) that create incentives for individuals, local agencies, health care organizations and professionals, and employers to adopt strategies that measurably advance health.

AHC recommendations

- AHCs, other health care delivery organizations, organized medicine, and the health professions should renew and, where necessary, realign their goals, values, and missions to better address societal needs and aspirations for our health care system.
- AHCs and other health care organizations should strive for the aims for health care delivery articulated by the Institute of Medicine (2001b) in its report, *Crossing the Quality Chasm: a New Health System for the 21st Century.* These include the need for a health care system that is safe, effective, patient-centered, timely, efficient, and equitable.
- AHCs should adopt and advocate the goal of transitioning our national health care system to a value-driven model of universal coverage and population health management through a combination of public and private mechanisms.
- In addition to participating in community or regional efforts to advance the population's health, each AHC should provide leadership through research, and education of current and future health professionals, on population

health management and a value-driven health system as fundamental strategies for health care delivery in the twenty-first century.

Universal coverage

The evidence in favor of universal health coverage is compelling and outweighs arguments for maintaining the status quo. Yet, the politics of the issue are complex, daunting, and, to date, have proven insurmountable. The financial costs of mounting a universal coverage program (even with limited benefits), competing budget issues, efforts to manage the federal budget deficit, the fear of big government, the impact on entrenched interests, past failures, and an ambivalent public have all made universal coverage a political morass.

Experience with state programs, however, shows that increases in effective coverage can occur, with the general acceptance of the population, with apparent improvement in health status, and without large increases in cost (Bodenheimer, 1997; Oregon Health Plan, 1997). Two separate analyses of proposals to expand health insurance coverage found that national health expenditures would increase by $23 to $57 billion or $34 to $69 billion, depending on the program, if universal insurance were implemented (Hadley and Holahan, 2003; Sheils and Haught, 2003). These additional medical service costs would only increase national health spending by 3 to 6 percent.

Universal health coverage can take many different forms, as is evident from the multitude of proposals for achieving universal coverage and the variation in approaches where it has been introduced (Collins, Davis, and Lambrew, 2004; Sheils and Haught, 2003). In some cases, these approaches are variations on the same theme, such as expansion of existing systems to cover the uninsured populations. In other instances, proposals are contradictory, such as incremental expansion of employer-based health insurance versus implementing structures to reduce the prevalence of employer-based health insurance.

Rather than advance a particular universal coverage plan, the Blue Ridge Group identified a set of principles for universal coverage that would support the development of a value-driven health system and could be applied to a variety of universal coverage approaches. These principles include:

- Each legal US resident has health insurance coverage for a basic set of effective health services. (This would likely require a mandate, perhaps on individuals.)

- The set of basic services includes preventive, health maintenance, acute, and chronic illness care. This set of services is regularly reviewed and adjusted according to ongoing research and evidence of effectiveness.
- Insured individuals are aware of the full costs of insurance and the costs of services they consume, and bear an appropriate share of those costs. Individuals are aware of how their behaviors contribute to their health and costs of their health care. Individuals are informed about the effectiveness of alternative treatments.
- Insurance coverage does not depend on employment status. Risk pools exist to provide all individuals access to insurance for basic health services. As a result, risk is shared among all stakeholders. The tax code treats health insurance costs equally across all kinds of employment. Subsidies are provided to low-income families.
- The performance (including costs) of the entire system, of individual providers, and of geographic populations can be objectively and accurately measured, and rewards are tied to performance.

These principles are consistent with those recommended by the Institute of Medicine to guide development of universal health insurance policies (IOM, 2004):

- Health care coverage should be universal.
- Health care coverage should be continuous.
- Health care coverage should be affordable to individuals and families.
- The health insurance strategy should be affordable and sustainable for society.
- Health insurance should enhance health and well-being by promoting access to high-quality care that is effective, efficient, safe, timely, patient-centered, and equitable.

The Blue Ridge Group's view of a value-driven health system emphasizes the need to reallocate existing resources rather than immediately add more resources to the system. For instance, reduction in overly intensive treatment of irreversible terminal illness could reduce total health care costs by 3 percent (Sloan and Taylor, 1999). In addition, health promotion and disease management programs show promise for improving health and reducing costs of medical services (Bodenheimer, Wagner, and Grumback, 2002; Fries et al., 1998; Weingarten et al., 2002). Their effectiveness does however depend on program design, and research on which designs are most effective is needed.

Direct reallocation of resources is most likely to be achieved by the federal and state governments, as funding that has supported the current piecemeal approach to providing care to uninsured individuals can be reallocated to new programs specifically designed to extend coverage and improve value. For example, a Florida program that provided insurance to children found that emergency visits dropped by 70 percent and saved $13 million in 1996 (Florida Healthy Kids Corporation, 1997). In addition, disproportionate share payments could be reconfigured and funds used to support uncompensated care pools could be shifted to pay for expanded insurance coverage.

With universal health insurance, physicians and health care delivery organizations that currently provide uncompensated care should and would be compensated for that care. This should reduce the need for cost-shifting (i.e., cross-subsidies and increased rates for insured patients) to cover uncompensated care costs. Additional resources to support universal coverage can be found in: increasing tobacco, alcohol, firearm taxes, and other user taxes; earmarking corporate taxes paid by for-profit health providers and plans; or collection of social responsibility contributions from employers that do not offer health insurance. In the long term, it is anticipated that new incentives for consumers and providers would enable cost management and improve the efficiency of health care programs thereby freeing resource for other uses within the health system. Other opportunities exist as well. For example, the growth of e-health in which personal health records maintained on computer connect patients with their providers improves efficiency both in the office and also with prescription services (see Chapter 6).

Actual implementation of universal coverage is likely to be accomplished through phasing, and incremental adoption by states and localities. Coverage expansion could continue the approach initiated by some federal and state programs of gradually including priority populations (e.g., women of childbearing age, people aged 60–64 years) as funding becomes available. Incremental expansion of coverage must, however, be accompanied by incentives for enrollees to pursue behaviors, and health care delivery organizations to adopt strategies, that advance health. Further, existing federal and state health insurance programs must be structured to promote value-driven practices (e.g., health promotion, investment in and use of information technology).

The challenges associated with designing an affordable, effective way to achieve universal coverage and gaining political support to implement the resulting programs should not be understated. Thus, legislative efforts should focus first on establishing universal coverage as a national priority. Subsequently, the specifics of how universal coverage should be achieved can be debated. Moreover, while extending health insurance coverage to all legal residents of the United States is an essential step toward improving the health status in this country, it must be accompanied by a set of equally important actions that will provide the foundation for a value-driven health system.

Population health

It might seem obvious that population health should be the primary focus of the public health system. Yet, during the twentieth century, this role was undermined by low levels of resources available for this purpose and diluted by other demands on public health agencies. Between 1981 and 1993, total US expenditures on health care oriented to individuals increased by more than 210 percent while funding for population-based health strategies, as a proportion of the health care budget, declined by 25 percent (Center for Studying Health System Change, 1996). According to the American Public Health Association, "only one percent of health dollars are spent on public health efforts to improve overall health" (American Public Health Association, 2003). Further, approximately two thirds of resources in the public health system were directed to personal health services, such as direct care to individuals rather than to core public health functions (Public Health Foundation, 1996). As a result, the public health infrastructure has been under-funded and public health was often considered to be the equivalent of publicly funded health care.

Public health itself was dwarfed by the enormous growth in the personal health care delivery system. Increasingly, and until quite recently, the health care system emphasized personal care over population care and diagnostic technologies and curative tactics over preventive strategies (IOM, 1988; Smith, Anderson, and Boumbulian, 1991). There are 3000 local public health agencies and myriad state and federal agencies working on public health in this country. Yet, until the bioterrorism scare of 2001, most Americans did not know what public health agencies do (Center for Studying Health System Change, 1996; Levy, 1998).

The need to bolster public health has been acknowledged by a variety of groups including the Centers for Disease Control, Robert Wood Johnson Foundation, Kellogg Foundation, Institute of Medicine, and the Public Health Functions Project (American Public Health Association, 2003; IOM, 1988, 2003c; Kindig, 1997; US Department of Health and Human Services, 1998). Specifically, to fulfill a pivotal role in managing population health, the visibility of public health must be heightened, alliances must be established or strengthened, the focus and allocation of resources within public health must be realigned, and funding for public health must be increased. If these requirements are met, then public health agencies will be positioned to be the nexus of the health care delivery system and community efforts to address the determinants of health.

A robust public health infrastructure will both contribute to and benefit from a value-driven health system. Once universal coverage is achieved, rather than providing services to the uninsured, public health agencies will be able to increase attention and resources to issues and activities that advance the health of the public. Moreover, as health care professionals and delivery organizations increase their focus on managing the health of populations, there is opportunity for collaboration among health care and public health professionals and for linking the medical model and public health model more visibly (Lasker, 1997). Ultimately, for a value-driven health system to function, public health and health care services must both be seen as integral parts of the health system.

Public health departments already serve population-based roles in environmental protection, public education, and outreach services to high-risk populations. Data collection and measuring population health improvement are logical extensions of public health agency functions. Further expansion could lie in coordinating efforts within communities and across the multiple determinants of health (Kindig, 1997). The continued development of the national health information infrastructure (NHII) – with its clear mission to support public health – is pivotal to progress in monitoring population health status (Detmer, 2003; National Committee on Vital and Health Statistics, 2002).

New methods and tools for tracking public health functions are needed. The proliferation of health and safety programs in nonpublic health government agencies challenges the coordination of public health functions and the ability of public health departments to demonstrate accountability for the resources allocated to them. Indicators are needed to track whether public health agency goals are being met and how those goals contribute to the health status of a community. Moreover, the public health community needs to be a major contributor to the development and ongoing monitoring of population-based outcome and performance standards.

Funding for public health activities should be evaluated to see how it could be optimally used to promote health. The level of, mechanisms for, and incentives created by public health funding need to be evaluated. Much of the funding for public health services and research has been provided in the form of categorical grants that address specific issues. As a result, there is little flexibility for public health professionals to address emerging or community-specific issues and little opportunity for public health researchers to pursue interdisciplinary or community-wide approaches to addressing public health issues. Past resources for the public health infrastructures (e.g., block grants structured on per capita bases, taxing insurers), as well as potential new sources, need to be catalogued and coordinated programmatically to maximize their potential. Again, value-driven, evidence-based policy can have significant impact through reallocation of existing resources.

Both the public and private sectors have begun working to strengthen public health capabilities and increase focus on population health. *Healthy People 2010* outlines the US health promotion and disease prevention agenda (US Department of Health and Human Services, 2000). In addition to 13 federal agencies, the Healthy People Consortium (with 400 national members and all state and territorial health departments) is working to meet the Healthy People goals. From 1997 to 2003, the Robert Wood Johnson Foundation and WK Kellogg Foundation co-funded the Turning Point Initiative to make public health more community-based and collaborative. One of the major lessons from this program is that "neighborhood/community work groups could be instrumental in generating and sustaining support for public health improvements" (Lewin Group, 2002).

Community health improvement

Many of the factors that contribute to health status lie outside the health system and are best addressed at the source rather than within the health care delivery system. In addition to insurance coverage, such factors include education level, literacy, employment status, income level, quality of housing, safety of neighborhoods, availability of transportation, and support networks for individuals and families. Since these factors largely lie within the realm of local and regional governments, it is appropriate and necessary that communities or regions be actively engaged in improving the health of citizens. This health emphasis will require action from a wide range of players responding to differing incentives. Examples of successful programs and strategies exist, but must be replicated throughout the country. Implementation will be fostered by appropriate measurement as well as collaboration and partnering of intellectual and economic capital.

According to the Institute of Medicine, "a community health improvement process that includes performance monitoring . . . can be an effective tool for developing a shared vision and supporting a planned and integrated approach to improve community health" (IOM, 1997). Such an effort must be iterative and evolving rather than a short-term, one-time event and should be based in a community health coalition or similar entity. The process provides a framework that allows communities or regions to take a comprehensive approach to maintaining and improving health, develop specific strategies to address the social and environmental determinants of health in the locality, and track progress over time. The basic steps of a community health improvement process include:

- Conduct a community health profile, such as demographic and socio-economic characteristics, health status, and health risks.
- Analyze health issues.
- Inventory health resources.
- Develop a health improvement strategy.
- Establish accountability for activities.
- Develop a set of performance indicators.
- Implement the improvement strategy.
- Monitor the process and outcomes.

The process will vary among communities as they consider their own health concerns, resources and capabilities, social and political perspectives, and competing needs in developing a health improvement program. Increasingly, community health improvement efforts will include the development of local health information infrastructures (LHII) to support data collection and analysis, enable evidence-based decision-making, facilitate communication among the diverse set of participants, and implement community-based strategies aimed at improving health (see also Chapter 5).

Any sector of a community or region can initiate collaborative efforts and lead a community health improvement process. Public health agencies, all health care delivery organizations, social service agencies, local government leaders, and individual citizens need to participate in the community health improvement process. Involvement by many sectors of a community is necessary to ensure that collaborative efforts focus on the ultimate goals of improving community health and maximizing the benefits derived from limited health care expenditures. Community health improvement efforts cannot be limited to the public sector. Private (including for-profit) health care delivery organizations also have a responsibility to participate (Schlesinger and Gray, 1998). Moreover, success is more likely to occur if objectives are reinforced throughout the community (e.g., physician offices, libraries, schools, employers). Employers are particularly suited to reinforce community health objectives through incentives for healthy employees and may reap direct benefits through a healthier and more productive workforce.

Successful programs and strategies will involve public accountability through appropriate measurement and public reports, as well as collaboration and partnering of human, intellectual, and economic capital. Revenues for such programs may come through a variety of strategies, including taxes, corporate contributions, new community conversion foundations, and philanthropic support. In addition, federal, state, and philanthropic programs that support community health improvement should be increased. Community issues other than health care and public health services such as education, safety, crime control, jobs, affordable and safe housing, and transportation should have guidelines (akin to HEDIS, the Health Plan Employer Data and Information Set developed by the National Committee for Quality Assurance) that foster accountability and contribute to the *Healthy People 2010* goals.

There is an increasing set of experiences and range of knowledge on how communities can address their health needs. Many of the lessons learned can be attributed to philanthropic support for community health initiatives. Both the Robert Wood Johnson Foundation and WK Kellogg Foundation have been leaders in using grants to stimulate and evaluate community health efforts.

The Turning Point Initiative (mentioned above) funded 41 communities in 14 states to develop partnerships that addressed public health needs at various levels of jurisdiction. These grants funded both planning and implementation and led to the formation of new organizations and health programs as well as new business practices and cooperative relationships between participants (Lewin Group, 2003). For example, to fill gaps in health services, the Central Kenai, Alaska partnership created medical transportation services and worked with the state health department and local hospital to establish a primary care clinic and collaborative funding agreements for future support.

To address an environmental health problem (i.e., leaf burning) that was identified as contributing to increased childhood asthma, the Decatur, Illinois partnership engaged support for a ban on leaf burning and then organized a community-wide effort of leaf removal – including distribution of leaf bags and volunteers raking leaves for elderly and disabled citizens. This effort has become an annual event and has broad-based financial support from the community. The Decatur Partnership also established a Family Enrichment Center to provide families with multiple community services under one roof. The available programs were selected by the community and include newborn health, youth development, Graduate Equivalency classes, a Hispanic community support group, a career-mentoring project, and a family investment project. To improve recreational and exercise opportunities in the community, the Twin Rivers, New Hampshire Partnership sponsored a project to create and maintain a bike path and recreational trail. Although the Turning Point Initiative is no longer funded, an analysis of the 41 partnerships concluded that many had created organizational structures capable of carrying on beyond the life of the grant (Lewin Group, 2003).

From 1994 to 2001, another major community health initiative – the Community Care Network (CCN) – supported partnerships focused on aligning resources with community health needs (CCN, 2001). CCN identified 49 partnerships that had begun to work to improve the health of their communities and provided information, technical support, and a framework for networking. Among the partnerships supported by CCN was Franklin Community Health Network (FCHN) based in Franklin County, Maine. This health network is based on a long tradition of community-based health care and was formed by the local nonprofit community hospital (Batt, Dixon, and Molloy, 1998). Among its many accomplishments, this network organized three community health "visioning" conferences, with the most recent one in 1998 focused on obtaining participation from previously under-represented groups such as the under-insured, uninsured, and nonprofessional populations. One of the most innovative, but somewhat controversial, activities pursued by FCHN was the design, funding, and implementation of the Greater Franklin Development Corporation to attract companies and new jobs to the area to offset the many job losses the region had experienced.

Community health improvement continues to be supported in a variety of ways. In 2002, three national community health initiatives – CCN, ACT (i.e., Accelerating Community Transformation) National Outcomes Network, and the Coalition for Healthier Communities and Cities – merged to form the Association for Community Health Improvement (ACHI). ACHI focuses its efforts on education, peer networking, and practical tools (e.g., health assessments and care models for disadvantaged populations). The Association of Academic Health Centers (AAHC) has established the American Network of Health Promoting Universities to increase the range of effectiveness of health promotion efforts at AHCs and strengthen partnerships between AHCs and local communities. Towards that end, the network has provided grants to four AHCs to convene community stakeholders as a first step in improving the health of their communities (American Network of Health Promoting Universities, 2003). For example, the University of Nebraska Medical Center project will address major disparities in health outcomes based on race, ethnicity, geography, socio-economic status, educational level, and other factors. In September 2003, the Department of Health and Human Services (DHHS) awarded 12 grants, totaling $13.7 million, to support community initiatives to prevent diabetes, asthma, and obesity (US Department of Health and Human Services, 2003).

Role for academic health centers

A value-driven health system creates both challenges and opportunities for AHCs. It requires AHCs to forge new partnerships outside their walls. It requires them to invest in long-term strategies that will yield benefits across the population rather than solely to their institution. It requires AHCs to apply their innovative capabilities to a new set of problems. Most importantly, it requires AHCs to view their mission in a new light and to place greater emphasis on advancing the health status of the community (IOM, 2003d). Virtually every activity within AHCs needs to be evaluated in terms of its consistency with a value-driven health system and its contribution towards value-driven health. Much of this effort will involve allocating more resources toward prevention, public health, and health evaluation sciences.

Academic health centers have a long tradition of providing patient care to the uninsured and playing a large part in the health care safety net. In 1999, major teaching hospitals constituted 6 percent of the nation's hospitals, but provided 50 percent of charity care in the United States – amounting to $4 billion (Association of American Medical Colleges, 2004). AHCs should transform this role into one of leadership in advancing universal coverage and a value-driven health system. Along with the Institute of Medicine, the Kaiser Family Foundation, the Commonwealth Fund, and a host of other organizations, the Association of Academic Health Centers (AAHC) and Association of American Medical Colleges (AAMC) advocate expanding health insurance coverage to all Americans. The AAHC and AAMC have ongoing initiatives to educate health professions, policy-makers, and the public about this pivotal issue. Leaders and faculty of individual AHCs can add their voices to this effort by helping to educate their local communities on the health impact and hidden costs of being uninsured and the need for national action on this issue.

Like all health care delivery organizations, AHCs need to assess how they can improve community health orientation within their own delivery systems and how they can assist in improving community or regional health status (Anderson and Boumbulian, 1995). Academic health centers can participate in a comprehensive community health improvement process as described above or respond to a specific need that affects the health of the population. The Health Promotion and Sports Medicine faculty at the Oregon Health Sciences University (OHSU), for example, tracked a substantial increase in steroid use among high-school football players in Portland, Oregon, between 1987 and 1991. To reverse this trend, OHSU faculty developed, implemented, and evaluated a steroid education program for high-school football teams. The analysis of this program concluded that it "enhanced healthy behaviors, reduced factors that encourage AAS (anabolic androgenic steroids), and lowered intent to use AAS" (Goldberg *et al.*, 1996).

The education of current and future health professionals, researchers, managers, and patients is a critical task for creating a value-driven health system. Each of these groups must develop a broad understanding of health, understand professional, personal, institutional, and community responsibilities for improving the health of the population, and acquire the competencies to succeed in a value-driven health system (Blue Ridge Academic Health Group, 2003; IOM, 2003d). Academic health centers must allocate sufficient time in the curriculum for health professional and public health students to master the skills necessary to manage the health of populations. These competencies could include understanding the illness burden of the population, epidemiology, health evaluation sciences, community action, and intervention. The AAMC has recommended that each medical school ensures that each student demonstrates knowledge of "the epidemiology of common maladies within a defined population and systematic approaches useful in reducing the incidence and prevalence of those maladies" (AAMC, 1998).

Medical schools should continue to explore ways to provide medical education in community settings, promote health, and be responsive to the needs of the at-risk population (Blue Ridge Academic Health Group, 2003). During the 1980s and 1990s, many AHCs successfully strengthened their primary care training programs. Several AHCs went beyond the primary care model to pursue community responsive medicine. The academic discipline of community-oriented primary care (COPC) incorporates traditional primary care with public health services (Smith, Anderson, and Boumbulian, 1991). COPC blends curative and preventative services, demographics, epidemiology, community organizations, and health education for defined populations. It is a denominator-driven system that assesses effectiveness through a formal epidemiological evaluation of the population at risk. Parkland Memorial Hospital in Dallas, Texas has successfully established a COPC network (see Case study, p. 62). This program provides unique inpatient and ambulatory teaching opportunities and enables continuity of care for both the COPC and inpatient settings (Smith, Anderson, and Boumbulian, 1991).

In 1997, the AAHC established the Center for Interdisciplinary, Community-based Learning (CICL) to strengthen AHC commitment to community-based learning, especially in under-served areas (AAHC, 2003). CICL provides expertise on model curricula, training sites, and relationships with community care facilities. It also supports a network of health professionals who are working to create an interdisciplinary, community-based curriculum.

Academic health centers could adopt other innovative approaches to prepare health professionals for community involvement as part of their practice. For example, AHCs could reassign specialty residency slots to "community" specialists or create opportunities for current generalists to assume a leadership role in community health. In addition, AHCs should assess the merits of establishing a new education track for health professionals (not necessarily physicians) who can fill needed roles in a value-driven health system. Further, AHCs can explore how funding mechanisms for clinical care and education should be restructured to support an emphasis on community health practice.

AHC research that supports population health (e.g., severity of health status, and effective strategies for promoting health within communities and regions) and other aspects of a value-driven health system should be expanded. Researchers can continue to explore the relationship between healthy populations and productivity, and refine calculations of the return on investment of spending to improve the health of the population. Academic health centers also can provide expertise as communities and public health agencies establish performance measures for their communities. Most importantly, AHCs must continue to strengthen the knowledge base that supports the practice of evidence-based medicine so that the effectiveness of health services is maximized across the health system. In particular, AHCs need to collaborate to develop and refine evidence-based decision-support systems to use within their electronic medical records to improve care safety and foster better outcomes. Further, AHCs need to provide stronger leadership for changing clinical practice patterns when indicated by evidence, so that unsupported variations within the system are eliminated (Wennberg, 2002). Federal agencies and private organizations can support this endeavor by supporting research and demonstration projects that advance the generation and dissemination of knowledge about cost-effective strategies for improving health.

Getting started

Although the need for dramatic change in the US health care sector is readily apparent, garnering sufficient interest and resources to transform the complex health care enterprise is no small task. Health is just one in a set of vital national interests – including education, the economy, the environment, defense, and homeland security – which require public investment and attention. Further, although fading in the memory of the public, the last experience with health care reform failed and policy-makers are likely to be wary of attempting a major overhaul.

Fortunately, the science of complex adaptive systems (CAS) provides guidance on how to introduce substantial change. CAS recognizes that complex systems (like health care) need "the freedom and ability to respond to stimuli in many different and unpredictable ways" (IOM, 2001b, p. 309). CAS research has determined that these systems move towards their goals by having a common purpose, internal motivations, and simple rules that guide individual behavior. These simple rules can lead to complex, innovative system behavior through self-organization. Thus, profound change in the US health sector can begin with a set of simple rules, a vision, and room for creativity at the local level.

Federal and state funding and policy decisions will play a pivotal role in creating an environment in which a value-driven health system will flourish. Health care organizations and professionals, employers, communities, and citizens do not, however, need to wait for government action. They can begin by refining, embracing, and sharing the vision of a value-driven health system within and beyond their organizations. They can recognize and reinforce practices and programs already in place that are consistent with a value-driven health system (e.g., efforts by the LeapFrog Group – see Case study, p. 69). They can expand the scope of value-driven practices by making future decisions and basing future actions on the value-driven framework or guiding principles.

As beneficiaries of substantial public investment and organizations with a unique set of resources, AHCs have both the responsibility and the means to help shape the health system of the twenty-first century. Academic health centers can translate the vision of value-driven health into clinical practice, research, and health professional education and in so doing help to spread that vision throughout the health sector.

Conclusion

The momentum for major health care reform in the United States has waxed and waned over the past decade. Meanwhile, quality, cost, and access problems persist, and in the case of access for the uninsured, the situation is deteriorating. The size and complexity of the uninsured problem means that many individuals and organizations must participate in the process of bringing the problem to the fore of the nation's political agenda. It is particularly important that both policy-makers and individual citizens understand the implications and hidden costs of the uninsured issue so that they do not view it simply as someone else's problem.

A value-driven health depends on and is essential to achieving universal coverage in the United States. It also increasingly appears to be critical to the nation's ability to manage its health care costs and keep its populace healthy and productive. The United States needs a new and broader approach to health care delivery. By establishing appropriate incentives, training decision-makers, investing in organizational information systems and a national health information infrastructure, building databases, measuring outcomes, and expanding knowledge about all the factors and interventions that improve health and productivity, policy-makers and health professionals will begin the long overdue transformation of the health care sector.

Through commitment, investment, collaboration, innovation, and appropriately structured incentives, the United States can make progress toward eliminating a fundamental weakness in its social structure and substantially improve the health of the nation. Undoubtedly, the challenge ahead is formidable, but the potential payoff is well worth the price. Total population health insurance coverage and a value-driven health system are good for the United States. It is time to assure them.

REFERENCES

Allison, D. B., Fontaine, K. R., Manson, J. E., Stevens, J. and VanItallie, T. B. (1999). Annual deaths attributable to obesity in the United States. *Journal of the American Medical Association*, **282**(16), 1530–8.

American Network of Health Promoting Universities (2003). Association of Academic Health Centers funds local health-promotion activities. *Health Searchlight*, **3** (1), 6.

American Public Health Association (2003). Prevention of leading causes of death. Underfunded, US health system in crisis. *News Release*. Washington, DC:

American Public Health Association. Online at http://www.apha.org/news/press/2003/leading_causes.htm.

Anderson, G. F. (1997). In search of value: an international comparison of cost, access, and outcomes. *Health Affairs*, **16**(6), 163–71.

Anderson, R. J. and Boumbulian, P. J. (1995). Comprehensive community health programs. In *Academic Health Centers in the Managed Care Environment*, ed. D. Korn, C. J. McLaughlin and M. Osterweis. Washington, DC: Association of Academic Health Centers.

Association of Academic Health Centers (2003). *Center for Interdisciplinary, Community-based Learning*. Washington, DC: Association of Academic Health Centers. Online at http:///www.ahcnet.org/programs/education/cicl.php.

Association of American Medical Colleges (1998). *Medical School Objectives Project Report II: Contemporary Issues in Medicine: Medical Informatics and Population Health*. Washington, DC: Association of American Medical Colleges.

(2004) *Protecting America's Uninsured*. Washington, DC: Association of American Medical Colleges. Online at http://www.aamc.org/uninsured/.

Ayanian, J. S., Kohler, B. A., Abe, T. and Epstein, A. M. (1993). The relationship between health insurance coverage and clinical outcomes among women with breast cancer. *New England Journal of Medicine*, **329**(5), 326–31.

Batt, R., Dixon, D. and Molloy, R. (1998). *At the Millennium: Successes of a Community-based Health System in Rural Maine 1994–2000*. Farmington, ME: Franklin Community Health Network. Online at http://www.fchn.org/FCHN/articles.AtTheMillenium.asp.

Blue Ridge Academic Health Group (2003). *Reforming Medical Education: Urgent Priority for the Academic Health Center in the New Century*. Atlanta, GA: Emory University.

Blumenthal, D. (1994). The vital role of professionalism in health care reform. *Health Affairs*, **13**(1), 252–5.

Bodenheimer, T. (1997). The Oregon Health Plan. *New England Journal of Medicine*, **337**(9), 651–5.

Bodenheimer, T., Wagner, E. H. and Grumback, K. (2002). Improving primary care for patients with chronic illness: the chronic care model, part 2. *Journal of the American Medical Association*, **288**(15), 1909–14.

Center for Studying Health System Change (1996). *Issue Brief Number 2: Tracking Changes in the Public Health System*. Washington, DC: Center for Studying Health System Change.

Christianson, J., Feldman, R., Weiner, J. P. and Drury, P. (1999). Early experience with a new model of employer group purchasing in Minnesota. *Health Affairs*, **18**(6), 100–14.

Collins, S. R., Davis, K. and Lambrew, J. M. (2004). *Health Care Reform Returns to the National Agenda: the 2004 Presidential Candidates' Proposals*. New York: The Commonwealth Fund. Online at www.cmwf.org.

Community Care Network (2001). *National Community Care Network Demonstration: About CCN*. Chicago, IL: American Hospital Association. Online at http://www.hospitalconnect.com/communitycare/about.html.

Custer, W. S. and Ketsche, P. (2000). *The Changing Sources of Health Insurance*. Washington, DC: Health Insurance Association of America.

Detmer, D. E. (2003). Building the national health information infrastructure for personal health, health care services, public health, and research. *BMC Medical Informatics and Decision Making*, **3**, 1. Online at http://www.biomedcentral/1472-6947/3/1.

Dixon, J., Lewis, R., Rosen, R., Finlayson, B. and Gray, D. (2004). Can the NHS learn from US managed care organizations? *British Medical Journal*, **328**, 223–5.

Feachem, R. G. A., Sekhri, N. K. and White, K. L. (2002). Getting more for their dollar: a comparison of the NHS with California's Kaiser Permanente. *British Medical Journal*, **324**, 135–43.

Florida Healthy Kids Corporation (1997). *Annual Report*. Tallahassee, FL: Florida Healthy Corporation.

Fries, J. F., Koop, C. E., Sokolov, J., Beadle, C. E. and Wright, D. (1998). Beyond health promotion: reducing need and demand for medical care. *Health Affairs*, **17**(2), 70–84.

Goldberg, L., Elliot, D., Clarke, G. N., MacKinnon, D. P., Moe, E., Zoref, L., Green, C., Wolf, S. L., Greffrath, E., Miller, D. J. and Lapin, A. (1996). Effects of a multidimensional anabolic steroid prevention intervention: the Adolescents Training and Learning to Avoid Steroids Program (ATLAS). *Journal of the American Medical Association*, **276**(16), 1555–62.

Gray, J. A. M. (1997). *Evidence-based Healthcare: How to Make Policy and Management Decisions*. New York: Churchill Livingston.

Green, R. M. (1976). Health care and justice in contract theory perspective. In *Ethics and Health Policy*, ed. R. M. Veatch and R. Branson. Cambridge, MA: Ballinger.

Hadley, J. and Holahan, J. (2003). Covering the uninsured: how much would it cost? *Health Affairs Web Exclusive*. Online at http://content.healthaffairs.org/cgi/reprint/ hlthaff.w3.250v1.pdf.

Heffler, S., Smith, S., Keehan, S., Clemens, M. K., Zezza, M. and Truffer, C. (2004). Health spending projections through 2013. *Health Affairs Web Exclusive*. Online at http://content.healthaffairs.org/cgi/content/ reprint/hlthaff.w4.79v1.

Holahan, J. and Pohl, M. B. (2002). *Changes in Insurance Coverage: 1994–2000 and Beyond*. Washington, DC: Kaiser Commission on Medicaid and the Uninsured. Online at www.kff.org.

Iglehart, J. K. (1998). Physicians as agents of social control. *Health Affairs*, **17**(1), 90–6.

(2002). Changing health insurance trends. *New England Journal of Medicine*, **347**(12), 965–2.

Institute of Medicine (1997). *Improving Health in the Community: a Role for Performance Monitoring*, ed. J. S. Burch, L. A. Bailey, and M. A. Stoto. Washington, DC: National Academy Press.

(1988). *The Future of Public Health*. Washington, DC: National Academy Press.

(1999). *To Err Is Human: Building a Safer Health System*. Washington, DC: National Academy Press.

(2000). *America's Health Care Safety Net: Intact but Endangered*. Washington, DC: National Academy Press.

(2001a). *Coverage Matters: Insurance and Health Care*. Washington, DC: National Academy Press.

(2001b). *Crossing the Quality Chasm: a New Health System for the 21st Century*. Washington, DC: National Academy Press.

(2002a). *Care without Coverage: Too Little, Too Late*. Washington, DC: National Academy Press.

(2002b). *Health Insurance is a Family Matter*. Washington, DC: National Academy Press.

(2003a). *Hidden Costs, Value Lost: Uninsurance in America*. Washington, DC: National Academy Press.

(2003b). *A Shared Destiny: Community Effects of Uninsurance*. Washington, DC: National Academy Press.

(2003c). *The Future of the Public's Health in the 21st Century*. Washington, DC: National Academy Press.

(2003d). *Academic Health Centers: Leading Change in the 21st Century*. Washington, DC: National Academy Press.

(2004). *Insuring America's Health: Principles and Recommendations*. Washington, DC: National Academy Press.

Kaiser Commission on Medicaid and the Uninsured (2002). *Underinsured in America: is Health Coverage Adequate?* Washington, DC: The Kaiser Family Foundation. Online at www.kff.org.

Kassirer, J. P. (1995). Managed care and the morality of the marketplace. *New England Journal of Medicine*, **333**(1), 50–2.

Kindig, D. A. (1997). *Purchasing Population Health: Paying for Results*. Ann Arbor, MI: The University of Michigan Press.

Knowles, S. and Owen, P. D. (1997). Education and health in effective labour empirical growth model. *Economic Review*, **73**(233), 314–28.

Lasker, R. D. (1997). *Medicine and Public Health: the Power of Collaboration*. New York: The New York Academy of Medicine.

Levit, K. R., Smith, C., Cowan, C., Sensenig, A., Caitlin, A. and the Health Accounts Team (2004). Health spending rebound continues in 2002. *Health Affairs*, **23**(1), 147–59.

Levy, B. S. (1998). Creating the future of public health. *American Journal of Public Health*, **88**(2), 188–92.

Lewin Group (2002). *Community Participation Can Improve America's Public Health System*. Battle Creek, MI: WK Kellogg Foundation. Online at http://www.wkkf.org.

(2003). *Communities Sustain Public Health Improvements Through Organized Partnership Structures*. Battle Creek, MI: WK Kellogg Foundation. Online at http://www.wkkf.org.

McGinnis, J. M. and Foege, W. H. (1993). Actual causes of death in the United States. *Journal of the American Medical Association*, **270**(18), 2207–12.

Miller, J. E. (1998). *Reality Check: the Public's Changing View of Our Health Care System*. Washington, DC: The National Coalition on Health Care.

Mokdad, A. H., Ford, E. S., Bowman, B. A., Nelson, D. E., Engelgau, M. M., Vinicor, F. and Marks, J. S. (2000). Diabetes trends in the US: 1990–1998. *Diabetes Care*, **23**(9), 1278–83.

National Committee on Vital and Health Statistics (2002). *Shaping a Health Statistics Vision for the 21st Century: Final Report*. Online at http://ncvhs.hhs.gov.

Oberland, J. (2003). The politics of health reform: why do bad things happen to good plans? *Health Affairs Web Exclusive*. Online at http://content.healthaffairs.org/cgi/reprint/hlthaff.w3.391v1.pdf.

Oregon Health Plan (1997). *The Uninsured in Oregon*. Salem, OR: Oregon Health Plan.

Pear, R. (2003). Big increase seen in people lacking health insurance. *New York Times*, September 30, A1 and A19.

Public Health Foundation (1996). *Measuring Expenditures for Essential Public Health Services.* Washington, DC: Public Health Foundation.

Ram, P. and Schultz, T. W. (1979). Lifespan, health, savings and productivity. *Economic Development and Cultural Change*, **27**, 399–421.

Reinhardt, U. E. (1998). Employer-based health insurance: R.I.P. In *The Future US Healthcare System: Who Will Care for the Poor and Uninsured?*, ed. S. H. Altman, U. E. Reinhardt and A. E. Shields. Chicago, IL: Health Administration Press.

Sackett, D. L., Rosenberg, W. M. C., Gray, J. A. M., Haynes, P. B. and Richardson, W. S. (1996). Evidence-based medicine. *British Medical Journal*, **312**(7023), 71–2.

Schlesinger, M. and Gray, B. (1998). A broader vision for managed care, part 1. *Health Affairs*, **17**(3), 2–10.

Sheils, J. and Haught. R. (2003). *Cost and Coverage Analysis of Ten Proposals to Expand Health Insurance Coverage.* Washington, DC: Covering America. Online at http://www.esresearch.org/covering_america.php.

Sloan, F. A. and Taylor, D. H. (1999). Essay: private and public choices in end-of-life care. *Journal of the American Medical Association*, **282**(21), 2078.

Smart, R. G., Mann, R. E. and Adrian, M. (1993). Health and productivity savings from increased alcoholism treatment in Ontario. *Canadian Journal of Public Health*, **84**(1), 62–3.

Smith, D. R., Anderson, R. J. and Boumbulian, P. J. (1991). Community responsive medicine. *American Journal of Medical Sciences*, **302**(5), 313–18.

Snyderman, R. (2002). Prospective health care planning: can it transform health care? *Enabling Prospective Health Care: 2002 Duke Private Sector Conference.* Online at http://conferences.mc.duke.edu/2002dpsc.nsf/contentsnum/ad.

Snyderman, R. and Williams, R. S. (2003). Prospective medicine: the next health care transformation. *Academic Medicine*, **78**(11), 1079–84.

Thompson, B. (1998). Trigger points. *The Washington Post Magazine*, 29 March, pp. 12–16, 23.

US Department of Health and Human Services (1998). *Description of the Public Health Functions Project.* Online at http://healthfinder.gov/phfunctions/project.htm.

(2000). *Healthy People 2010: Understanding and Improving Health*, 2nd edn. Washington, DC: US Government Printing Office. Online at http://www.healthypeople.gov.

(2003). *News Release: HHS Awards $13.7 Million to Support Community Programs to Prevent Diabetes, Asthma and Obesity.* Washington, DC: US Department of Health and Human Services. Online at http://www.hhs.gov/news/press/2003press/20030918.html.

Vinni, K. (1983). Productivity losses due to illness, disability and premature death in different occupational groups in Finland. *Social Science and Medicine*, **17**(3), 163–7.

Weingarten, S. R., Henning, J. M., Badamgarav, E., Knight, K., Hasselbad, V., Gano, A. and Ofman, J. J. (2002). Intervention used in disease management programmes for patients with chronic illness – which ones work? Meta-analysis of published reports. *British Medical Journal*, **325**, 925–8.

Weissman, J. S., Gatsonis, K. C. and Epstein, A. M. (1992). Rates of avoidable hospitalization by insurance status in Massachusetts and Maryland. *Journal of the American Medical Association*, **268**(17), 2388–94.

Weissman, J. S., Stern, R., Fielding, S. L. and Epstein, A. M. (1991). Delayed access to health care. *Annals of Internal Medicine*, **114**(4), 325–31.

Wennberg, J. E. (2002). Unwarranted variations in healthcare delivery: implications for academic medical centers. *British Medical Journal*, **325**, 961–4.

Wennberg, J. E., Fischer, E. S. and Skinner, J. S. (2002). Geography and the debate over Medicare reform. *Health Affairs Web Exclusive*. Online at http://www.healthaffairs.org//WebExclusives/WennbergWebExcel021302.htm.

Wolf, A. M. and Colditz, G. A. (1998). Current estimates of the economic costs of obesity in the United States. *Obesity Research*, **6**(2), 97–106.

World Health Organization (WHO) (1996). *European Health Care Reform Analysis of Current Strategies*. Copenhagen: WHO Regional Office for Europe.

Case study

A community-oriented primary care network: Parkland Health and Hospital System

Ron J. Anderson, M.D. and Sue Pickens M. Ed.

Parkland Health and Hospital System in Dallas, Texas is one of the largest publicly funded teaching hospitals and health care systems in the United States. It has been serving the citizens of Dallas County for over 110 years as a major safety net provider of health care. This year Parkland will provide over 43 000 admissions and over 16 000 births, representing 40 percent of all babies born in Dallas County. Parkland provides over 70 percent of Dallas County's major trauma care, as well as over 60 percent of the county's AIDS-related services. Total outpatient visits reached one million visits in 2002.

Parkland developed a community-oriented primary care (COPC) network to improve care for both individuals and communities. In 1986, Parkland completed the plan for the development of the COPC system, *Community Oriented Primary Care, A Plan for Dallas County*, and opened the first clinics in 1987. Today, services are provided through a system of nine COPC health centers and specialty programs from which care is extended in non-traditional settings including 18 homeless shelters, 10 schools, 11 churches, and 1 senior citizen center via multidisciplinary teams composed of a mix of midlevel practitioners and primary care physicians. The 173-member physician staff for the network belongs to a group practice, is board certified or board eligible, and has clinical faculty status. Several staff members have advanced degrees in public health or a subspecialty board. Sixty percent are African-American, Hispanic, or Asian, 54 percent are women; approximately half are bilingual. Nonphysician staff include: nurse practitioners, physician assistants, nutritionists, health educators, outreach workers, translators, social workers, psychologists, and dentists. The scope of primary care service includes pediatric, adolescent, adult, and geriatric medicine.

Ron J. Anderson is President and Chief Executive Officer at Parkland Health and Hospital System. Sue Pickens is Director of Strategic Planning and Population Medicine at Parkland Health and Hospital System.

Outreach prevention programs for cancer, AIDS and Healthy Start (a grant-funded program that targets high-risk pregnancies to lower neonatal and infant mortality rates in underserved communities) have been implemented. COPC cooperates with existing public health programs in addressing immunizations, sexually transmitted diseases, disease surveillance, health education, maternal and child health, and health maintenance examinations for public school students. Community partnerships include: family planning services operated by the University of Texas Southwestern Medical Center co-located with COPCs in four sites; Women, Infants and Children's public health services co-located with COPCs in seven sites; Parkland's women's health prenatal care clinics co-located in five sites and two freestanding sites, and dental services provided by a nonprofit agency (Dallas Dental Health, Inc.) and funded in partnership with the city of Dallas, Parkland, and various philanthropic sources.

Parkland also works closely with the Dallas Housing Authority to provide medical services in two of the Dallas Housing Authority low-income housing developments. The Injury Prevention Center of Greater Dallas was established as part of the community's response to a 38 percent increase in trauma hospitalizations from 1990 to 1991. The Center was established in 1994 and is supported by the major hospitals, foundations, and government grants. The Violence Intervention and Prevention Center, which is funded by federal grants and financial support from private organizations, provides Dallas County victims and their families access to medical and psychological assessment, medical follow-up, intervention and prevention services, and legal advocacy.

Parkland has conducted numerous evaluation and outcome studies that have shown a decrease in Emergency Room utilization by COPC pediatric patients, a reduction in length of stay with lower costs for COPC inpatients, and infant mortality rates better than the Texas or the United States for minority populations. Parkland received the prestigious Foster McGaw Award from the American Hospital Association in 1994 for excellence in community service in recognition of its community-oriented primary care program.

Dallas County experienced tremendous growth through the 1990s. The uninsured and indigent are now diffused through Dallas County. Many of Parkland patients no longer come from the traditional inner city neighborhoods. Many now come from suburban and near suburban communities. As a result, Parkland has identified a need for six new COPC sites as well as community-based subspecialty services. As in the past, it is expected that many people accessing care through these new services will have significant medical problems resulting from lack of access and deferred maintenance. Thus, although the system may achieve cost savings at the individual service level, the increased number of patients and increased level of services they will initially require will delay overall "system" savings. Such results have significant political ramifications for community funding options since Parkland, owned and operated by the Dallas County Hospital District, receives tax funding for indigent care.

Commentary

Enriqueta C. Bond, Ph.D. and Peter O. Kohler, M.D.

This chapter calls for fundamental change in the American health care delivery system, as have many recent prestigious reports, including the Institute of Medicine's *Crossing the Chasm: a New Health System for the 21st Century* (Institute of Medicine, 2001). The Blue Ridge Academic Health Group, whose work underpins the chapters in this volume, calls for universal health coverage (whether private or public), more rationale and effective use of the trillion-plus dollars currently spent on health care, and a shift to community-oriented and population-based approaches to health.

Unfortunately, we believe universal coverage will be exceedingly difficult to achieve and, without universal coverage, movement towards community-oriented and population-based approaches to health appear unlikely to happen. One of the major blocks is our American cultural emphasis on the rights of the individual versus the good of the community. This emphasis on the individual is a fundamental principle in the delivery of health care today in the United States and shows itself in an overwhelming concern for privacy that is far higher than in many other parts of the world. In addition, there is lack of agreement about whether health care is a basic human right or the personal responsibility of each individual. As we attempt to reshape our system of care, these factors further complicate the enormous and complex political challenge of rationing health care spending in order to put our health care dollars to best use. We will discuss each of these issues in turn.

The prevalent view of contemporary medicine is that of a physician caring for an individual patient. This is the result of years of focus on the physician doing everything possible for the patient, no matter how futile or how great the cost. This attitude is changing somewhat, but the greatest expenditures on health are still made in the last years of life. Perhaps the most strongly held American core value is the freedom of individual choice, which results

Enriqueta C. Bond is President of The Burroughs Wellcome Fund. Peter O. Kohler is President of Oregon Health & Science University.

in the nearly impossible task of trading individual, or even marginal benefit for the greater good. An example graphically illustrates this point. A decade ago, a physician senator in Oregon believed that with a limited state budget, more good would result from prenatal care for hundreds of pregnant women than from treating a single young boy with a bone marrow transplant for leukemia. This became a notorious example of the "Rule of Rescue" and led to enormous media attention on the young boy. Yet, the public could not see the damage done by the lack of insurance for coverage of prenatal care to literally hundreds of women.

Another important concept is that either now or at some point in the future, budgets for health care will necessarily be limited. This brings up the need for a global budget or a series of global and limited budgets. Health care providers appropriately focus on their individual patients and strive mightily to find ways to cover needed treatments. Some of the more recent pharmacological agents carry an enormous price tag. As costs for either drugs or devices increase, the cost of health care and therefore insurance rises will push as yet undefined limits. Common sense dictates that there is a limit beyond which this will become unbearable financially, and therefore the global budget concept will likely need to be accommodated. Currently, insurers utilize upper limits for payments, but care providers must cover the costs by spreading it to all payers.

A series of reports on the uninsured from the Institute of Medicine demonstrate that the lack of health insurance is widespread and enduring in the United States and that there are adverse health, psychosocial, and economic impacts on uninsured individuals and members of families with even one uninsured member (Institute of Medicine, 2003). In order to achieve universal coverage, government must mandate that individuals either purchase or be eligible for public programs. Coverage would not only benefit the individual and his or her family, but also the community. Another report in this IOM series shows that the adverse effects of a lack of health care insurance spill over to the community.

Given technological advances, our aging population, and unhealthy lifestyles in much of our population, there is not enough money in the United States treasury to pay for everything that could be provided in the way of health care. This raises the specter of the "R"-word or rationing. Currently, our society rations by not providing adequate and appropriate care to those without insurance coverage. We need to adopt a system or systems in which a budget forces discipline in providing the most cost effective and appropriate care for the target population. The Veterans Administration is one example of a system with a set, constrained budget as is the state Medicaid budget. A single payer system with all its attendant political difficulties is another possible model. Such a system could be privatized for a region as an alternative to government, with a biennial bid process. Without a budget, our health care system will not be able to force decisions between population approaches and individual patient decisions or between prenatal care and costly cancer treatments that would only provide an additional six months of life.

Chronic conditions are now the leading cause of illness, disability, and death in the USA, and affect almost half of the US population. Obesity affects over 30 percent of the population and, together with a sedentary lifestyle, contributes to the looming epidemic of diabetes in the United States. How can we provide both positive and negative incentives to individuals to take responsibility for adopting healthier lifestyles?

One negative approach would be to increase insurance premiums for those who persist with unhealthy lifestyles. A positive approach can be found in the annual report of WellPoint, a large insurance company (WellPoint, 2002). WellPoint's data show that member participation in health improvement programs for chronic illnesses such as asthma, diabetes, and heart disease improves clinical outcomes and quality of life while reducing costs. For WellPoint members participating for three years in the company's diabetes program, average Emergency Room visits dropped 27 percent and average blood sugar levels decreased 15 percent. Unfortunately, only 25 percent of the 300 000 WellPoint members who have been diagnosed with diabetes participate in the diabetic health improvement program. We might achieve more widespread participation in such programs by working with employers and physicians, and providing incentives to physicians for delivering the services and to employees who take advantage of such services. This will require creating a culture of health in our schools, workplaces, and communities that expect individuals to take personal responsibility for healthy behaviors. Also for this to be effective at a societal level, any uninsured individual would have to be a participant.

In our view, the key to the sweeping change called for in this chapter has everything to do with how we pay for health care. Such change will require universal coverage, rationing by establishing a budget for the care of a population, using evidence to guide what we pay for, and creating incentives that foster individual responsibility for health.

REFERENCES

Institute of Medicine (2001). *Crossing the Quality Chasm: a New Health System for the 21st Century*. Washington, DC: National Academy Press.

(2003). *A Shared Destiny: Community Effects of Uninsurance*. Washington, DC: National Academy Press.

WellPoint (2002). *Wellpoint by Design: Annual Report*. Thousand Oaks, CA: Wellpoint. Online at http://www.wellpoint.com/investor_info/annual_reports/.

Commentary

Integrating personal *values* into *value*-based health care

Robert Galvin, M.D.

As health care remains at the top of the national agenda, it is timely to re-visit what it is we want out of our trillion-dollar annual expenditure in this sector. The Blue Ridge Academic Health Group has developed a vision of what they call a "value-driven" system, designed to deliver cost-effective, high-quality medical care to a fully insured population. Their vision stresses evidence-based medicine, population health, and a nation engaging in a dialogue about rationing and resource allocation. While there is broad agreement among policy experts on many of these principles, making them operational will require decisions that will prompt debate. Three pivotal issues must be addressed. First, what do we mean by value? Second, how do we achieve efficiency while still providing incentives for innovation? Third, how do we decide where to begin?

What do we mean by value?

Value, as defined by the Blue Ridge group, is high-quality, medically appropriate care delivered at optimal cost. However, only occasionally does the scientific clearly guide day-to-day decisions by doctors and patients. More often, differing treatment options all have some marginal benefit, data on quality are lacking, and neither physician nor patient knows the costs resulting from their decisions. The choices that determine *value* are, therefore, based on the *values* of those that receive and deliver care. Understanding the values of users of the US health care system, and integrating them in a framework for reform, is critical. The lack of their integration in prior reform efforts may explain why Americans continue to reject social insurance models of health care, as they did with proposals for federally funded catastrophic health insurance coverage in the 1980s and the Clinton health reforms of the 1990s. Although there is no

Robert Galvin is Director of Global Healthcare at General Electric Company.

69

disagreement that the European social insurance model delivers care to more people at lower per-capita cost, and with superior measures of broad population health, there are clearly features of those systems that Americans continue to reject. A successful framework for reform must reflect the values of the public.

The Blue Ridge model is an exemplary system as seen from the perspective of academic clinicians. But if a restructured system is to succeed, the *values* of customers, patients and payers must be integrated into the definition of *value*. Although it is not completely clear what these values are, Americans seem to want a system that focuses on innovation, high technology, excellent customer service, and only very limited rationing for those who have coverage. Surveys of dissatisfaction with our system and willingness to change have to be read very carefully. There is an old saying that to understand what people really believe, watch what they do, not what they say. While a majority of the population may state that our system needs a complete overhaul, and that they would be willing to pay more to reduce the number of uninsured, in the past this same group has been reluctant to sacrifice what they have. Although many may be uncomfortable with what this says about American values, the fact is that no lasting reform will occur unless these values are understood and addressed.

Innovation

Reforming the health care system while preserving incentives for innovation is a major challenge. In fact, no nation has figured out how to do this. The European models provide little capital to incentivize innovation in diagnostics or treatment, yet this is probably the characteristic of the US system that the population most values. However, encouraging innovation must be balanced with assessing cost-effectiveness and having clinicians and patients bear some responsibility for the cost of their decisions. Slowing down innovation would be unpopular with the US population, and is a predictable consequence of reimbursement systems that either arbitrarily establish global budgets or restrict access to services. Developing models in which professionals, whose responsibility it is to balance scientific evidence and patient preferences, are incentivized and held accountable for their use of new treatments is a direction more consistent with American values. Consumers and patients also need to be involved in the decisions they make, and creative health benefit designs need to be developed to address this.

Innovation also occurs in the way that people pay for and receive care. A clear conclusion from the past 30 years of experimentation in the US delivery system is that experimentation is good. The population has been clear that it wants choice, information, caring clinicians, and customer service. Health care markets segment like any other consumer market, and these same attributes mean different things to different people. Some people want integrated systems like Kaiser Permanente, others want to control their own health care, and still others favor alternative medicine. A system which encourages customization has led to creative experiments such as managed care, physician practice management companies, pharmacy benefits managers, specialty hospitals, centers of excellence, decision-support software, and others. While many would argue that these experiments represent wasted administrative expenses, others would say exactly the opposite. A dynamic market that continues to create innovative delivery models best serves a population that demands choice and customization.

The chapter is very candid about the weaknesses of the US health care system, but does not spend as much time on its strengths. The lack of a central authority that administratively sets prices is also the basis of the pluralism that leads to innovations and creativity. Some of the dollars expended on what turn out to be marginally effective new technologies are also the fuel that drive the research and development necessary for true break-through products. There is a central problem of access that our system must address: the argument in this commentary is that it should be addressed not by choosing models that reflect values of other populations, but by building on the values of our current system and continuing to innovate.

Where to begin

Deciding how to get started in driving improvements in the areas of access, cost, and quality can be a paralyzing exercise. Private sector payers, who also believe in a value-driven system, are focusing on quality as a first step. The Leapfrog Group, comprising 160 employers and representing 33 million covered lives, was founded to use the purchasing power of its members to drive "leaps" in quality improvement. The underlying concept is that quality can be improved by educating and incentivizing consumers and patients to seek it, while simultaneously reimbursing clinicians for delivering it. The employer community believes that overall quality reduces costs, and that the savings from increased quality can be used to expand coverage to the uninsured.

These employers believe that the best way to educate consumers about quality is to publicly release scientifically accurate performance measures that consumers care about. Evidence from multiple sectors demonstrates that this kind of performance transparency improves quality and efficiency. The Leapfrog effort began with three hospital safety "leaps", developed by physician experts. Over 1000 hospitals have reported their results and 25 million consumers have been shown the results. The Leapfrog Group is working closely with Medicare and other government purchasers of health care to make sure that a standardized set of performance measures is developed, so that providers will not be unduly burdened with data collection. The private and public sectors are also collaborating to develop reporting formats that are salient to consumers and beneficiaries.

Summary

The Blue Ridge vision for health care reform is comprehensive and outlines an ideal, value-driven health system. Further integrating the values of the payers and end-users, which include preservation of incentives for innovation in treatment and delivery systems, is critical for success. Reform will not be attainable or sustainable unless American values in health care, which may be substantially different from European values, are the foundation on which a uniquely American health care system is built. The Leapfrog Group, composed of private and public sector payers, has attempted to integrate these values in its strategy. More cooperation between purchasers and academic health centers represents an opportunity to accelerate the reform agenda.

3 Stronger leadership in and by academic health centers

Introduction

Leaders of academic health centers (AHCs) have always experienced a wide range of formidable challenges during their tenure. AHCs are complex organizations to lead because of their multiple missions, substantial size, highly specialized products and services, diverse internal and external constituencies, and culture marked by autonomy of faculty and departments. They operate as academic, business, and (in many cases) public organizations simultaneously, in an industry that is in the midst of evolving its production modes (i.e., from cottage to manufacturing to knowledge-based). Across AHCs, financial threats abound as a result of reduced government support and declining clinical revenues.

In many cases, governance structures are being or need to be modified because governing boards do not always facilitate needed change and internal decision-making processes are not always efficient. Moreover, the career path of AHC leaders is often antithetical to the development of skills necessary for effective leadership. Further, a coherent strategy to build future leaders is lacking in most AHCs. Planning for future leadership is often equivalent to establishing a search committee when a key position becomes vacant.

An array of societal, economic, and technological forces is creating a new and as yet uncharted terrain for AHCs. Academic health center leaders must address demographic shifts, new capabilities arising from information and communications technology, and growing consumer expectations for speed and customized products and services. These changes require that organizations assume new roles, acquire new capabilities, develop new business models, and interact with both customers and staff in new ways.

Academic health center leaders face a new frontier where they need the ability to cope with a different landscape from week to week. An organizational vision that motivates staff is more important than ever. Leaders need to predict and direct change rather than just react to it. They need to interpret myriad messages from the environment and convert them into a framework that guides both long-term strategies and routine operations. They must forge an organizational culture that embraces constant change and successfully adapt and transform their organizations while preserving core values.

Leaders have no option but to assess and refine their own skills to keep pace with the changing environment and to facilitate excellence in their organization. For example, electronic connectivity and greater reliance on relationships beyond organizational lines require new technical and communications skills and knowledge. Changes in the composition of the workforce, consumer expectations, and interactions with the media are increasing the importance of humanistic dimensions of leadership (i.e., leaders must be proficient in managing more than the bottom line). Organizational members not only need to participate in shaping their jobs and developing clearly defined performance expectations, but they must also be offered opportunities to develop the skills needed to meet their job requirements and expectations.

If these already complex organizations are to succeed in meeting these new challenges, adroit leadership is essential at a variety of levels, not just at the top. Formal and informal leaders throughout the enterprise need to be given opportunities to make decisions as a means of developing and practicing leadership skills. Otherwise organizations risk a shortage of future leaders or discontinuity during inevitable leadership transitions.

The Blue Ridge Academic Health Group (Blue Ridge Group) believes that AHCs:

- can and should provide greater value to society,
- must transform themselves in response to the changing needs of society and changing market forces,
- can achieve the needed transformation by taking greater advantage of business practices used in other industries, leveraging the capabilities of information technology and electronic commerce, expanding their focus on managing population health, and partnering with a range of external parties within their regions,
- should be active participants in the effort to build a value-driven health system.

To achieve these objectives AHC leaders will need to possess the full set of essential leadership skills for contemporary organizations and to apply those skills to transforming their organizations for success in the twenty-first century. Moreover, AHCs will need a cadre of individuals throughout the organization with these leadership skills.

This chapter explores the issue of what AHC leadership should look like today and in the coming decade. It addresses three questions. What notable challenges do AHC leaders face? What are the relevant leadership skills for AHC leaders? How can AHCs cultivate leadership skills within their organizations? During the course of its study of leadership, the Blue Ridge Group concluded that effective leadership within AHCs requires that AHCs learn from and help to shape the environment in which they operate by also providing leadership beyond their organizations. Thus, not only does the Blue Ridge Group call on AHCs to strengthen leadership within their institutions, it also encourages AHCs to demonstrate value-driven leadership within their communities, regions, and the entire health care sector.

For purposes of this discussion, the senior ranking AHC official (e.g., vice president or dean) is considered to be the AHC leader. The leadership of AHCs is considered to include the senior ranking AHC official, other senior administrators, the governing board, and president of the parent university (if applicable). At the same time, leaders exist throughout all levels of AHCs. Some of these are formally appointed (e.g., department chair); others assume their position by default; still others appear in the form of teams or individual work units. In addition, the AHC as an organization is recognized as having the potential to be a leader because of the number and size of its spheres of influence. Despite the dominance of market forces, and accompanying increased visibility of third-party payers in shaping the health care sector, AHCs continue to influence the health care community through their roles as developers and disseminators of new knowledge, educators of future health professionals, and providers of highly specialized care. Moreover, many AHCs represent a significant share of their parent university's budget and personnel, qualify as large employers, and provide significant percentages of patient care within their communities and regions.

The AHC leadership milieu

At least some AHCs are experiencing significant management gaps and lack of leadership continuity. Medical school deans are serving an average of 2.8 years, down from an average 3.6 years between 1980 and 1992 (Aschenbrener, 1998; Petersdorf, 1997; Sheldon, 2000). In 2000, an estimated 20 percent of medical schools were without deans (Sheldon, 2000). Department chair positions were in a similar situation with approximately 40 chairs of surgery being vacant and some being open for long periods of time. These disconcerting statistics are not surprising when viewed in terms of the nature of the job. AHC leaders face high expectations, multiple roles (i.e., clinician, scientist, educator, administrator, entrepreneur, fund raiser, organizational merger specialist), a diverse constituency, responsibility without commensurate authority and resources, and a faculty that is not easily led (Petersdorf, 1997).

Academic health center leadership challenges are complicated by eroding revenue streams which have resulted in some AHCs experiencing budget deficits, staff turnover and reduction, and organizational restructuring (Commonwealth Fund Task Force on Academic Health Centers, 2000; Pardes, 2000). All AHCs face difficulties in finding resources to make needed investments. Those AHC educational structures that lag developments in the clinical arena require overhaul. Greater demands on health care professionals to manage an ever-growing base of knowledge and apply new methodologies (e.g., evidence-based medicine or population health management) create new challenges for both health professional school curricula and investment in information systems that support the clinical enterprise.

Funding is not the only challenge facing AHC leaders. Some schools are experiencing difficulty recruiting faculty to teach core undergraduate courses and finding ambulatory placements for their students (Blumenthal, Weissman, and Griner, 1999). Schools also face uncertainty surrounding the appropriate numbers mix, as well as appropriate training for and availability of future health professionals (e.g., applications for medical school decreased each year between 1996 and 2002) (Association of American Medical Colleges, 2002; Pardes, 2000). Like all health care organizations, AHCs must respond to the need for significant changes in the clinical arena (Institute of Medicine, 1999, 2001). Growing competition for research funding from private industry along with demands for better accountability are driving efforts to manage the research enterprise (for the first time in many institutions). Finally, AHCs must confront issues of collective responsibility (e.g., excess capacity) and competition from new sources or risk cutbacks and outcomes imposed by regulation or competition (Fein, 2000).

AHCs are part of an industry whose production modes are still evolving (see Table 3.1). While retaining aspects of its original cottage or craft production mode, health care has adopted and continues to adopt elements of a manufacturing production mode. Simultaneously health care is being driven into a knowledge or learning production mode by advances in information technology and consumer expectations (Maccoby, 1999). As a

Table 3.1 Transformation of health care

	Craft →	Manufacturing →	Learning
Structures/roles			
• Organization	Cottage industry	Factory/bureaucracy	Interactive system
• Economic role of	Sole proprietor,	Employee	Large-system
physician	Small partnerships	Entrepreneur	stakeholder
• Physician role in team	Authority	+Provider	Partner-teacher
• Patient role	Submissive, trusting	Customer-client	+Partner-learner
Values	Caring	Efficiency	Knowledge creation
	Personal trust	Scale	Individual development
	Expertise	Uniformity	Social development
Model of care	Biomedical	+Prevention	+Epidemiological
	Individual skill	+Outcome measures	+Psychosocial
Focus	Individual	+Institutional	+Community → global
Technology	Hand tools	+Electromechanical	+Information
		+Chemical	+Biogenetic
Systems			
• Quality control	Peer review	+Statistical process control	+Continuous improvement
• Cost control	Unregulated	Profit-based	Shared responsibility
• Learning	Individual	+Organizational	+Community
Organizational skills	Mentoring	Monitoring	Team competence
Leadership model	Master-apprentice	Administration	Distributed leadership
	Functional expertise	Visionary-interactive	dialogue
Leadership thinking	Analyzer	Energizer	Humanizer

Note: The + symbol indicates that the characteristic in the column to its left also holds true for this column.
Source: Reprinted with permission from the Association of Academic Health Centers. Originally published in M. Maccoby, On creating the organization of learning, in *Creating the Future: Innovative Programs and Structures in Academic Health Centers*, C. H. Evans and E. R. Rubin, editors, Washington, DC: Association of Academic Health Centers, 1999, p. 7.

result, like all health care organizations, AHCs are confronting changes in the means of their work, values, definition of quality, and roles of health professionals, as well as organizational structures, systems, and skills. Organizations in the learning production mode are likely to be interactive rather than bureaucratic, rely on cross-functional teams rather than hierarchy, use interactive dialogue and shared goals rather than top-down commands, and require leaders who are synthesizers and socializers rather than analyzers or energizers.

AHC leadership challenges

Academic health centers clearly need to embrace, adopt, and sustain profound changes for long-term success. They are, however, diverse organizations and at varying stages of preparedness to embark upon large-scale and deep organizational change. Thus there is no single strategy or set of strategies that will assure success for all AHCs. It is essential that AHC leaders identify needed changes, assess their organizations' capacity for transformation, and evaluate their personal readiness to lead such an effort. Reflecting upon the state of AHCs (to the extent that they can be generalized) and the framework provided by the Leadership Mirror (described below), the Blue Ridge Group identified specific challenges that AHC leaders face as they plan and implement desired changes.

Shared values and a clear vision provide a sense of purpose and continuity, motivate staff, and contribute to organizational success (Collins and Porras, 1994). These foundational elements of the organization are growing in importance as organizations move away from command and control style operations toward decentralized decision-making as a means of being responsive to customer needs through both speed and ability to customize. Yet, in many AHCs, core values may seem to be contradictory or under siege from external forces.

As identified in Table 3.1, the values associated with the three production modes evident within health care differ (e.g., personal trust and expertise versus efficiency and uniformity versus knowledge creation and social development). AHCs operate in both the business and academic realms. Faculty members are often troubled when the market views the fruit of their labor as commodities and are uncomfortable when patients are called customers. Autonomy and academic freedom are second nature to most faculty, but they are being asked to demonstrate accountability and respond to organizational enterprise needs. Health professionals, particularly physicians, are taught to assume responsibility and function independently. Meanwhile, health care is evolving toward patient-centered, interdisciplinary services.

Identifying and articulating core values is a necessary task for AHC leaders. During a Johns Hopkins Medicine leadership retreat, senior executives were divided into five groups and asked to identify core values of the organization. Working independently, each group identified the same set of values – integrity, honesty, collegiality; excellence (being number one in all that we do);

innovation; transmitting knowledge to the world; and alleviating suffering by translating basic information. This exercise provided the AHC executive with a means of determining how well established and clear the organization's values were at that point in time. It also reinforced the institution's values among senior leaders.

The process of identifying or clarifying AHC core values may require considerable effort. Academic health center leaders can begin by initiating dialogue about the organization's true core values versus habits or norms erroneously assumed to be core values. Subsequently, AHC leaders and staff can focus on identifying new approaches that can be used to achieve core values in the changing environment. For example, improving health might be an AHC core value. Excellence in the clinical arena previously relied upon a great deal of physician independence and focused predominantly on care given to individual patients without consideration of aggregated results. Now it is far more likely to depend on teamwork, interdisciplinary approaches, patient involvement, explicit assessment of satisfaction as well as a focus on value and population health outcomes. Achieving this core value will depend on actions of AHC staff and AHC investment in training and information technology.

Once identified, core values provide the foundation for the organization's vision and mission and underlie all of its strategies and policies. Values and vision need to be shared throughout the organization. Continued promotion of the vision has been linked to the success of collaborative projects and will become more important as collaboration becomes more prevalent within AHCs (Bland *et al.*, 2000). The high rate of routine turnover among students and residents makes articulating core values and vision an ongoing task for AHC leaders. Moreover, as the AHC workforce becomes more diverse, greater effort is needed to bridge generational and cultural differences among staff to achieve shared values throughout the institution. Some AHC leaders are using new communication approaches that provide both timely information as well as opportunity for input (e.g., town meetings involving faculty and staff, electronic bulletins) (Griner and Blumenthal, 1998a).

Achieving a shared vision among top leaders – including the governing body – increases the likelihood of securing creative change (Bulger, Osterweis, and Rubin, 1999). For example, the board and university president along with the vice president of the University of Cincinnati Medical Center provided a united front in advocating large-scale changes that placed corporate need over that of individual units. This joint commitment overcame well-entrenched departmental resistance and provided a springboard for future enterprise-wide changes (e.g., privatization of the hospital and closing of one facility).

Although a solid relationship with the AHC governing body is pivotal for the AHC leaders, AHC experience with effective governance varies widely. Private institutions often have the opportunity to build the boards that preside over them. In contrast, public AHCs or universities do not have the same level of influence over governance. Although governing boards are expected to serve as trustees, acting to protect and preserve the institution for future generations, boards of public institutions may see themselves not as guardians of the institution but as representatives of the special interests that led to their appointment (Duderstadt, 2000).

The current climate increasingly requires quick decisions from governing bodies that are often accustomed to acting with great deliberation rather than speed. An important challenge for public higher education today is assuring lay boards of the experience, quality, and clarity of role necessary to govern complex institutions. Each AHC needs a core of influential trustees who understand the institution, can provide useful criticism, and support its efforts.

Achieving a more "sophisticated level of governance" may require continued educational efforts by the senior AHC executive and university president (Bulger, Osterweis, and Rubin, 1999). Alternately, it might entail creating a sub-board of the overall university that has specific responsibility for overseeing the AHC (Commonwealth Fund Task Force on Academic Health Centers, 2000). Some AHCs have sought to strengthen governance and improve the flexibility and speed of decision making by reducing the role of the state or parent university through restructuring. For example, Oregon Health Sciences University (OHSU) has become a quasi-public corporation (Blumenthal, Weissman, and Griner, 1999). (See also case study on OHSU in Chapter 4).

Equally important, AHCs require rational organizational structures that facilitate internal decision-making (Griner and Blumenthal, 1998b). Both changing organizational configurations (e.g., mergers or alliances with external partners) and the need for enterprise-wide decision-making are driving changes in AHC organizational structures. For example, Emory Healthcare was created through the consolidation of Emory's clinical facilities (including The Emory Clinic, The Children's Center, Emory University Hospital, Crawford W. Long Hospital, Emory/Adventist Hospital, Wesley Woods Center of Emory University, and a limited partnership with Columbia/HCA's metropolitan Atlanta facilities) (Saxton et al., 2000). This structure provides administrative consolidation and coordination, but allows each entity to operate as a distinct business unit. Emory's Woodruff Health Sciences Center (WHSC) has implemented a new governance structure that is headed by the executive vice president for health affairs and WHSC director, who is also chairman and chief executive officer of Emory Healthcare. Within the clinical enterprise, Emory has also implemented a decision-making structure comprised of 10 teams of 15 members (e.g., operations, clinical performance improvement, marketing, managed care, clinical research). These teams serve as a resource to business units, have decision-making authority on matters within their purview, and make recommendations on broader issues to senior leadership.

Academic health centers often fail to deliberately develop, communicate, or apply their operating model (i.e., the concrete plan of how the organization will operate in the marketplace). Rather than articulating how leaders want the organization to behave, the kinds of relationships they want to establish with business partners, how they will interact with staff, and what they want to be known for in the marketplace, AHCs may have relied on traditional practices as the basis for their operations. As a result, translating strategies into daily activities and defining the organization's culture become more difficult within these organizations. Moreover, AHC organizational structures (e.g., clinical departments or financial reporting systems) may inhibit implementation of the chosen operating model (e.g., multidisciplinary curriculum or an enterprise-wide approach to resource allocation).

The University Health System Consortium Funds Flow Project enables AHCs to make explicit use of an operating model. This initiative enables AHCs to identify the flow of funds between the divisions of their enterprise and in so doing align their business practices with mission-driven initiatives. As part of this process, AHCs articulate an operating model and identify how various organizational characteristics need to be transformed (see Table 3.2). As AHCs implement the model, they must educate their organizations on the need for change as well as implement new processes (e.g., routine use of performance measures) to support their new operating model (Garson, 1999; Geheb, 1999, 2000; Harrison, 1999). (See also discussion of this methodology in OHSU case study and commentary by Garson in Chapter 4.)

The Blue Ridge Group identified three cultural issues that will likely impede AHCs' ability to implement profound changes. First, AHC leaders need to continue to promote the shift away from "a loose confederation of independent faculty members and autonomous departments" toward an organizational culture that "acknowledges the exquisite interdependence of diverse

Table 3.2 Changing AHC operating model

Characteristics	Tradition	Transformation
Accountability	Individual personal goals	Individuals with personal goals aligned with enterprise goals
Governance	Individual units (school, departments, hospital, practice plan)	Common oversight to establish and oversee enterprise goals
Culture	• "Religious" defense of noble work • Individual objectives • Cacophony (multiple voices) • Innovation with inconsistent application • Entitlement	• "Business-like" defense of noble work • Common objective • Polyphony (multiple voices) • Innovation with consistent results • Risk
Organization	Fiefdoms	Collaborative units
Finances	• Independent financial models • Variable accounting standards • Risk held centrally • Deal making • Unclear view of funds flow • Secrecy • Confusion	• Common financial language • Single accounting standards • Risk at operating unit • Strategic investment (return on investment) • Clear view of funds flow • Openness • Clarity
Other metrics	Poorly defined	Defined by mission
Decision-making	Slow, imprecise, chaotic, idiosyncratic, and nonstrategic	Deliberate, precise, organized, paced, and strategic

Source: Reprinted with permission from University Health System Consortium. Originally published in M. Geheb, *Transforming AHCs: Operating in a New Economic Environment*, Oak Brook, IL: University Health System Consortium, 2000, p. 4.

units" and an organization focused on the needs of the enterprise (Kirch, 1999). By increasing collaboration among and accountability from individuals and units, AHC leaders will reduce the time spent mediating disputes. To do so, however, AHC leaders will need to create and communicate a vision that appeals to the common interests among diverse disciplines so that they will be willing to cross traditional barriers.

In some instances, AHC leaders can take advantage of external factors to shape organizational culture. The University of Massachusetts Medical Center (UMMC) developed "a genuine sense of community" among its faculty and administrators from its inception as a result of external skepticism about its formation (Bulger, Osterweis, and Rubin, 1999). This hostile environment combined with intense political and public scrutiny resulted in both depart-ment leaders and faculty members being more team-oriented than those at some AHCs. This team orientation has proved to be a strategic strength for the institution. In addition, UMMC understands and is driven by its mis-sion to educate health professionals for the state and provide care to central and western Massachusetts. It recognizes that it is different from medical schools in the Boston area and does not seek to copy them. Clarity of mission and an institutionally focused organizational structure have provided a solid foundation for innovation and robust performance at UMMC.

The attitudes and styles of leaders within an AHC can promote or impede a collaborative culture. Although never mandated to do so, the primary care departments at the University of California, Irvine, College of Medicine (i.e., family medicine, general internal medicine, and general pediatrics) cooperate extensively in education, patient care, and research (Scherger et al., 2000). This model evolved gradually over many years. As faculty experienced success collaborating on multidisciplinary medical school courses and eventually residency programs, they realized that "working together not only makes sense educationally, but also saves crucial amounts of time and resources" and serves as a model of professionalism for students. Today the primary care faculty "share educational resources, a research infrastructure, and clinical systems, thus avoiding duplicative use of valuable resources while maximizing collective negotiating abilities and mutual success."

Second, AHC leaders need to foster a learning environment for all organi-zational members. Beyond being educational institutions, AHCs need to be "organizations where people continually expand their capacity to create the results they truly desire . . . where people are continually learning how to learn together" (Senge, 1990). To achieve sustained high performance, AHCs need to take full advantage of their organizational knowledge and provide sufficient opportunities for all staff to develop fully. This issue is particularly important in the learning production mode where organizations need to learn "how to change and adapt to competition, information technology, and new values of customers and employees" (Maccoby, 1999). In this mode, front-line staff focus on meeting customer needs while their supervisors focus on translating front-line experiences into organizational learning.

Both formal training and informal incentive programs can contribute to success in this area. Emory Healthcare formed the Learning Council to antici-pate and coordinate the learning needs of the components of its integrated delivery system (Franklin and Moore, 1999). The Learning Council created a competency assessment feedback program to facilitate learning among staff.

This program is based on a 360-degree feedback approach and includes a survey tool, a survey feedback report, a guidebook, and a coaching process to assist participants in formulating and completing a personal strategic plan. The Mayo Clinic established the Clinician–Educator award to promote educational innovation and scholarship by funding the development of educational projects (Viaggiano, Shub, and Giere, 2000). Similarly, the University of Virginia Health System provided grants to faculty to encourage informatics development and innovative use of information resources (Watson, 1997).

Third, strengthening institutional citizenship is another important cultural shift for AHCs. Academic health center faculty need to develop strong identification with their institutions and not just with their disciplines. Academic health center success requires that faculty support the enterprise and contribute to its advancement. While AHC leaders need to provide a shared vision around which the organization can rally, individual members need to be ready to be a part of the team.

These cultural shifts can be reinforced through development and use of explicit performance measures at the organizational, unit, and individual levels. Faculty performance evaluations are becoming routine in many AHCs and appointment letters are becoming more explicit about the institution's expectations for faculty performance (Griner and Blumenthal, 1998a). To influence culture and desired behavior, robust evaluations need to incorporate the full set of desired behaviors (e.g., institutional citizenship, mentoring, establishing external relationships) and not just those criteria traditionally considered for promotion and tenure decisions. In addition, these cultural issues can be incorporated into educational curricula for students and health professionals. For example, medical schools can expose their students to the need for institutional citizenship when they address professional values in the curriculum. (See Chapter 4 for more discussion of cultural change.)

The complexity of leadership is growing in contemporary organizations, yet "few people who become leaders in academic medicine aspire to, plan for, or seek training to develop leadership skills" (Daughtery, 1998). Unlike the corporate world, past experiences of AHC leaders do not necessarily translate into leadership preparation. The traditional route for AHC leadership is through academic achievement rather than business experience or training. Young faculty may be discouraged from pursuing mid-level management positions that provide needed experience for future leaders because of a perception that management is "something that academics do when they can no longer cut it as investigators or clinicians" (Commonwealth Fund Task Force on Academic Health Centers, 2000). Moreover, some of the attributes and cultural processes associated with a skilled clinician or researcher may be counterproductive in the leadership arena (Schwartz *et al.*, 2000).

For example, most vice presidents and deans were medical students who trained to be assertive, independent physicians. These same leaders were likely medical school faculty in an environment that traditionally values individual autonomy and rewards individual achievement, not behavior that supports a larger community of interests. Many AHC leaders were practicing physicians who experienced the autonomy of decision making and emphasis on the singularity of the physician–patient relationship. Once in a leadership position, however, these same individuals must be skilled at collaborative behavior. Academic advancement and recognition usually comes with achievements in a specialized research or clinical domain. After ascending the ladder of academic reward and recognition, however, AHC CEOs find themselves in a web of relationships and in need of breadth to relate to diverse constituencies, not depth of medical specialization. As a result, typically AHCs are not known for having strong leadership habits, the vocabulary of leadership does not pervade these institutions, and leaders often learn on the job.

Training can play a significant role in leadership development when it focuses on conceptual ability, teachable interpersonal skills, and personal growth. Attempting to develop leadership skills is not likely to yield significant benefits while learners are focused on mastering their discipline or before they have professional experience on which to draw (Chow, Coffman, and Morjikian, 1999). Yet, undergraduate health professional education can contribute to leadership development through student contact with faculty who model effective leadership behaviors and varying leadership styles, discussions of the nature of professionalism and values of health professionals, and assignment of projects that require use of leadership skills (e.g., communication, collaboration, understanding diverse perspectives). A limited number of medical schools offer dual-degree programs in medicine and business, but these students appear to be most interested in careers directing hospitals and insurance companies rather than the public sector (Sherrill, 2000).

Several AHCs have leadership programs focused on residents. The University of Washington School of Medicine developed a course that helps senior residents to refine teaching and supervisory skills. Participants explore leadership, problem-solving, managerial techniques (e.g., setting goals and providing feedback), and communication among various team members through sample cases and videotaped vignettes of situations likely to be encountered (Wipf, Pinsky, and Burke, 1995). The University of Minnesota Internal Medicine Residency Program offers the Physician Management Pathway (PMP) (Paller *et al.*, 2000). The PMP exposes interested residents to management concepts, provides them the opportunity to begin developing leadership skills, and provides career mentoring through a monthly seminar series, a preceptorship with a physician-executive, and a supervised project.

A variety of leadership and management development programs are offered nationally and internationally for organizational leaders in health care generally and AHCs specifically (Association of American Medical Colleges, 2003; Cambridge University, 2000). The Council of Deans (COD) of the Association of American Medical Colleges (AAMC) offers a fellowship program for senior faculty members who are interested in being considered for deanships in the near future (Gabriel, 2002). The program provides exposure to a dean mentor and requires a research project and participation in COD activities.

Some institutions have developed in-house programs to meet the needs of their faculty and staff. The University of Virginia (UVA) Darden Graduate School of Business Administration developed a program for department chairs in the UVA School of Medicine. Participants meet one weekend per month for a year and cover topics such as strategic thinking, marketing, finance, operations, organizational behavior, leadership skills, and managing education. The University of Iowa's Institutional Leadership Development Program is described in the case study accompanying this chapter.

It is important to assure that such programs are consistent with the starting point and culture of learners and align with strategic organizational priorities, desired work force competencies, and the planned work products of the organization (Morahan *et al.*, 1998). In particular, leadership training should relate knowledgeably to the health professions and their evolving societal roles. For example, the Johnson and Johnson-Wharton Fellows Program in Management for Nurse Executives focuses on developing the leadership skills needed for collaborative and innovative partnerships. Toward that end, it addresses self-knowledge, strategic vision, risk taking and creativity, interpersonal skills and communication effectiveness, and managing change (Chow, Coffman, and Morjikian, 1999).

Coaching and mentoring of individuals and teams of faculty and staff are necessary to prepare them for future leadership opportunities but are more often used for technical skills than leadership skills. Both coaching and mentoring offer AHC leaders an opportunity to convey organizational values and emphasize desired cultural attributes (e.g., collaboration) while responding to the specific needs of individuals (Henry and Gilkey, 1999). The most effective mentoring occurs through example (e.g., solve problems as a team with leader as head). Departments that do not have regular departmental meetings or in which attendance is irregular are missing an important opportunity for the chair and senior faculty to mentor younger staff.

Succession planning is critical to the continued development of leadership capability and the ability of an organization to sustain high performance. Rarely do successful large corporations recruit their leaders from outside the firm; they groom their own leaders and, in so doing, maintain and align institutional vision and goals (Collins and Porras, 1994). Yet with rare exceptions succession planning does not occur within AHCs. Typically, AHCs conduct national searches to fill key vacancies and emphasize "intellectual fire power" over understanding of culture or interpersonal skills (Commonwealth Fund Task Force on Academic Health Centers, 2000). This kind of tactical decision-making can lead to a lack of continuity of institutional vision or goals. In contrast, Baylor College of Medicine has a strong leadership tradition (Bulger, Osterweis, and Rubin, 1999). It relies heavily on internal appointments for leadership positions, actively plans for leader succession, and uses former CEOs as advisors to ensure smooth, short transitions with minimal uncertainty.

The need for AHC leaders to reach beyond their organizations has been growing over time. They have gone from gathering data about their markets, to working on targeted community projects, to establishing informal and formal relationships with a variety of groups (such as employers, third-party payers, industry, other parts of the university). It is increasingly important that AHCs not only respond to but also influence their environments. External structural barriers that inhibit internal collaboration (e.g., accreditation requirements that do not keep pace with changing clinical care structures) require attention by AHC leaders. It is also important that AHCs attend to the development and strengthening of external relationships. A 1997 study by the Association of Academic Health Centers concluded that "the relationship between an AHC and its community is a critical leverage point as the AHC undergoes transformational change" because that relationship "can facilitate or sidetrack efforts by the academic health center to create partnerships, increase cost effectiveness, reshape the workforce, introduce new products, or modify the class sizes or composition of health professions schools" (Bulger, Osterweis, and Rubin, 1999).

The shape of leadership

There are myriad definitions of leadership. Senge describes it as "the capacity of a human community to shape its future, and specifically sustain the significant processes of change required to do so." He believes that leadership grows from the "energy generated when people articulate a vision and tell the truth (to the best of their ability) about current reality" (Senge *et al.*, 1999). Thus, leadership entails "defining a vision that people can rally around, developing a strategy to achieve the vision, and motivating a group of people to achieve the vision" (Kotter, 1996). Some scholars link the purpose of leadership with specific kinds of change such as reducing the gap between a group's values and its practices or increasing social capital (i.e., the communal bonds, moral resources, and collective goods that people invest in one another as members of a community) (Couto, 2002).

Organizations typically have three kinds of leaders (Senge *et al.*, 1999). Local line leaders focus on creating better results within their unit. They have "accountability for results and sufficient authority to undertake changes in the way that work is organized." Network leaders or community builders move about the organization carrying ideas, support, and stories. They participate in broad networks of alliances with other like-minded individuals, help line leaders directly and by putting them in contact with others from whom they can learn, and remind executive leaders of their ongoing role in supporting change initiatives. Executive leaders have overall accountability for organizational performance but less ability to influence work processes directly. Their primary role is to create an organizational environment for continual innovation and knowledge creation. They do so by investing in new infrastructure, encouraging inquiry, and leading by example through the norms and behaviors within their own teams.

Leaders who seek change that extends beyond organizational lines or confront diverse groups within their organization require additional capabilities. Innovative leaders use stories that permit organizations to build new practices or fundamental beliefs and values. Their stories may also question taken-for-granted assumptions that stifle any organization's ability to adapt to a changed environment. Their stories and values may be taken from one domain (such as faculty meetings) and told in simpler fashion in another (such as legislative hearings).

Leaders teach a wide range of groups most successfully by framing their stories to appeal to basic concepts common to different domains (Gardner, 1994). The more diffuse a group, the more a leader must reach for common ground. For example, Albert Einstein could not administer Princeton University based on a shared knowledge of theoretical physics. He would need to know the minds and motives of administrators, faculty, students, board members, alumni, and other organizational constituents. Genius does not make this leap from one domain to another; leadership does.

Transforming leaders shape and are shaped by their followers in the pursuit of significant change. They raise expectations for themselves and others. Transforming leaders achieve success by conveying new stories to, and learning new stories from, others (Couto, 2000, 2002). Innovative, transforming leadership uses "new stories about the nature of problems and solutions that permit people to conduct tasks of significant change" (Couto, 2002). It attempts to raise the level of a group's practices to its values and may increase the amounts and improve the forms of social capital. Innovative, transforming leadership expresses old and new truths through familiar and new stories. Such stories move us from exchanges of mutual benefit that further common interest to willingness to sacrifice for a new state of affairs. This form of leadership is particularly relevant for AHCs in light of the challenges and changes they face (such as achieving a shared vision among diverse constituencies, strengthening the AHC through enterprise-wide decision-making, or creation of a value-driven health system).

Whatever their end goal, effective leaders use tangible processes and behaviors to convert their vision into reality and manage the conflict and collaboration needed for change (Couto, 2002). Leaders seeking to transform their organization face both organizational and personal development activities as well as leadership and management tasks. Generally, these activities comprise:

- setting direction for the organization through vision, strategy, an operating model, and stretch goals,
- shaping the culture,
- ensuring competency development (including both technical and leadership skills for staff and self),
- establishing connections to the environment,
- providing sound management of routine operations and new initiatives.

The Leadership Mirror is a model that identifies 14 elements that are part of successful business transformation. The Blue Ridge Group found this model, developed by John Nackel, to be a useful construct in assessing the many facets of AHC leadership. (See full description at end of chapter.)

New dimensions of AHC leadership

Expectations for leaders are growing. A series of consumer focus groups concluded that leaders in the twenty-first century should have integrity, provide genuine attention to the customer and employees, be constantly learning and updating technology and expertise, and offer adequate and useful information for employees and customers. In addition, health leaders are expected to demonstrate caring and compassion, involvement in the community, and financial health for their organizations (Health Forum, 1999).

Academic health center leaders also face growing expectations. For example, deans previously ensured that educational programs met accreditation standards, distributed resources (without having to disclose how much was given to whom), aided department chairs in recruiting faculty, attempted to keep people happy, promoted the school, and rewarded outstanding achievement (Aschenbrener, 1998). Today, deans must design educational programs to address societal and workforce needs, reduce costs, right-size the faculty, establish direction and encourage collaboration, promote integration with other AHC units and outside partners, and foster institutional alignment.

Similarly, in addition to bearing responsibility for the performance, reputation, and success of academic and clinical programs, department chairs are now expected to:
- share collective responsibility for success of the AHC (by being well-informed about the environmental context, participating in strategic planning, and modeling core values of the AHC),
- assume more responsibility for managing the cost of education and research,
- explore new relationships with industry, health care partners, or community agencies,
- develop people (i.e., select people whose competencies match the needs of the organization, set expectations for performance and assess productivity

in relation to those expectations, and ensure that faculty and staff have the coaching, mentoring, and opportunities for learning necessary to continue their professional and personal growth),

• participate in succession planning (Aschenbrener, 1998; Johns and Lawley, 1999).

Not surprisingly, these new expectations are driving the need for leaders to possess additional skills. Whereas in the past, academic and clinical achievement were primary selection factors for AHC leaders, interviews with current and former deans revealed that interpersonal skills and personality characteristics as well as management training and experience contributed to success in their roles (Yedidia, 1998). These findings are consistent with research by Goleman, who found that although technical skills and cognitive abilities are threshold capabilities, effective leaders are distinguished by their emotional intelligence (Goleman, 1998a, 1998b). Analysis of the literature on successful educational curricular change and organizational change identified a series of leadership characteristics and actions that contribute to success. These include advocacy of the vision by the leader, promotion of a cooperative environment, assurance of real participation, ongoing evaluation of a project, and using human resource development effectively (i.e., training and aligning rewards with desired behaviors) (Bland *et al.*, 2000).

Analysis of the leadership literature from the perspective of AHCs reveals several themes (see Table 3.3). First, the confusion generated by the rapidly changing environment requires that leaders orient their organizations through articulation of core values and motivate their staff through creation and effective communication of a creative vision. Second, collaboration within and beyond AHCs will continue to increase and requires specific skills for AHC leaders and organizations. Third, ongoing personal development or transformation is a component of effective leadership (Goleman, 1998a, 1998b).

As our knowledge of the biological mechanics of health continues to deepen and our understanding of the social components of health continues to broaden, the US health sector faces the opportunity to achieve a significantly higher standard of performance. This opportunity arises amidst a multitude of existing shortcomings and emerging technological capabilities that point to the need for and potential to achieve a new vision for health in the twenty-first century. The continued existence of a large population of uninsured citizens, varying levels of quality and safety achieved by health care provider institutions, and continued escalation in costs of health care without

Table 3.3 Leadership competencies and characteristics identified in the literature

Source	Health leader competencies and characteristics
Goleman (1998a, 1998b) on Emotional intelligence	Self-awareness: knowing one's preferences, resources, and intuitions Self-regulation: managing one's internal states, impulses, and resources Motivation: emotional tendencies that guide or facilitate reaching goals Empathy: awareness of the feelings, needs, and concerns of others Social skills: adeptness at inducing desirable responses
Eastwood (1998) on Leadership in AHCs	Blend of "visionary, prophet, analyst, manager, coach, and mediator with skills informed by practical knowledge" Strongly motivated Possess a great deal of energy Self-knowledge Self-confidence Broad perspective Integrity Other directedness (including respect and ability to assess the abilities and motivations of others) Ability to communicate Ability to listen Ability to select good people Ability to handle uncertainty Ability to handle praise and criticism Ability to act and take risks Ability to use power Ability to make difficult decisions
Yedidia (1998) on Qualities to be considered in selecting a dean	Academic and clinical achievements Personality traits: • patience with process • openness to diverse points of view • capacity to act decisively • penchant for taking pride in the accomplishments of others Management experience: • prior experience in addressing complex, cross-cutting issues • ability to attend to a variety of issues at once • capacity to incorporate a view of institution-wide needs in decision-making • insider status (both potential asset and potential liability)
Franklin and Moore (1999) on Skills needed to lead integrated delivery systems	Capacity to amass critical resources quickly Ability to cross traditional boundaries and form alliances Cognitive flexibility Ability to integrate and interpret information Ability to develop creative vision and convey it using stories

Table 3.3 (*cont.*)

Source	Health leader competencies and characteristics
O'Neil (1999) on Physician leaders	Ability to align organizational efforts with vision through communication, focus, and continued involvement Ability to develop partnerships, alliances, and acquisitions Ability to manage change, including: • self-knowledge • ability to resolve conflict • create a culture that recognizes diversity of ability, provides training and environment, and ensures that people grow in their professional work • link the leadership agenda to the developing ability of its members • develop a diverse executive team that is aligned with the vision and strategy of the organization
Chow, Coffman, and Morjikian (1999) on Nursing leaders	Systems perspective as well as competencies in vision development, taking risks, innovating, and managing change
Bland *et al.* (1999) on Leadership of collaborative curricular changes in medical school	Ability to build a shared vision and keep it visible Ability to bring diverse partners together Ability to negotiate and handle conflict Project management capabilities (e.g., organizational skills, accountability systems) Knowledge about various domains involved in the project including the traditions and politics of each
Halverson (1999) on Skills needed for an integrated community health system	Inclusiveness: bring everyone who is part of problem or part of solution to the table • be willing to share control • seek out new and different people to participate • listen carefully to community perceptions • gain common vision and agreement on goals Innovation: overcome constituent traditions, harness collective ingenuity to arrive at new approaches • explicitly discuss value of innovation • create an innovations fund • create structured ways to learn from failure Integrity: provide the basis for trust and support among diverse participants • communicate • use a policy of full disclosure • ensure actions are consistent with words

accompanying improvement in health status of the population signal needed changes (Institute of Medicine, 1999, 2001).

The health care community is just now beginning to reap the benefits of advances in information and communications technology, nanotechnology, robotics, tissue engineering, genomics, and pharmacogenetics. New models of health care management are emerging with growing involvement of patients in their own care. Increasing connectedness in the health care sector and the economy at large reduces (although by no means eliminates) the difficulty associated with developing a systematic approach to managing the health of individuals and populations and creates opportunities for significant administrative cost savings (Goldsmith, 2000). The potential to monitor population health, customize diagnostic and therapeutic services for individual patients, and offer facile routine interaction between health care professionals and patients could stimulate the next major transformation in the delivery of health care (on a par with the introduction of sanitation techniques and the discovery of antibiotics).

Yet, along with significant potential to improve health, these developments raise a complex set of issues (e.g., equity, efficacy, and funding) that must be addressed. The health sector will need to determine how to balance allocation of resources among these highly sophisticated technologies and primary health needs such as nutrition, screening, or immunization. Health care in the future will be more than the illness care, illness prevention, and public health of the past. It will also include identification and treatment of the determinants of health at the societal level as well as value-driven services that meet the care needs of individuals. As the production modes of health care evolve, the industry will be able to draw upon the strengths offered by each. Ultimately, health care may successfully combine the trusting physician–patient relationship of the craft mode, outcome measures and efficiency of the manufacturing mode, and transformation of information and experience into useful knowledge in the learning mode (Maccoby, 1999).

Such profound change within the health care domain is, however, inhibited by limited and diffuse leadership of a sector populated by many diverse constituencies with well-entrenched interests. Thus, there is an urgent need to assimilate cutting-edge theories and proposals with nascent technological capabilities into a coherent vision that will motivate the myriad groups to coalesce and work collaboratively toward a radically different and dramatically improved future health system. In short, innovative and transforming leaders are needed to take full advantage of imminent technological achievements to improve health in the United States.

As discussed in Chapter 2, progress is evident in some of the areas that would provide an infrastructure for a value-driven health system (e.g., tools for population health management, evidence-based medicine, robust information systems, health professionals as proficient knowledge managers). Considerable work remains, however, in other areas such as:

- universal coverage,
- reimbursement mechanisms that offer health maintenance incentives to both health professionals and patients,
- expanded understanding of professionalism to include care of population as well as care of individuals,
- willingness to shift resources away from medical applications toward other factors that contribute directly to the health of a population (e.g., housing, education, nutrition, employment).

Moreover, there is not yet a sustained effort to create a true health care system in the United States. To drive such an effort, AHCs must articulate the vision for a new health system, define and communicate the framework needed for a value-driven system, become value-driven organizations, model and assess value-driven behaviors, educate value-driven health professionals and patients, and advocate for value-driven health policies. First and foremost, AHCs need to envision the future clearly and convey it in different ways to reach a variety of audiences so that others can embrace it and will be motivated to create a "new world order" for health care.

Progress will also require that AHC leaders cultivate a culture of change within their own institutions so that their enterprises can be transformed into value-driven organizations. As such, they can develop, model, and evaluate health organization and professional behaviors consistent with value-driven health care. They can identify skills needed to practice in such a system, educate future health professionals about those behaviors and skills, and disseminate knowledge about best organizational practices across the entire health sector.

By providing innovative, transformational leadership in the health sector, AHCs necessarily position themselves amongst those at the forefront and sustain their ability to train future health professionals and develop future health leaders. Alternatively, when AHCs respond in an ad hoc manner as forces buffet them, they risk damage to their organizations and to the public's health interests. Although this endeavor represents a huge stretch goal, AHCs are well positioned to create a coherent platform for change and align the various interest groups for action. Their traditional role as educators, innovators, and thought leaders provides them with influence in the health community through connections to and credibility with many different constituencies.

Although AHCs can make significant contributions to the development of a value-driven health system, they cannot and should not seek to bear the full burden of leadership. One of the key concepts of value-driven health is that risk and responsibility are shared by all participants and that contributors to the health system are defined broadly and extend to civic and business leadership as well as health leadership. Academic health centers should work with their communities and regions to communicate the concept of a value-driven health system, to develop strategies for increasing responsibility among local citizens for maintaining their health, and to share leadership opportunities associated with building a value-driven health system. Working collaboratively on this endeavor will increase the social capital of all participating parties with ultimate benefit accruing to the community as a whole. Success in this arena will depend on AHCs being open to ideas from their collaborators and seeking innovative approaches to community issues. The American Network of Health Promoting Universities, established by the Association of Academic Health Centers, can contribute to progress on this front as it seeks to raise health promotion on the agendas of AHCs, increase the effectiveness of AHCs' health promotion efforts, and strengthen partnerships between AHCs and local communities (Association of Academic Health Centers, 2003).

Leadership recommendations

There are many ways that AHCs can strengthen the leadership capabilities within their organizations. The Blue Ridge Group focused its recommendations on four areas likely to yield notable benefits: careful selection of AHC leaders, development of leadership skills among organizational members, working with governing bodies, and collaborating with communities to build value-driven health systems.

Leadership selection

Academic health centers should seek leaders with the ability (i.e., qualities and experience) to transform their organizations and to work with their communities to build value-driven health systems.

Developing organizational leadership

Academic health centers should develop the leadership skills of their professionals and students to build stronger organizations and value-driven health systems for their communities.

Academic health centers can make progress toward strengthening their internal leadership capabilities in the following ways.

- Articulating skills and characteristics critical for successful leadership and incorporating those criteria into recruitment and promotion efforts for all faculty and staff.
- Providing continual development opportunities for AHC professionals oriented to meeting both the needs of the organization and the individual's professional development plan.
- Identifying and nurturing potential future leaders through explicit mentoring, comprehensive appraisals with direct feedback from both supervisors and peers, and opportunities for both individuals and teams to attend leadership development programs.
- Developing team leader skills through mentoring, educational opportunities, and low risk projects.
- Attending to leadership abilities in the selection of faculty and staff who participate on committees, task forces, and project teams.
- Attending to succession preparation as part of strategic planning for the institution.
- Fostering institutional citizenship in faculty, staff, and students through educational programs, communication opportunities, explicit expectations, and performance evaluations.
- Strengthening formal and informal mentoring (e.g., include as part of performance expectations) and acknowledging individuals who serve as role models.
- Encouraging and rewarding collaboration across departments and disciplines.
- Considering leadership potential in the admissions process for health professional school candidates.

Academic health centers can make progress toward strengthening their collaborative leadership capabilities and advancing the development of a value-driven health system by:

- Drawing upon experiences of a wide range of community representatives (e.g., community health, public health, and education professionals; public officials; philanthropic agencies; and other parts of the university).

- Participating in assessment of community or regional health needs to determine how the AHC can contribute to the effort to advance the health status of the population (e.g., provide resources for development of a regional health database).
- Advancing efforts to improve population health status through educational programs for students, professionals, and patients.
- Allocating institutional resources to encourage research on population health issues.
- Initiating health policy debate on the need for and requirements of value-driven health care at local, state, and national levels.

Strengthening governance

Academic health centers should work with and develop the capacity of their governance bodies to provide strong leadership, sound guidance, and effective decision making for their institutions.

To make progress in this area, AHC leaders can:

- Continue and strengthen efforts to educate governing boards about immediate and longer-term challenges facing AHCs (e.g., visit other AHCs or attend national meetings together).
- Initiate conversation with board members on their respective roles in the changing economic climate and boundary conditions that enable leaders to act effectively.
- Ensure that all members of governance bodies and the AHC leadership team clearly understand and acknowledge conflict of interest laws and issues.
- Continue the development and use of performance measures that provide effective assessment of organizational and leadership performance.
- Encourage board members to play an active governance role while supporting the management team in its designated role as managers of the enterprise.

Collaborating with communities

Academic health centers should partner with professional organizations and specialty societies to strengthen leadership skills of their faculty and students, to help create and support needed change within AHCs, and to advocate for necessary changes in the health care system.

To make progress in this area, AHCs and their partner organizations can:

- Review curricula of existing leadership and related programs to determine if they are consistent with the current climate and needs of AHCs (e.g., do the programs address relevant leadership skills and tasks and offer a balance between leadership and management issues?).
- Determine if the focus of leadership and management programs should be broadened to include emerging developments in health care and the evolving nature of professionalism within health care (e.g., interdisciplinary care, population health management, knowledge management, health informatics including e-health and bioinformatics).
- Include institutional citizenship in both undergraduate and professional education programs.

Conclusion

Today AHC leaders need more than technical expertise, extensive managerial experience, and strong people skills. They must have vision for where health care should be in the twenty-first century, be able to share that vision effectively with diverse audiences, and be able to develop alliances that will work toward that vision. They must also have a vision for where their organization fits in that future health system and be able to transform their organization for future success. Thus, they must attend to leadership tasks of:

- developing an operating model and implementation strategies
- forging a culture supportive of team learning
- establishing stretch goals and performance measures for the organization, for themselves as individuals, and for their staff
- ensuring that professional development opportunities address both technical and leadership capabilities
- building solid relationships with their governing boards
- planning for continued organizational success through future leaders.

Needless to say, energy, commitment, staying power, and a sense of humor are also prerequisites for the job.

Academic health centers face the challenge of transformation across each of their missions. They cannot, however, transform themselves within a vacuum. They must strive to shape the environment in which they operate so that they are better able to reach their ultimate goal of improving health in this country. The current climate requires that AHC leaders extend their role from their organizations to their community and health care generally. AHCs need to help define the attributes of the future health sector. The Blue Ridge Group believes that the potential to create a health system for the nation has never been greater and that AHCs should act on the opportunity to shape a system that truly meets the needs of the public.

Despite its daunting nature and considerable risks, the role of the AHC leader offers the potential to shape the future of health in this nation. By leading instead of reacting, AHC leaders can take advantage of the unique set of opportunities presenting itself to this generation of health professionals. The US health sector needs transformation. With inspired leadership, AHCs can help to make it happen. Leaders can transform their organizations to achieve sustained high performance through a set of leadership and management tasks that require action at both the organizational and personal levels.

REFERENCES

Aschenbrener, C. A. (1998). Leadership, culture, and change: critical elements for transformation. In *Mission Management: a New Synthesis*, Volume 2, ed. E. R. Rubin. Washington, DC: Association of Academic Health Centers.

Association of Academic Health Centers (2003). *American Network of Health Promoting Universities*. Online at http://www.ahcnet.org/programs/leadership/ahhpu.php.

Association of American Medical Colleges (2002). Medical school applications may be on the rise. *AAMC Reporter*. Online at http://www.aamc.org/newsroom/dec02/medschoolapps.htm.

(2003). Leadership training programs for medical school department chairs. *The Successful Medical School Department Chair: a Guide to Good Institutional Practice*. Online at http://www.aamc.org/members/msmr/successfulchair/module2/leaderprograms/national.htm and http://www.aamc.org/members/msmr/successfulchair/module2/leaderprograms/inhouse.htm.

Bland, C. J., Starnaman, S., Hembroff, L., Perlstadt, H., Henry, R. and Richards, R. (1999). Leadership behaviors for successful university-community collaborations to change curricula. *Academic Medicine*, **74**, 1227–37.

Bland, C. J., Starnaman, S., Wersal, L., Moorhead-Rosenberg, L., Zonia, S. and Henry, R. (2000). Curricular change in medical schools: how to succeed. *Academic Medicine*, **75**, 575–94.

Blumenthal, D., Weissman, J. S. and Griner, P. F. (1999). Academic health centers on the front lines: survival strategies in highly competitive markets. *Academic Medicine*, **74**, 1037–49.

Bulger, R. J., Osterweis, M. and Rubin, E., eds. (1999). *Mission Management: a New Synthesis*, Volume 1. Washington, DC: Association of Academic Health Centers.

Cambridge University (2000). *Cambridge International Health Leadership Programme*. Online at http://www.cpi.cam.ac.uk/courses/health/html.

Chow, M. P., Coffman, J. M. and Morjikian, R. L. (1999). Transforming nursing leadership. In *The 21st Century Health Care Leader*, ed. R. W. Gilkey. San Francisco, CA: Jossey-Bass.

Collins, J. C. and Porras, J. I. (1994). *Built to Last*. New York: HarperCollins.

Commonwealth Fund Task Force on Academic Health Centers (2000). *Managing Academic Health Centers: Meeting the Challenges of the New Health Care World*. New York: The Commonwealth Fund.

Couto, R. A. (2000). Community health as social justice: lessons on leadership. *Journal of Family and Community Health*, **23**, 1–17.

(2002). *To Give their Gifts: Community, Leadership, and Health*. Nashville, TN: Vanderbilt University.

Daugherty, R. M. (1998). Leading among leaders: the dean in today's medical school. *Academic Medicine*, **73**, 649–53.

Duderstadt, J. J. (2000). *A University for the 21st Century*. Ann Arbor, MI: The University of Michigan Press.

Eastwood, G. L. (1998). Leadership amid change: the challenge to academic health centers. In *Mission Management: a New Synthesis*, Volume 2, ed. E. R. Rubin. Washington, DC: Association of Academic Health Centers.

Fein, R. (2000). The academic health center: some policy reflections. *Journal of the American Medical Association*, **283**(18), 2436–7.

Franklin, E. and Moore, R. M. (1999). Developing organizations by developing individuals. In *The 21st Century Health Care Leader*, ed. R. W. Gilkey. San Francisco, CA: Jossey-Bass.

Gabriel, B. A. (2002). The COD fellowship program: training tomorrow's medical school leaders today. *AAMC Reporter* March. Online at http://www.aamc.org/newsroom/reporter/march02/codfellowship.htm.

Gardner, H. (1994). *Leading Minds: an Anatomy of Leadership*. New York: Basic Books.

Garson, A. (1999). A report card for faculty and academic departments on education, research, patient care services, and finance. In *Creating the Future: Innovative Programs and Structures in Academic Medicine*, ed. C. H. Evans and E. R. Rubin. Washington, DC: Association of Academic Health Centers.

Geheb, M. A. (1999). Combining funds flow, analysis with financial goal setting. In *Creating the Future: Innovative Programs and Structures in Academic Medicine*, ed. C. H. Evans and E. R. Rubin. Washington, DC: Association of Academic Health Centers.

(2000). *Transforming AHCs: Operating in a New Economic Environment*. Oak Brook, IL: University Health System Consortium.

Goldsmith, J. (2000). The Internet and managed care: a new wave of innovation. *Health Affairs*, **19**(6), 42–56.

Goleman, D. (1998a). *Working with Emotional Intelligence*. New York: Bantam Books.

(1998b). What makes a leader? *Harvard Business Review*, November-December, 93–102.

Griner, P. F. and Blumenthal, D. (1998a). New bottles for vintage wines: the changing management of the medical school faculty. *Journal of the American Medical Association*, **73**, 719–24.

(1998b). Reforming the structures and management of academic medical centers: case studies of ten institutions. *Academic Medicine*, **73**, 817–25.

Halverson, P. K. (1999). Leadership skills and strategies for the integrated community health system. In *The 21st Century Health Care Leader*, ed. R. W. Gilkey. San Francisco: Jossey-Bass.

Harrison, D. C. (1999). The Cincinnati funds flow study. In *Creating the Future: Innovative Programs and Structures in Academic Medicine*, ed. C. H. Evans and E. R. Rubin. Washington, DC: Association of Academic Health Centers.

Health Forum (1999). *Leadership for a Healthy 21st Century: Creating Value Through Relationships, Executive Summary*. Chicago, IL: American Hospital Association.

Henry, J. D. and Gilkey, R. W. (1999). Growing effective leadership in new organizations. In *The 21st Century Health Care Leader*, ed. R. W. Gilkey. San Francisco, CA: Jossey-Bass.

Institute of Medicine (1999). *To Err is Human: Building a Safer Health System*. Washington, DC: National Academy Press.

(2001). *Crossing the Quality Chasm: a New Health System for the 21st Century*. Washington, DC: National Academy Press.

Johns, M. and Lawley, T. (1999). Leading academic health centers. In *The 21st Century Health Care Leader*, ed. R. W. Gilkey. San Francisco, CA: Jossey-Bass.

Kirch, D. G. (1999). Reinventing the academy. In *The 21st Century Health Care Leader*, ed. R. W. Gilkey. San Francisco, CA: Jossey-Bass.

Kotter, J. P. (1996). *Leading Change*. Boston, MA: Harvard Business School Press.

Maccoby, M. (1999). On creating the organization from the learning age. In *Creating the Future: Innovative Programs and Structures in Academic Health Centers*, ed. C. H. Evans and E. R. Rubin. Washington, DC: Association of Academic Health Centers.

Morahan, P. S., Kasperbauer, D., McDade, S. A., Aschenbrener, C. A., Triolo, P. K., Monteleone, P. L., Counte, M. and Meyer, M. J. (1998). Training future leaders of academic medicine: internal programs at three academic health centers. *Academic Medicine*, **73**, 1159–68.

O'Neil, E. (1999). Core competencies for physicians. In *The 21st Century Health Care Leader*, ed. R. W. Gilkey. San Francisco, CA: Jossey-Bass.

Paller, M. S., Becker, T., Cantor, B. and Freeman, S. L. (2000). Introducing residents to a career in management: the physician management pathway. *Academic Medicine*, **75**: 761–4.

Pardes, H. (2000). The perilous state of academic medicine. *Journal of the American Medical Association*, **283**(18), 2427–9.

Petersdorf, R. G. (1997). Dean and deaning in a changing world. *Academic Medicine*, **72**, 953–8.

Saxton, J. F., Blake, D. A., Fox, J. T. and Johns, M. M. E. (2000). The evolving academic health center: strategies and priorities at Emory University. *Journal of the American Medical Association*, **283**(18), 2434–6.

Scherger, J. E., Rucker, L., Morrison, E. H., Cygan, R. W. and Hubbell, F. A. (2000). The primary care specialties working together: a model of success in an academic environment. *Academic Medicine*, **75**(7), 693–8.

Schwartz, R. W., Pogge, C. R., Gillis, S. A. and Holsinger, J. W. (2000). Program for the development of physician leaders: a curricular process in its infancy. *Academic Medicine*, **75**, 133–40.

Senge, P. M. (1990). *The Fifth Discipline: the Art and Practice of the Learning Organization*. New York: Doubleday Currency.

Senge, P. M., Kleiner, A., Roberts, C., Ross, R., Roth, G. and Smith, B. (1999). *The Dance of Change: the Challenges to Sustaining Momentum in Learning Organizations.* New York: Doubleday Currency.

Sheldon, G. (2000). Personal communication.

Sherrill, W. W. (2000). Dual-degree MD-MBA students: a look at the future of medical leadership. *Academic Medicine*, **75**, S37–S39.

Viaggiano, T. R., Shub, C. and Giere, R. W. (2000). The Mayo Clinic's clinician-educator award: a program to encourage educational innovation and scholarship. *Academic Medicine*, **75**, 940–3.

Watson, L. (1997). *University of Virginia Health Sciences Center Health Informatics Enhancement Program (HIEP) Evaluation.* Charlottesville, VA: University of Virginia.

Wipf, J. E., Pinsky, L. E. and Burke, W. (1995). Turning interns into senior residents: preparing residents for their teaching and leadership roles. *Academic Medicine*, **70**, 591–6.

Yedidia, M. J. (1998). Challenges to effective medical school leadership: perspectives of 22 current and former deans. *Academic Medicine*, **73**, 631–9.

Appendix

The Leadership Mirror

John G. Nackel, Ph.D.

Leaders can transform their organizations to achieve sustained high performance through a set of leadership and management tasks that require action at both organizational and personal levels. The Leadership Mirror is a model that identifies 14 elements of successful business transformation and divides those elements between leadership and management as well as between personal and organizational activities (see Figure 3.1). Pivotal leadership activities for sustained high performance by an organization include the following leadership and management components and actions.

Build the organizational transformation platform

The transformation platform is the first necessary component of profound organizational or personal change (see Figure 3.2). It defines the what, why, and how of an organization's role within a market, industry, or community. By detailing the kinds of behaviors necessary to achieve internally established goals, it provides the basis for an organization's culture. The platform comprises five levels as described below. Virtually all organizations contain these levels, but vary in how well they articulate and execute the performance at each level. Defining a vision, mission, and operating model does not ensure that the leaders will be able to transform their organization. They must attend to all of the leadership and management functions detailed in the Leadership Mirror.

The **vision** is an important source of an organization's (or individual's) identity and purpose and defines the desired future state. The vision should be based on the core values or set of beliefs and concepts that represent the ideal state for an organization or person. Both vision and values are long term and largely unmalleable. They should be sustained by the business transformation process and provide a sense of continuity and purpose for actions that result from enterprise change.

John G. Nackel is Executive Vice President of US Technology Resources, Aliso Viejo, California, USA.

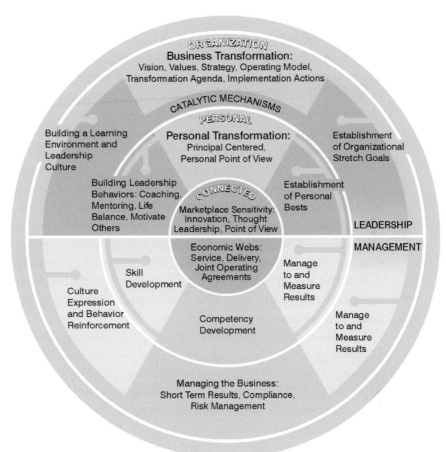

Figure 3.1   The leadership mirror

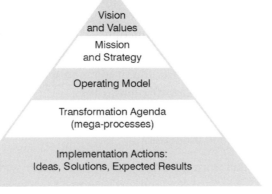

Figure 3.2   The transformation platform

The **mission** is a clearly articulated statement about an organization's or an individual's current direction. It is the expression of the vision for a period of time. It is more dynamic, fluid, and often shorter lived than the vision. The mission describes an organization's current business including the kinds of goods and services it offers. The mission will change over time in light of market influences and economic changes.

Strategy stems from the vision and mission to inform how the organization will act. It translates the mission into an operating model. Both the mission and strategy should change as an organization transforms its business.

The **operating model** is a concrete plan of how an organization will act in the marketplace. It outlines how organizational leaders want the organization to behave, what they want the organization to be known for in the marketplace, how they want to interact with employees, and desired relationships with business partners. The operating model converts strategy into daily activities and helps leaders to define processes that support the desired culture. It plays a pivotal role in business transformation and is often the point of breakdown in a transformation effort.

The **transformation agenda** defines which of the organization's functional areas will be involved in implementing the operating model, illustrates how the mega-processes fit together to support the operating model, and identifies which individual competencies are required to enact the operating model. It does not, however, prescribe how the organization should be structured.

Implementation actions are highly detailed plans of how individuals will operate on a day-to-day basis as they strive to execute the other levels of the pyramid. As a set, they are a more granular version of the operating model and describe the high-level activities needed to fulfill the transformation agenda. Implementation actions detail the relationships among competencies, solutions, and expected results but do not prescribe how an organization ought to be structured.

Catalytic mechanisms are policies and practices that are simple, easy to comprehend, and result in substantially raising the bar over current levels of performance. These simple procedural edicts are a potent way of reinforcing or achieving desired behaviors (Collins, 1999).

Develop a personal transformation framework

Change must occur within people before it can occur within an organization, therefore a framework to support personal transformation is a critical element of creating an organization with sustained high performance. Such a framework is similar to the organizational transformation platform and includes a personal vision, mission, values, understanding of strengths, goals, and implementation actions to achieve personal goals. It helps leaders clarify what they want to achieve and ensures that decisions and actions are based on a clearly articulated set of core values. ·

Establish connections to the market

Sensitivity to the environment and a framework for linkages to the marketplace enable sound decision making, provide the basis for future external relationships, and are critical for high-performing organizations. Organizational leaders should not only scan the environment constantly, but also generate thought leadership for their organization by generating and sharing new ideas, striving to be innovative, communicating with important players outside the organization, and developing a "point of view" on the marketplace.

Establish organizational stretch goals

Organizational stretch goals are long term, easy to understand, and flow from an organization's vision and values. They are the stratospheric heights to which all organizations who want long-term performance should aspire and drive business transformation by motivating the organization to examine where it needs to change to achieve those goals. Creating these goals is an important part of leadership because it provides a tangible target to achieve while pursuing the organization's vision. These goals should be achievable, but require substantial energy.

Establish personal bests

Personal bests are organizational stretch goals on an individual level – long-term, easy to grasp, and vision-centered goals that individuals strive for as part of their own personal transformation process. Personal bests require an assessment of individual processes. They challenge individuals to consider how they currently operate and to determine how they need to change to reach their goals. Personal bests should be aligned with the organization's stretch goals. Leaders should not only develop their own set of personal bests, but also encourage other individuals to formulate and accomplish their own personal goals.

Create a leadership culture and a learning environment

The combination of a leadership culture and a learning environment provides both the reason and means of constant organizational renewal. A leadership culture is one in which an organization's beliefs, behaviors, norms, and standards are centered on transforming the work of the organization to address its opportunities effectively. It is an organization's identity as an entity that is principled, proactive, and continually changing and prepared for changes in the marketplace.

Effective leadership cultures are constituted by diverse individuals with a shared understanding of the organization's vision or purpose, values, and mission. This shared understanding disperses responsibility to achieve the permanent aspects of the business-transformation pyramid and guides actions without the requirement of managerial oversight. Diversity in the professional, experiential, and cultural background of staff is an organizational asset since it is likely to broaden the range of approaches to problems thereby increasing speed in designing solutions that ultimately strengthen the organization.

A leadership culture is characterized by balance among the various segments of the Leadership Mirror and commitment to long-term success. It is also balanced in terms of the ability to implement organization-wide changes quickly while attending to human needs and sustained behavior reinforcement. Finally, a leadership culture assesses progress toward the vision and mission on a regular basis through established goals and measures and provides mechanisms to address shortcomings or develop needed competencies.

A learning environment is one that is structured around the generation, acquisition, and application of new knowledge. Such an atmosphere stimulates learning about an organization's environment and thus strengthens an organization's capacity to change by connecting the individual and organization to the marketplace. It also empowers individuals to examine how they act and where they need to change as part of their personal transformation. Moreover, a learning environment provides staff with the skills necessary for change and helps to create the mindset for continual change.

Model personal leadership behaviors

Personal leadership behaviors – including mentoring, sponsoring, coaching, and work-life balance – are important for the development of a learning organization and therefore contribute to the development of a sustained high-performing organization. These activities encourage learning, reinforce the vision, mission, and organizational goals, and build trust between a leader and individuals within the organization (Tichey and Cohen, 1997).

Manage the business

Ultimately, whether or not an organization is successfully transforming itself can be determined through its day-to-day operations and the actions that create short-term results. Tactical necessities must closely involve the elements of the transformation agenda. They are the concrete actions and tasks associated with fulfillment of the mission and vision. They include producing valued products and services as well as establishing and meeting quarterly earnings or other business projections.

Develop competency

Competency development is a means to ensuring that leaders and others in the organization possess the managerial skills necessary for the achievement of the vision and values. By fostering competency development in themselves and in others, organizational leaders reinforce the learning environment at the same time as they acquire needed skills. Competency development is critical for ensuring the completion of tactical necessities and success in key business processes. Such competencies may include specific technical expertise, process enhancement, product development, sales and marketing, or service delivery.

Establish economic webs

Leadership is interconnected and must not only link the personal and organizational spheres, but also the organizational and external spheres. Leaders must connect the organization to the economy through both its suppliers and customers and strive to cultivate new partnerships that support the transformation agenda.

Manage to, and measure, organizational results

Robust performance measures allow leaders to determine if the organization is transforming successfully and whether it will reach its stretch goals. Leaders need to develop the correct set of performance measures (i.e., measures that matter and are aligned with an organization's goals) and ensure that these measures are continually assessed and acted upon. Some standards are traditional and fairly easy to measure, such as revenues or profitability. Others reflect more intangible, but increasingly crucial elements of success (e.g., use of intellectual capital). Effectively used, performance measures provide accountability and communicate expectations to the organization, thereby shaping how organization members behave and providing the objective data needed to make judgments about how people, processes, and technology can be best aligned to achieve the organization's vision.

Manage to, and measure, personal results

Personal performance measures enable individuals to track their progress toward personal stretch goals. These measures should be aligned with personal goals, identify desired behaviors, and include expectations for results. Organizational leaders can influence the development and use of personal performance measures through both voluntary (e.g., encouragement) and involuntary (e.g., requirement of employment) means.

Reinforce behaviors and cultural expression

Behavior reinforcement entails the development of systems that support a learning environment on a daily basis. Such systems typically include human resources, communications and knowledge transfer, pay for performance or other reward systems, and educational and training programs. Both financial and nonfinancial mechanisms support behavior and contribute to employee satisfaction, so a combination of systems should be implemented to encourage employees to strive for excellence.

Develop behavior reinforcement skills

In addition to business and technical competency, leaders need personal and social competencies such as self-awareness, self-regulation, motivation, empathy, and social skills. These soft skills include adaptability, commitment, optimism, understanding others, communication, team building, conflict management, and change catalyst, among others (Goleman, 1998a, 1998b). Developing and using these skills is more subtle and complex than developing and applying technical skills. Moreover, leaders must not only possess these skills, but also be willing to use them as part of the organizational change.

REFERENCE

Collins, J. C. (1999). Turning goods into results: the power of catalytic mechanisms. *Harvard Business Review*, July. Online at http://harvardbusinessonline.hbsp.harvard.edu.

Tichey, N. M. and Cohen, E. (1997). *The Leadership Engine: How Winning Companies Build Leaders at Every Level*. New York: HarperCollins.

Case study

Building an institutional leadership development program: the University of Iowa Hospital and Clinics

Douglas S. Wakefield, Ph.D., Michael G. Kienzle, M.D., R. Edward Howell and Robert P. Kelch, M.D.

Background

Academic Health Centers (AHCs), like all health care organizations, face a growing complex of challenges to their traditional tripartite missions of teaching, research, and patient care. Critical to the success of AHCs is the development of stronger and more capable leaders at all levels. Despite this pressing need, effective strategies for creating successful leaders at AHCs have not been well defined.

The CEO of University of Iowa Hospitals and Clinics and the Dean of the Roy J. and Lucille A. Carver College of Medicine formed a partnership to jointly address one segment of the leadership continuum – the so-called middle managers who are vitally important in their current roles and a group from which future senior leadership will emerge. Thus the Institutional Leadership Development Program (ILDP) was created in 1998 with the goal of enlarging the size and enhancing the quality of the leadership pool available to the institution through faculty and staff participation in a specially designed program. The ILDP participants would potentially benefit the institution by:
- strengthening mid-level management,
- serving future leadership roles,
- solving multidisciplinary issues, problems, and conflicts,
- acting as change agents in leading and managing the necessary, cultural evolution.

Douglas S. Wakefield is Professor and Head of the Department of Health Management and Policy in the College of Public Health at the University of Iowa. Michael G. Kienzle is Special Assistant to the Dean and Director of Economic and Business Development in the College of Medicine at the University of Iowa. R. Edward Howell is Vice President and Chief Executive Officer at the University of Virginia Medical Center. Robert P. Kelch is Executive Vice President for Medical Affairs at the University of Michigan.

112

Early on we needed to clarify the primary focus of a leadership program. The fundamental question was whether our focus should be preparing individuals to be successful leaders anywhere or preparing individuals to be successful leaders in our institution. The ILDP adopted the institutional leadership focus, using the following basic program design features:

- Focus would be on both individuals and teams within the institution.
- Focus would be on the middle management group comprised of emerging clinical and managerial leaders rather than the senior management group.
- Curriculum would be a blend of broadly applicable and institutionally specific content.
- Faculty would include both internal and external academic/consultant experts and leaders from inside the institution.
- Emphasis would be on internal network development.
- Each class would be a heterogeneous mixture of physicians, other clinicians, and administrators.

The ILDP development included three major activities. We began by identifying the general content of the program. During this phase we created a shared language and perspective on which management, leadership, and policy-specific content and skills were to be included in the ILDP curriculum. These areas include: Human Resources Management, Communications, Financial Management, Decision Support/Information Systems, Process Improvement and Safety, and Strategic Planning.

Our second task was to assess the adequacy of internal and locally available resources and determine whether we should buy or build the program in-house. Developing the general content allowed for a specification of tasks and responsibilities and the initial budget development. Locally available resources and the high degree of linking curriculum to actual decision and production processes within UI Health Care made it more logical to develop the ILDP curriculum internally. Our last development task was to develop the topic content. During this step the specific curriculum and teaching plan for each general content area and individual sessions were developed.

Outcomes

To date, 6 class cohorts, for a total of 180 participants drawn from both the College of Medicine and the University Hospitals and Clinics, have completed the ILDP training. In addition, an active Alumni Network has been developed and continues to receive periodic educational infusions and assignment to high-profile strategic tasks outside of their home departments or original areas of responsibility. The major outcomes include:

- Responses of "students" and their supervisors (including academic and hospital department heads) have been overwhelmingly positive.
- Growing management language shared between the College and the Hospital.
- Enhanced understanding of both the external and internal "big pictures."
- Expanded internal networking and communications.
- The emergence of a new learning culture.
- ILDP Alumni assuming new job titles and responsibilities within the enterprise.
- Increasing requests by staff to participate in ILDP.
- Development of an internal Nursing Leadership Academy modeled on ILDP.
- ILDP influence showing up in new service experience and clinical initiatives.
- Senior staff increasingly interested in serving as ILDP faculty.
- Unknown effect on bottom line.

Lessons learned

In the course of our work we have learned a number of very important lessons on program organization, content development, motivating participants, sharing information, alumni development, and ongoing evaluation.

Organization

- Direct reporting relationship to top management is critical.
- Program must have its own budget and be sufficiently funded.
- Involve key senior leaders as faculty to get buy-in, expertise, and to enhance vertical networking.

Content development

- Identifying content areas is a critical step. This represents a key learning process for all involved. This may be time-consuming since there are many different interpretations and uses of the same management and leadership concepts.

Motivation to participate

- Using a formalized, visible, and competitive selection process helped to differentiate ILDP from other educational activities.
- There is widespread intellectual hunger within AHCs for new ideas, information, and skills. This is often unrecognized as an opportunity to maximize the organization's intellectual capital.

Sharing information

- Sharing new internal data, information, and insights was critical because it helps to decrease information hoarding and reinforces the importance of being selected for the development program. It also forces the organization to acknowledge the value of information and the benefit of making it accessible to those at all levels of decision making.

Alumni development

- Developing an alumni identity is critical; otherwise this type of program just becomes one of the "fads tried by management."
- The real value to the organization comes from new and innovative assignments for the alumni who share a common professional development experience.
- Support of the Alumni Network demonstrates a continuing commitment to and expectation for personal and professional growth.

Ongoing evaluation

- Improvement can only come through rigorous evaluation and application of what works well and what needs to be improved.
- There must be a commitment to evaluate, adjust, and communicate the adjustments at each step.
- Everything (e.g., accommodation, atmosphere, content, satisfaction) in every class session should be evaluated. The most important evaluation is what happens to the alumni after graduation.

Commentary

Edward D. Miller, M.D. and Steven Lipstein

As we reflect on the content of this chapter, we acknowledge right up front that the issue of leadership in academic health centers (AHCs) remains a vexing problem. On the one hand, leaders of AHCs are chosen because of their talents in research, clinical care or education. Many, however, have only managed small groups of individuals and modest operating budgets. The person chosen is often selected because the faculty respects the individual and the trustees believe that the person has the appropriate skills, but those skills have often not been tested. On the other hand, the skills that are necessary for success in such a position are the ability to grasp broad concepts, to interact effectively with a variety of people in groups and as individuals, to develop a sufficient resource base to finance institutional objectives, and then to make reasoned decisions and execute them. We offer three overarching themes on leadership to consider.

First, leaders have to stand for something. As this chapter points out, senior leaders must adopt a clear sense of the core values of the institution and a vision for an organization. Why does anyone aspire to be a dean? A hospital president? Can you articulate why you love your job? Or do you? Are you in it for the money? For the power? For the prestige? Or some other calling?

Often times, senior administrative and faculty leadership fail to recognize how important shared values are. Shared values influence the choice of new department heads. Shared values influence the promotion process and shared values influence the hiring or retention of key administrative leaders. At Johns Hopkins, leadership examines these values every other year in a formal retreat away from campus. There is no ambiguity and it helps set the tone of the organization. At BJC HealthCare, health system leadership meets with the

Edward D. Miller is Chief Executive Officer for Johns Hopkins Medicine and Dean of the Medical Faculty at Johns Hopkins University. Steven Lipstein is President and Chief Executive Officer at BJC HealthCare.

Board of Directors twice annually in an off-campus retreat format to revisit and reinforce the vision and direction of the organization.

Second, leadership development and succession planning are not the same thing. At both of our institutions, we continue to place more emphasis on decentralization, what the folks at BJC HealthCare call "distributed autonomy with congenial controls." Alignment of responsibility and authority at lower levels within the organization allows not only for accountability to be clearly recognized, but it helps grow the next generation of leaders. Growth of leaders within AHCs needs to be continuously stressed. Hopkins has started a formal leadership development program, which includes faculty and administrative staff. Departments there are allowed to nominate two people from their ranks and hospital vice presidents also get to nominate individuals whom they think will benefit. After three years of this program, new leadership has been recognized and given significant responsibility. It also serves to foster retention of key individuals.

At the same time, we need to carefully evaluate whether or not it is always appropriate for today's leaders to groom their successors. Do we do so to sustain the culture? To keep the momentum? To demonstrate that today's leaders are good mentors? Keep in mind that there is nothing wrong with new blood, a fresh start, and a truly new vision. Be careful not to entrench the status quo.

Both of us come to our respective organizations from elsewhere in academic medicine. Unlike corporate America, academic medicine has a rich history of developing tomorrow's leaders, even when they move on to other "competing" organizations. The very best leaders for your organization are not always "inside the company."

Third, leaders don't always know what they're doing. But do they have to? Is it more important to know the right answer, or to be able to lead a process that enables others to find it? Knowing the right thing to do is much easier than getting it done. Successful leaders need to be able to execute a vision, not simply create one. Sustained leadership over the years can only be achieved by demonstrated success. People within the organization are willing to be held accountable for their actions as long as the leader will be held accountable to the same dimensions of performance.

The leader of an AHC must set priorities, establish milestones, and report back to the organization successes and failures. Over time, board members, physicians, employees, and the community grow to respect the leader and the organization. As a result, they will make sacrifices for the organization and can stake a claim in its success.

The challenges that AHC leaders face are daunting. Financial pressures, academic pressures, public expectations, and judicious use of limited resources tax the best of minds. A clear vision of where the organization needs to move and how to measure the appropriate speed of change is the task of an AHC leader. This chapter offers valuable insight into that task.

4 Pursuing organizational and cultural change

Introduction

The academic physician, academic medicine, and the health professions in general are in the midst of an extended period of organizational and professional turbulence. Beginning with the explosive growth of managed care in the 1980s, the relatively closed, professionally self-regulated health services sector has been pushed into a more classically competitive marketplace. The 1990s brought additional impetus for change with shifting public policy, changing demographics, increasing consumerism, and the growing influence of information technologies. Further, the turn of the century brought renewed public concern with deficiencies and inconsistencies in the quality of health care services.

The health care sector is clearly laboring under the strains of this changing and demanding environment. The new marketplace is squeezing the financial resources and compensation available to health professionals and organizations. Societal needs, expectations, and aspirations for the health care system have changed and are growing. Academic health centers (AHCs), in particular, continue to face great challenges in adapting their multiple service and academic missions to changing societal, financial, and service requirements.

Academic health centers have adopted measures to improve service, cut costs, and increase productivity. They are learning how to do more with less. They have also worked to develop new capabilities and revenue streams in an attempt to shore-up strained academic and clinical resources. These efforts increase the service and performance expectations for faculty and staff who find it increasingly difficult to pursue research and teaching goals. In almost every aspect of the changing health care environment, strategies for competitiveness and fiscal discipline have been in contest with long-established organizational structures, processes, norms, values, and traditions of the health professions. The ensuing conflicts have been difficult to manage. As a result, AHCs are experiencing significant internal turmoil. Faculty morale and loyalty to the institution are being affected. Traditional AHC organizational structures and management solutions are fast becoming insufficient, if not obsolete.

In the face of this difficult environment, AHCs must address the cultural and organizational barriers to professional and institutional success in the health system of the twenty-first century. They must update their missions (as identified in Chapter 2), restructure their organizations, and adopt new approaches to supporting and motivating their staff. This chapter explores four key areas – enterprise management, organizational innovation, knowledge workers, and cultural archetypes – that are key elements of value-driven organizations.

Enterprise management

Academic health centers are often characterized as conglomerates of mini-fiefdoms. They comprise highly autonomous units that have varying degrees of financial independence and frequently divergent goals. The AHC organizational structure typically maximizes a wide range of activities and freedom for individual units and faculty members alike. Financial risk has typically been concentrated at the top of the organization, with individual clinical faculty members or health professionals bearing little or no risk for the decisions they make. Their income is ensured in the short run, regardless of how the institution fares. This structure has made AHCs exceedingly difficult to manage and lead. Moreover, the typical AHC is part of or affiliated with a university, an association that brings another layer of complexity to its environment and management.

Academic health center operations and revenue flow have often been determined more by history than by institutional needs. In the precompetitive era, when revenue streams were strong, AHC executives, deans, and hospital directors could afford to "cut deals" with department chairs and program leaders to attract or retain key faculty and build recognized programs. This culture of deal-making was pervasive throughout academic medicine. As a result, funds flowed and often still flow through the organization based on past negotiations rather than on maximizing return on investment or supporting a current institutional priority.

To survive in the new environment, however, an AHC must function as a common enterprise in which individuals and units support shared objectives and participate in the risks and rewards of working toward those goals. Thus, AHC faculty must go beyond stating that teaching, research, and patient care are interrelated. They must understand that enterprise-wide decisions such as investing in information systems, reallocating space in research laboratories, integrating billing systems, developing capacity in primary care or other emerging disciplines, reducing numbers of residents, or closing beds are not done to or for an individual unit but to strengthen the entire enterprise.

Enterprise-wide management involves managing all pieces of the AHC enterprise toward a common objective. It does not imply a particular organizational structure and may take various forms of ownership such as affiliations, contractual arrangements, or asset mergers. It does, however, require a collaborative and unified approach to governance whether or not the AHC owns all of the major units – including the school of medicine, hospital, and practice plan.

Success in enterprise-wide management requires influencing what is in the system to achieve a common set of goals. For clinical services, from the market's perspective, there must be a single unified voice for the institution, a centralized authority for contracting, and the ability to make timely decisions. Academic health center leaders need to create an environment in which each unit understands that its long-term success is intricately tied to the success of the whole enterprise. Accordingly, enterprise-wide goals will be considered more important than goals of individual units, and individual unit goals that conflict with enterprise goals should be revised or eliminated. For example, individual clinical departments traditionally have maintained control over cash reserves that accrue over time from their services. An enterprise-wide approach would enable each department to retain some cash reserves, but would also enable the AHC to have access to a pool of reserves obtained from all departments to serve as strategic capital and support AHC-wide investment needs.

In the past, success was measured at the unit level by faculty size, amount of space allocated, volume of clinical activity, level of research funding, revenue generated by faculty, percentage of residency matches, publications, and individual reputations. Today, success must be measured by how those elements contribute measurably to the individual unit and to the entire enterprise. This shift must not come at the expense of innovation by units and individuals, and it must not lead to a centralization of economic risk within the organization. In fact, it is essential that risk be distributed throughout the enterprise by clearly defining accountability and responsibility and by aligning incentives (including personal recognition and compensation) with budget and operational performance. Ultimately, enterprise-wide performance, including all economic activity of the AHC mission, must be measured to ensure long-term academic viability.

In addition to common goals, enterprise-wide management requires shared policy and appropriate infrastructure support, including clearly defined governance and management structures, and integrated financial and information systems. Regular communication with various stakeholders is fundamental to building trust in the enterprise. So, too, is the commitment to act on credible data. The culture shift that is needed to manage the enterprise can be facilitated through specially designed training programs for targeted audiences. These programs should focus on the skills needed at the individual and unit levels in this new kind of organization. Routine "town meetings" aimed at keeping the entire organization abreast of changes should ease the transition as well. Among the stakeholders to be involved in the evolution of the enterprise will be the relevant governing board and senior executives of the university so that they will understand and support AHC efforts.

To establish enterprise-wide management, AHCs need transparency. All parties must be able to see credible performance information for measurement and accountability of all parts of the organization. Only with such information will individual components be able to compare their performance, and AHC leadership be able to make rational decisions on allocating resources. For example, a comprehensive budget that identifies all revenue sources and documents all cross-subsidies within the organization is essential for AHCs to track their true performance. This approach need not mean a loss of control for individual units; rather, it means increased accountability and potential for greater gains.

Measuring performance of the enterprise

Performance measures serve multiple purposes within an organization; they support rational resource allocation, provide clear expectations to staff, and provide a mechanism for demonstrating accountability within the enterprise and to external stakeholders. Performance measures should be linked to the organization's strategic objectives and applied at each level of the organization including enterprise or aggregate measures, department or unit measures, and individual staff measures.

Academic health centers must use a quantitative and analytical approach to allocating their resources as they strive to achieve their missions with quality and efficiency. Traditional financial performance measures such as return on investment and internal rate of return should be part of the set of data points routinely tracked by AHCs to aid decision-making. The measures need to be balanced with other measures of quality, service, and productivity, which are tied to the organization's mission, vision, and strategies.

Table 4.1 presents sample performance measures for AHCs and the Appendix presents performance metrics adopted by Baylor College of Medicine. Among the performance measures in use by AHCs, those related to productivity, such as gross revenues generated per faculty full-time equivalent and direct cost per case, are more developed than those related to quality, innovation, or societal value. Looking across the AHC missions, productivity measures related to patient care and research tend to be more developed than those related to education. During the 1990s, however, there was increased interest in calculating the cost of undergraduate medical education, and several methodologies have been developed and used by schools of medicine (Franzini, Low, and Proll, 1997; Goodwin, Gleason, and Kontos, 1997; Jones and Korn, 1997; Rein *et al.*, 1997). As federal graduate medical education (GME) financing changes and competition grows from contract research organizations, AHCs will likely face greater incentives to manage the processes of GME, and research will therefore need more sophisticated measures in these areas.

Two kinds of performance measures are needed: a common set of performance measures relevant to all AHCs, such as research dollars per square foot for a given discipline or productivity ratios for various specialties to allow comparison with other organizations; and performance measures unique to specific institutions or applicable only to a specific subset of AHCs, including urban versus rural, research-oriented versus clinically oriented, and domestic programs versus international programs. To ensure continued innovation, appropriate metrics – reduction in adverse reactions or dollars saved from the introduction of new clinical protocols or patents granted – must be developed so that this unique AHC characteristic is preserved. Further, AHCs should include performance measures that assess their impact on the community.

As described by Tim Garson in his Commentary that accompanies this chapter, before introducing performance measures, attention should be given to the process of initial development and ongoing refinement. In particular,

Table 4.1 Sample performance measures for AHCs

	Productivity	Quality	Innovation	Societal Value
Patient care	Clinical revenue per medical doctor	Health-related functional and outcomes assessments	Savings from introduction of new clinical protocol	Amount of indigent care provided per year
	Outpatient encounters per hour	Satisfaction with experience of care	Revenues generated from introduction of new service	Improvements in community health markers
	Cost per case	Health status of the community		Local economic impact of clinical activities
Research	Direct grant revenue per faculty full-time equivalent (FTE)	Publications per faculty FTE	Increased revenue from new institutional practices to capture financial benefits of research	Health impact of new diagnostic or treatment capabilities (e.g., projected lives saved)
	Indirect grant revenue per faculty FTE	Patents per faculty FTE	Reduction in grant preparation time	Cost impact of new diagnostic or treatment capabilities (e.g., projected dollars saved)
	Research revenue per net assignable square foot	Royalties per faculty FTE		Local economic impact of research activities
		Rank in federal research funding		
Education	Clerk weeks per department	Student satisfaction with support services	Improved student access to knowledge sources from introduction of online resources or tutorials	Percentage of students who enter primary care or other needed disciplines
	Contact hours per faculty FTE in teaching activities (e.g., lectures, labs, small groups, grading)	Student evaluations of faculty	Improvement in student satisfaction, board scores, or faculty productivity from curriculum reforms	Balance of health professionals within a region
	Cost per student	Percentage of students who pass boards		Local economic impact of educational enterprise
		Percentage of students who graduate		

faculty, staff, and leadership should be jointly educated on the intent, validity, and planned application of the measures and should be consulted in the definition of the measures. Failure to build trust in these tools among faculty and staff will undermine their effectiveness.

Organizational innovation

Reform with change

The AHC, like all provider organizations, seeks to adopt competitive practices and the fiscal discipline to compete in the medical marketplace. At the same time, AHCs must provide an environment that encourages people to pursue quality, foster creativity, promote discovery, and nurture future health professionals, scientists, and educators. Academic health centers have had limited success in achieving this balance, in part because traditional AHC organizational structures and management approaches are unable to meet contemporary challenges.

Academic health centers and teaching hospitals have employed a variety of organizational and personnel management strategies to improve their competitiveness and fulfill academic and service obligations. Organizational strategies have included vertical and/or horizontal integration of clinical units and departments, large institutional and hospital mergers, acquisition and development of primary care "feeder" practices, aggressive cost reductions at owned or affiliated hospitals, various forms of administrative process consolidation, reorganization of care processes and policies, expansion of outpatient capacity, and improvements in information technology and organizational communications. In some instances, they even became insurers through creation of health care plans. Personnel management strategies have included various forms of individual and clinical unit productivity goals and incentivization schemes tied to salaries and bonuses, departmental and hospital discretionary funds, dean's funds and dean's taxes (Commonwealth Fund Task Force on Academic Health Centers, 2000). Some AHCs have experimented with, and adopted, a "mission management" approach to organizational and personnel management. With this approach, AHCs attempt to develop systems appropriate for organizing work and managing personnel within each separate mission: research, education, patient care and, sometimes, community service (Bulger, Osterweis, and Rubin, 1999).

A major and unintended consequence of these new organizational and management initiatives is that faculty are buffeted by shifting and sometimes conflicting professional and institutional expectations and responsibilities. Traditional areas of faculty responsibility, authority, and autonomy are being circumscribed (Eisenberg, 1999; McKinlay and Arches, 1985). Unable to devote sufficient time or effort to research, teaching, or professional self-development – goals and activities that are fundamental to their professional identity and personal values – many faculty, especially clinical faculty, feel devalued and disillusioned (Kataria, 1998). Recently published research confirms that clinical faculty satisfaction is below that of other medical school faculty (Blumenthal *et al.*, 2001). Many question whether academic values and missions are being replaced wholesale by "corporate" values (Blake, 1996; Relman, 1994). One respected commentator has suggested that medical schools are neglecting their university missions and appear to be regressing toward the proprietary school model that was the subject of Abraham Flexner's scathing report on the status of medical schools in 1910 (Ludmerer, 1999).

Further, despite these and other ambitious initiatives, a substantial number of AHCs continue to struggle to maintain operating margins. A report to the Commonwealth Fund Task Force on Academic Health Centers found in the year 2000 that 14 of 17 research-intensive AHCs experienced an operating loss, a bond downgrade, or a negative bond rating (Weissman and MacDonald, 2001). This seriously affects the financial strength of AHCs and limits the traditional utilization of clinical revenues to cross-subsidize education, research, and administrative costs within the AHC and throughout the university.

It has become increasingly clear that many strategies being employed by AHCs, including most "mission management" strategies, are designed primarily to improve the efficiency and effectiveness of traditional systems rather than to define new ones. This is a typical response that a leading medical sociologist has aptly identified as the pursuit of "reform without change" (Bloom, 1998). The process of reform without change is likely a major reason why, after years of various implementations, most AHCs continue to experience turmoil and uneven progress in balancing missions and achieving goals.

One of the many tests of leadership in this new environment, following on the need to revisit and realign values and missions, is to lead necessary organizational change. The Institute of Medicine (IOM) 2001 report, *Crossing the Quality Chasm*, provides important guidance. In articulating the growing public and professional dissatisfaction with the status, trajectory, and priorities of the health care system, *Crossing the Quality Chasm* reaches a conclusion at once bold and yet almost intuitively obvious by now to professionals and the public alike:

The current care systems cannot do the job. Trying harder will not work. Changing systems of care will. (IOM, 2001)

This is a pivotal conclusion in the public dialogue concerning our health care system: the quality of health care and access that Americans deserve and desire cannot be achieved by driving higher productivity in existing systems of care – or by further consolidating, streamlining, or expanding these systems. Instead, new systems must be designed.

Health care has safety and quality problems because it relies on outmoded systems of work. Poor designs set the workforce up to fail, regardless of how hard they try. If we want safer, higher-quality care, we will need to have redesigned systems of care, including the use of information technology to support clinical and administrative processes. (IOM, 2001)

It is vitally important that AHCs (and all other organizations involved in health delivery) take the measure of this assertion. It is likely that many existing organizational structures within AHCs – their schools, clinics, and hospitals – are inadequate. The ability of health professionals and the health care system to perform to their potential depends upon the development of more appropriate organizational, informational, and related systems. This, of course, does not make the existing organizations and processes easy to redesign or to replace. But difficult or not, reform with change is imperative.

Barriers to change

One of the fundamental impediments to optimal performance within AHCs is the organization of faculty in traditional, discipline-based departments. Whether seen as an accident of history or as a rational development within twentieth century medical and academic structures, it is clear that the traditional departmental organization is often a barrier to the achievement of twenty-first century missions and goals.

On the clinical side, the departmental structure reflects training regimens regulated by well-established specialty certification boards that grew as new technologies and discoveries in biomedical science encouraged the proliferation of subspecialties. Clinical departments evolved as faculty-centered structures designed to promote traditional faculty and professional values, priorities, and rewards. In the majority of medical schools, and certainly in those considered to be (or striving to be) elite, departmental "silos" have long served as mechanisms to ensure freedom of inquiry and protected time for reflection, research, and related academic activities.

Autonomy and authority are primary values that have permeated the entire profession. Historically, nonacademic physicians carried and structured these values into their work environments by setting up solo or small, single-specialty group practices, setting their own hours and career goals, developing informal patient referral networks, and establishing individual hospital privileges and affiliations. For both academic and nonacademic physicians, often their most meaningful institutional ties have been to their professional (usually medical or surgical specialty) organizations.

On the basic science side, the departmental structure has served very much the same functions. Academic health center and medical school basic science departments developed along classical divisions dating back to the origins of the biomedical and behavioral sciences: first chemistry, biology, and the physical sciences, and later proliferating into subspecialties, including microbiology and molecular genetics, cell biology, neurobiology, molecular pharmacology, pathology, biomedical statistics, biomedical engineering, and most recently genetics. These basic science departments, too, evolved as structures designed to promote traditional values, priorities, and rewards. Individual creativity and achievement in research, including success in winning extramural research funding, have been most highly valued and rewarded.

The middle of the twentieth century until the early 1980s was an era of expanding health care expenditures, increasing rates of fee-for-service reimbursement, and relatively robust federal and philanthropic funding for basic science research. It was also an era when both basic and clinical sciences developed largely through differentiation and subspecialization. It can be argued that the traditional faculty-centered departmental structure was a rational and effective organization by which biomedical science and medicine could make significant strides in such an era. But both the game and the playing field have now changed.

Public policy and market dynamics have forced all providers and provider organizations to become far more market-centered. In health care, as in other service industries, the market demands quality services at a competitive price. This requires that service organizations have an entrepreneurial and competitive spirit, and demonstrate their ability to meet customer (here patient and increasingly purchaser) needs.

Few would disagree that, while some departments are adapting better to the demands of the market than others, taken together, clinical departments of AHC medical schools have been reluctant change agents. Departments were not designed to enable more than relatively ad hoc and contingent forms of cross-department or cross-disciplinary cooperation in either their service or their academic missions. Despite significant efforts to integrate many administrative functions within integrated faculty practice plans, clinical departments continue to pose barriers to improving clinical operations and implementing delivery innovations. As a result, the marketplace (and by proxy, usually the medical school dean) is causing unprecedented stress on the departmental structure by asking it to pursue goals and undertake functions for which it is not designed. More than one commentator has remarked that the clinical department chair's job is becoming almost untenable (Aschenbrener, 1998; Korn, 1996).

In the basic sciences, the causes of stress on the departmental structure are of somewhat different origin. It is largely the progress of science itself that has begun to break down previous divisions between disciplines. The convergence of biomedical science around the methods of cellular and molecular biology has made these methods relatively ubiquitous. Therefore, over the last decade, the importance of departmental affiliation in differentiating the basic science faculty has diminished. Departments are becoming more alike in the questions being addressed, in the science being applied, and in the training being provided. Also serving to loosen these structures are collaborative service laboratories needed to perform analyses such as high-end computation. Even though academic advancement still requires investigators to demonstrate independence and originality, cross-disciplinary and cross-departmental collaboration have become routine, if not necessary, for successful work.

Yet, while academic departments are under great strain, they continue to have relevance and to serve important functions in structuring and protecting the academic life of faculty, in education, and in the organization and administration of many other institutional goals. And many external systems and structures remain in place that make departmental divisions still important. Among these are academic and professional societies and journals, as well as public and private research funding agencies, many of which still look to support work initiated within specified disciplines by individual investigators.

The challenge for AHCs, therefore, is to develop new organizational arrangements, systems, and processes that can meet two fundamental objectives. First, they must draw from and strengthen important academic and administrative roles traditionally played by the departments. Second, they must overcome departmental barriers and enable the appropriate organization of faculty to meet pressing new missions and goals. A survey of such efforts suggests some principles and approaches that can guide leaders in the effort to reform with change.

Change in research

The Program in Biological Sciences (PIBS) at the University of California, San Francisco (UCSF) Medical School represents one approach to reforming organizations around research. The PIBS was created in 1985 to leverage the methodological convergence in the basic biological sciences. The UCSF concluded that progress might best be achieved through programs rather than departments. The goal was a new organization that would not replace the departmental structure, but overlay it with a research and training organization that would enable faculty and students to easily cross departmental boundaries to pursue work and collaboration. The PIBS has been very successful and UCSF is currently developing an entirely new biomedical sciences campus and pursuing clinical reorganization initiatives based on this model.

Extrapolating from this effort, the principles most important to the success of this model appear to have been to:
- Ensure the integrity and continuing viability of individual basic science departments by preserving their roles in the administration of research and education programs.
- Create a new mechanism through which departments can align their interests and optimize their resource utilization and performance in the pursuit of common goals.

This was accomplished by a strategy that included:
- Strong leadership in building a consensus among chairs and departments for the need and opportunity to pursue such a model.
- Establishing an organizing mechanism – the PIBS Executive Committee – made up of all basic science chairs and elected faculty members.
- Centralizing responsibilities for faculty recruitment, admissions, curricular, and core facilities largely with the PIBS Executive Committee.
- Securing departmental control over their full-time employees or full-time equivalents (FTEs), space, appointments, and promotions.
- Making each department the home of one or more research or graduate programs, so that multidisciplinary research and graduate training programs continued to be administered by individual departments as a resource for all departments.

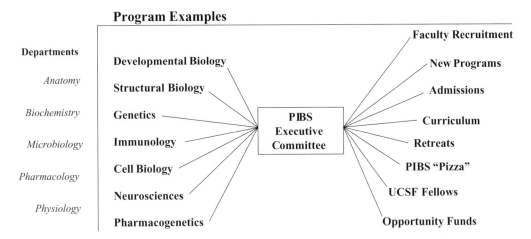

Figure 4.1   Anatomy of PIBS

The result is an organizational structure that reinforces mutual incentives and reciprocal responsibilities (see Figure 4.1). It is a model that enables faculty to cooperate to achieve common and converging goals. It allows for small new teams of talent to develop new programs and projects that can function as new "businesses" within the larger organizations. The important roles of the departmental structure are maintained for faculty. Department chairs are empowered to address both departmental and broader institutional goals. Students have access to the entire basic science faculty for research and doctoral work. But larger perspectives are possible and new "micro-organizations" can also form and flourish.

Change in clinical care

In clinical care, there has been progress in developing new organizations and systems that cross departmental barriers. These primarily involve the development of "centers" for either disease- or demographic-specific care. Many AHCs, community hospitals, and other providers have developed specialized centers for cross-disciplinary, comprehensive care. These include spine, diabetes, eye, mental health, and cancer centers, as well as children's, women's, and geriatric health centers and others. There is growing consensus in the provider community that such centers offer a more patient-centered environment than the traditional multi-site, multi-department approach.

Also becoming more widely understood is the prevalence and impact of chronic disease on population health status and on health care costs. Chronic conditions affect almost half the population and account for a majority of health care costs (Hoffman, Rice, and Sung, 1996). Both professionals and the public are increasingly aware of the inadequacy of fragmented and episodic care for the management and treatment of chronic illness or disability (Wagner, 2000). The Medical Expenditure Panel Survey (MEPS) of the Agency for Healthcare Research and Quality (AHRQ) and the National Center for Health Statistics identified 15 common chronic conditions as the leading causes of morbidity and mortality in the nation. These include: cancer, diabetes, emphysema, high cholesterol, HIV/AIDS, hypertension, ischemic heart disease, stroke, arthritis, asthma, gall bladder disease, stomach ulcers, back problems, Alzheimer's disease and other dementias, and depression and anxiety disorders (MEPS, 2000).

Within AHCs, by far the most well developed centers for multidisciplinary care are the comprehensive cancer centers. The best of these, particularly those that have achieved National Cancer Institute (NCI) comprehensive cancer center designation, are examples of what it is possible to achieve within the AHC environment – and only within that environment. These centers combine the best in advanced care, research, and training. They bring together expertise from many disciplines, including medicine and surgery, nursing, nutrition, rehabilitation, and others. They also bring together a wide range of diagnostic and treatment resources. They enable faculty and staff to develop systematic approaches to particular diseases and customized approaches to individual patients. Teams of care providers and staff routinely organize and reorganize to meet various demands and to pursue new courses of research, treatment, or training. Patients are accommodated and their families are supported by facilities and services centrally and conveniently located. At their best, they allow new subgroups to develop and pursue new ideas coming from research efforts discovered within or external to the organization.

These centers are vitally important to progress in the diagnosis and treatment of cancer nationwide. They are prime examples of patient-centered health services and a compelling model for similar efforts around other chronic diseases. They are a leading paradigm for how AHCs can be the foundation for progress across their multiple missions in research, education, and care. The most innovative centers are constantly looking to leverage new ideas and technologies, such as the Internet, to further improve patient management and research activities. Yet comprehensive centers like these are not yet the standard approach for delivering complex care. Why?

The most important factors normally described are limited federal funding and payer reimbursement systems that do not recognize or reward collaborative care. Regardless of other issues and barriers, the inability to fund the creation of such centers, or to receive appropriate payment for health services provided within them, severely limits the capacity of health professionals and organizations to develop the coordinated systems of care they know would better serve their patients. It is time to break down these barriers. And, it is time for AHCs to lead the way in suggesting and pressing for specific policies and reforms that will address these barriers.

The existing organization of AHC providers and health services in departmental units is insufficient for the task of organizing and delivering comprehensive disease-focused, patient-centered care. Although the departmental model may be viable for episodic care, that model cannot support the transition to a value-driven health system that includes population health management. It is imperative, therefore, that AHC and health profession leadership come together to forge, embrace, and aggressively advocate a new leadership agenda. *Crossing the Quality Chasm* strongly urges major health system stakeholders to adopt the 15 leading chronic conditions identified by the MEPS as "priority conditions" around which to focus efforts to reorganize the health system. The Blue Ridge Group supports that recommendation.

A new leadership agenda must aggressively pursue the expansion of federal support for the establishment of patient- and disease-centered efforts. It must also pursue reform in public and private reimbursement systems. Payments must be aligned with desired practices and outcomes so that health professionals and provider organizations can transition to more functional structures and organizations. Finally, a new leadership agenda must support a dramatic increase in our capacity to assess, measure, and improve quality and outcomes in health care.

We now know that discovery of new treatments is not the cure. Research has shown that valuable innovations require, on average, 17 years before they are picked up and generally applied (Balas, 2001). Even then, substantial variations in performance persist. Strong advocacy must be undertaken to generate the federal funding resources that can support new research on quality and outcomes metrics and the development and application of information technology needed to measure quality and assure improvement in managing outcomes.

Change in education

The educational and training missions within the AHC are no less in need of organizational redesign. Even though the medical school has long been the organizational center of the AHC, starting with the Flexner report of 1910, medical schools have been regularly criticized for allowing their education programs to take a back seat to other missions. In the decades following the establishment of federal funding for research through the National Institutes of Health (NIH) and other agencies, medical schools were criticized for valuing faculty contributions (and funding support) in research over contributions towards medical student educational goals. In more recent years, they were criticized for valuing contributions (revenue generation) in clinical care over educational service (Ludmerer, 1999).

It is not surprising that educational programs might take a back seat to other mission imperatives. There have been strong financial incentives for medical schools to encourage and reward faculty achievement in research and productivity in clinical care. Significant programs for funding of biomedical research are provided through the federal government, philanthropies, and the private sector. Clinical revenues, in particular, have been used to cross-subsidize the costs of medical education. Very few such financial resources, public or private, have ever existed for the direct support or incentivization of teaching. Yet even a sudden flood of new funding would not be enough to address the need for educational reforms. As it has in the other mission areas, the faculty-centered departmental structure has defined and increasingly limited educational innovation.

Until some significant reforms undertaken in the last decade of the twentieth century, most medical school curricula were organized into two to three years of large lecture courses in the biological sciences followed by one to two years of clinical rotations. This structure enabled the vast majority of faculty to avoid any teaching obligations, and for those with such duties or aspirations to teach only one to two courses per year. Many "teaching" faculty taught (and many continue to present) only one or two lectures per semester or per year, with many clinical teaching duties handled by "voluntary faculty" preceptors in the community.

Nevertheless, a critical mass of extremely dedicated teachers developed in all schools. Though sometimes held in poorer esteem by research-driven colleagues and passed over for promotion, they have managed to structure supportive learning environments. Often spurred by the national accrediting body, the Liaison Committee on Medical Education (LCME), medical schools have devoted the resources necessary to meet and exceed traditional professional standards.

In the late 1980s and early 1990s, a medical educational reform movement swept medical schools. Medical education, characterized by the large lecture format and minimal interaction with faculty, was subject to much critique.

Molecular biology was changing and vastly expanding the knowledge base. Medical practice was changing as the new market-driven environment began to impinge on the organization of care. Gender and cultural issues in the delivery of care grew more prominent. It was no longer enough for medical students to learn primarily through memorization and recitation. They had to become problem solvers.

The new model developed and adopted by many schools was the small group seminar and problem format. Many large lecture classes were replaced, or more often augmented by small group seminars, journal clubs, and problem-solving sessions. The basic science curriculum was redesigned to reflect the cross-disciplinary convergence around the new methods of molecular biology and genetics. Students also were offered courses on medical ethics, medical economics, and other relevant topics. New clinical rotations were added in nontraditional outpatient and ambulatory settings.

Deans and department chairs were creating flexible teaching funds and working to adjust promotion criteria that would weigh teaching contributions more heavily. Just as faculties and departments were pledging a renewal of support for the teaching mission, the market and public policy tide turned and resources began to tighten. Deans and departments now faced the prospect of having to fulfill significantly increased commitments of faculty time and departmental resources to the teaching mission at a time when they faced increased clinical demands and the reduction of departmental financial resources.

While new curricula are being implemented to favorable reviews in AHCs around the nation, the increased expectations and resource requirements have heightened the strains within and between departments. Clinical departments and faculty are affected more than those in the basic sciences. Departments trying to fulfill teaching obligations press faculty to teach. Clinical faculty who like to teach increasingly are pressed to generate revenues and meet clinical productivity goals and measures. Most departments struggle with even minimal teaching time and resource requirements. Many clinical faculty argue that they should be separately compensated for time away from the clinic.

Once again, the limitations of the departmental structure are implicated in the problem of meeting mission goals in this new era. That traditional departmental structures would have difficulty with the educational mission might seem surprising. It should not. The educational mission must draw on the same constellation of inter- and cross-disciplinary resources as the other missions. Institutional expectations, environmental factors, faculty commitments, and departmental priorities and resources are not aligned. Department chairs, individually or collectively, do not have the real or organizational resources to meet the demands of this new environment.

Aligning the teaching function with the research and care missions within the imperatives of the current environment can only be achieved with the proper organization of faculty and resources. As with the other missions, this requires mechanisms for cross-disciplinary and interdepartmental cooperation and reciprocation.

A great many efforts are underway within AHCs as well as among professional and industry associations to develop rational responses. Most AHCs have developed special departmental or institutional teaching funds to provide awards and bonus incentives for faculty teaching. Many have developed salary adjustment and other compensation formulas based upon the relative valuation of teaching and other mission fulfillment activities (Rouan and Wones, 1999; Sussman *et al.*, 2001). At the same time, the drop in medical school applicants that occurred in the late 1990s and the shifting distribution of students seeking postgraduate training is causing increased reflection within the various specialties as they too look at their "market" of consumers. While many of these approaches are extremely laudable and quite sophisticated, most are progeny of the "reform without change" approach. Most will fail because they are aimed at reforming the processes of a structure that can no longer support its function.

Real and necessary change will require more. At UCSF, a novel program to support teaching is the Academy of Medical Educators. The Academy is an interdepartmental network of master teachers who are selected by a peer review process. Membership in the Academy is a special honor that can be supported by a five-year endowed chair. The Academy has been replicated in at least one other AHC and others are studying it.

The advantage of this approach is that a new organization is being created and populated by master teachers who will represent the best in educational commitment throughout the organization. The Academy's effectiveness will, however, depend on how it is organized and developed. If the Academy develops simply as a faculty-centered network of gifted and dedicated teachers, this approach could turn out to be simply another form of incentive and reward system, or a new institutional mandate competing with traditional departments for resources. These outcomes would signal a reform without change. To be a reform with change, the Academy will have to develop into an organization that involves departmental leadership and that has the power to effect the marshalling and reorganization of some departmental functions and resources into cooperative programs structured to achieve student-centered educational goals.

Enabling knowledge workers

Optimizing performance

For more than a century, social scientists and, more recently, business management experts have studied the effects of organizational change and dislocation and have developed sophisticated models of process and personnel management. French sociologist Emile Durkheim laid the foundation for this work at the turn of the twentieth century. Durkheim wrote a path-breaking treatise on a major and growing fact of modern societies, the phenomenon of suicide. He described a new schematic of causes of suicide in modern societies and introduced, among others, the concept of "anomic suicide" (Durkheim, 1966). Durkheim described anomie as a condition of personal dislocation and anxiety often caused when social conditions (usually social or economic upheaval) cause individuals or classes of individuals to lose their sense of the importance or value of their contributions to society. Traditional values and definitions of success are called into question. New values and normative expectations are not yet well defined and may be years or decades from full social articulation and codification.

As a result, affected individuals or classes of individuals essentially lose their way. They lose their motivation. They lose the frame of reference necessary to solve problems, or even define success. They become discouraged and disillusioned. At the extreme, they commit suicide. In an earlier work, *The Division of Labor in Society*, Durkheim identified anomie as a problem inherent to the ever-changing, increasingly complex division of labor and fragmentation of traditional communities in modern societies (Durkheim, 1964). He went on to suggest that a critical role for society, including leaders in government, industries, and all professions, was to develop common goals (based on humane values) and systems by which affected individuals and groups could renew and sustain the motivation to understand and contribute in times of significant change.

Through successive waves of technological, organizational, and marketplace changes during the twentieth century, most industries, companies, governments, and organizations of any significance have developed in-house human resource and organizational management capabilities. Catalyzing, organizing, and responding to the many human resource challenges of change has become a significant core competency; however, neither the medical profession nor universities and their AHCs have kept pace with the development of such capacities. Academic faculty, especially AHC faculty, have pursued academic and service functions in a relatively protected, self-regulated, and unchanging environment. They have operated with relative autonomy in host institutions under well-established and stable systems of academic and professional conduct, expectations, and goals.

With the changed health care environment, universities and their AHCs can no longer operate as simply host institutions. They are now like other large and complex organizations that must support and manage system-wide change involving large numbers of professionals and staff. Academic health centers must quickly learn, and incorporate as a core organizational competence, the art and science of managing the "knowledge worker."

An ever-growing percentage of people are "knowledge workers": information and knowledge are both the raw material of their labor and its product . . . It's not only that more people do knowledge work; also increasing is the knowledge *content* of all work, whether it's agricultural, blue collar, clerical, or professional. A physician today armed with antibiotics, magnetic-resonance imaging, and microsurgery techniques brings far more knowledge to his work than his pre-World War II predecessors, whose principal tools were boiling water and a kindly manner. (Stewart, 1997, p. 41)

The university and the AHC are the paradigmatic employers and creators of knowledge workers. Most of the organizational structures within these institutions, including the traditional departments, have been extremely well adapted for knowledge work. Two distinguishing characteristics of these professionals are that they are self-directed and motivated, provided they have an opportunity to apply their knowledge effectively. Unlike manual laborers or other "directed" workers, they expect their work to be defined not by its quantity or its costs, but by its results (Drucker, 1996). They are best employed and managed as "associates" rather than "subordinates" – the way a conductor directs an orchestra. Following Durkheim's early observations, contemporary research confirms that if knowledge workers are mismanaged and lose their sense of being effective within an organization, they will lose direction and motivation.

Drucker identifies six factors for organizations and professionals to consider as they seek to strengthen knowledge worker productivity (Drucker, 1999, p. 142):

- Knowledge worker productivity demands that we ask the question: "What is the task?"
- It demands that we impose the responsibility for their productivity on the individual workers themselves. Knowledge workers have to manage themselves. They have to have autonomy.
- Continuing innovation has to be part of the work, the task, and the responsibility of knowledge workers.
- Knowledge work requires continuous learning on the part of the knowledge worker, and equally continuous teaching on the part of the knowledge worker.
- Productivity of the knowledge worker is not – at least not primarily – a matter of the quantity of output. Quality is at least as important.
- Finally, knowledge worker productivity requires that the knowledge worker is both seen and treated as an "asset" rather than a "cost." It requires that knowledge workers want to work for the organization, in preference to all other opportunities.

Drucker starts with the question, "What is the task?" because, unlike manual work, where the task is given and obvious, in knowledge work, the task often is not obvious to anyone except the relevant knowledge workers. Having responsibility for defining the tasks, including how the work should be done, enables and motivates knowledge workers to take responsibility for structuring effective solutions.

While at first blush this might seem somewhat utopian or unrealistic, there are innumerable examples of knowledge workers assuming such responsibility with great success (Drucker, 1999). However, it might be enough to contemplate the differences in productivity and motivation between a clinical faculty member in a department for whom significantly higher clinical output targets have been set, and a clinical faculty in a comprehensive cancer center setting faced with the same new goals.

In general, faculty measured against departmental productivity targets will likely be less motivated than those working in a more comprehensive clinical care setting. A faculty member in the first situation will have few choices but to see more patients. She or he will have little chance of affecting the goals or defining the "task," and is reduced to reacting as a subordinate, rather than engaging as an associate. A faculty member in the second situation will have better opportunities to work with colleagues and teams to define the task and to refine work processes and/or resource utilization to achieve institutional goals. She or he will be able to redefine the task in order to achieve higher quality outputs that can affect financial performance. The faculty member treated (however inadvertently or indirectly) as a subordinate will not perform as well as the faculty member able to engage and define the task as an associate and team member.

Clarifying expectations

Virtually all AHC faculty and staff are knowledge workers. Management of AHC faculty is legendary in its difficulty. Even before the era of market-driven change, it was often sardonically described as "herding cats." Now, however, the sardonic grins have disappeared and a new sense of urgency in managing these particular knowledge workers has taken its place. Many AHCs have embarked on comprehensive programs designed to bring new management discipline and performance expectations to their faculties (e.g., University of Alabama at Birmingham, Washington University) (Blue Ridge Academic Health Group, 1998). Most AHCs have worked to redefine faculty and staff performance goals and metrics and realign them with changing environmental and organizational missions and expectations.

For instance, more than five years ago, the Baylor College of Medicine initiated a process of faculty evaluation. The effort stemmed from a strategic plan initiated out of the realization that the organization had to understand and then change and adapt to new market conditions in all three missions. Vitally important to this effort has been the development of new standards and metrics by which faculty can calibrate their expectations and contributions and by which those contributions can be measured, assessed, adjusted, and rewarded. Critical to this entire process has been the gathering and organizing of data from and about all aspects of patient care, education, and research.

Important lessons can be gleaned from Baylor's effort about how a change process affects those directly involved. One lesson is that the very process of collecting data can itself be a significant change and cause significant stress within the organization. Data collection is not a value-neutral process. It is an activity that signals and represents important information about how missions, values, and goals are being (or are likely to be) redefined. Every new bit of data requested and collected is likely to signal implications for the roles and expectations of those from, or about, whom the data are collected or provided.

It is therefore important to manage the data-collection process as carefully as any other aspect of the change process. Affected faculty and staff must be incorporated into, and informed of, the change process, beginning with the definition of relevant parameters, data needs, and data collection processes.

Baylor has also addressed faculty concerns by ensuring that individual faculty data remain confidential between faculty and chairs, with only departmental-level data shared with deans or the board.

The Baylor initiative has led to the development of a sophisticated set of financial metrics used to measure effort, contribution, and success in each mission area (see the Appendix for an in-depth description of these metrics). These and similar measures have been developed by other AHCs, many with the assistance of consulting firms, such as Cap Gemini Ernst and Young (CGE&Y) and in collaboration with the University Health System Consortium (UHC). These metrics are necessary and important tools that promote the alignment of faculty and staff efforts with new market realities.

Nevertheless, despite a great deal of faculty participation in the development of such metrics, Baylor and all other AHCs report significant faculty dissatisfaction with them. Although still early in the process, common complaints are that they epitomize the "commoditization" of health care and diminish the status and role of the health professional in the care process (Johns and Niparko, 1996). While they quantify and enable measurement (often for the first time) of faculty and staff productivity and its financial impact, these measures may be limited by what they measure accurately as much as by what they do not measure accurately. Most difficult to assess are measures of the quality and outcomes of faculty and staff effort along each mission focus.

For faculty, professionals, and knowledge workers in general, who have high and very specialized levels of expertise and knowledge, judgments and measurements of quality are usually the most important metrics. Admittedly hard to quantify, they are nevertheless routinely acknowledged and measured by peer respect and esteem. Academic health center management and productivity enhancement measures that fail to adequately develop and factor-in quality metrics, however, may be fated to fail. Most are likely to be only minimally effective in orchestrating the change and performance required. Baylor has taken the position that there are core metrics that help chairs and deans to lead and manage, recognizing that certain individual contributions are best assessed qualitatively by the relevant chair or supervisor (Garson, 1999).

Measuring quality and outcomes

In clinical care, quality and outcomes measures incorporated for faculty evaluation are often limited to patient satisfaction surveys. These are helpful and useful, but are only a first step in capturing, quantifying, and measuring the quality and outcomes of care. Since quality and outcomes are what matter most to the knowledge worker, it is absolutely critical that such measures become integral and primary in faculty commitment and evaluation metrics.

Understanding that the current status of development of such metrics is universally acknowledged to be rudimentary, how can this problem be addressed? The first step, as Drucker suggests, is to ask the question: "What is the task?" If the task is to understand how to measure and evaluate quality and outcomes of clinical care, then who is in the best position to answer that question? Primarily (though not exclusively) it is the clinical care professional. The second step is to give the responsibility of answering this question to the clinicians. When asked what quality is, clinicians often respond, "I don't know how to explain it, but I know it when I see it." If they are not motivated to go beyond that explanation, then their clear knowledge of what constitutes quality will remain within the knowledge base shared by their relatively small group of professional peers. If, however, these clinicians are teamed with other knowledge workers who are experts at developing metrics for intangible measures, progress can surely be made. As simple as this might sound, these two steps have yet to be taken seriously. They should be.

In research, quality and outcomes metrics are better grounded. They are embedded within the peer-review process that serves as the foundation for awarding research support to investigators. There is also, within each field of research and scholarship, a hierarchy of journals, invited lectures, and other forms of "publication" that assess contributions along the hierarchy. This is a firm foundation, though more can be done.

For instance, over many years in Great Britain, a complex bibliometrics algorithm has been developed and continually refined, which assigns weighted values to all professional publications. This effectively creates a hierarchical ranking based on reputation. The publishing record of individual scientists and faculty in the universities is tracked and weighted by these metrics and can be accessed for the purposes of evaluating the quality of scientific work of candidates for promotion and hiring. Though understandably difficult to calibrate precisely and subject to some debate, there is growing interest in the adoption of this, and related quality metrics in the United States (Holmes *et al.*, 2000). Since scientists, too, will claim to know quality when they see it, efforts to quantify and make such knowledge accessible seem a reasonable and important project to shore-up a new focus on knowledge-worker support and management.

Equally important is the acceleration and expansion of quality and outcomes metrics for teaching faculty. A variety of metrics exist, including, but not limited to, student evaluations, peer review through observation and review of pedagogical methods, performance of students on standardized tests, and scholarly contributions in the field and in the development of pedagogical methods. Yet, broadly accepted standards by which to measure relative strengths of faculty in teaching are lacking (Blumenthal, 1997). This gap exists because teachers face a moving target. Student populations change over time and present different learning needs. Content requirements are constantly evolving and new technologies create new pedagogical opportunities. Moreover, comparisons across disciplines are complicated. Different subjects, departments, and schools attract students with differing abilities, motivations, demographics, prior preparation, and experience. Additionally, the development of standardized metrics is impeded by limitations on access to needed data.

For instance, a leading researcher and his collaborators, conducting research on training outcomes and quality, asked all specialty certification boards for data on their board certification examination pass rates. All but one specialty board declined or failed to provide this information. Analysis of what limited information was obtained raises a range of important questions about training outcomes that, among other things, could aid in developing quality and outcomes metrics that could be applied to evaluating, designing, and improving clinical training (Blumenthal *et al.*, 2001). In education, as in clinical care and research, significant progress in developing quality and outcomes data and metrics is both possible and essential.

Academic health centers, academic society, and health professions leadership must become the leading advocates for the development of quality and outcomes metrics in every mission area. Renewed federal funding for research and development of such metrics is essential. The full cooperation of all academic, professional, and institutional stakeholders in accommodating such research and development is also essential. For example, all certifying boards should publish their board pass rate data by program, as has been the policy of the American Board of Internal Medicine since 1996.

Bringing good things to life

We spend all our time on people. The day we screw up the people thing, this company is over. (Jack Welch, Former Chief Executive Officer, General Electric Company)

The General Electric Company (GE) is a global corporation with dozens of enterprises in hundreds of locations around the world (Lynch, 2001). During

Jack Welch's 30-year tenure as Chairman and CEO, GE grew from a $28 billion to a $130 billion company The vast majority of GE's 350 000 person workforce consists of knowledge workers, some of whom are dedicated research scientists, engineers, and high technology professionals. The challenge of managing this large, diverse, international workforce is daunting. While much about the GE situation is not directly analogous or applicable to AHCs today, there are a number of knowledge worker management practices and policies that deserve emulation.

General Electric considers its dedication to "People, Processes and Performance" as key to its success. These three elements are driven through the organization by a strong leadership process that continuously evaluates, articulates, and then reinforces organizational priorities and values. The organization is defined by the need to constantly drive change so that it is always seeking and creating new growth opportunities. Change is driven through a combination of organizational structures and processes built around:

- hiring great people,
- creating a performance culture,
- linking results with rewards,
- demanding shared values,
- believing everyone counts.

Professional and leadership development are primary functions of the organization and new talent is constantly sought after and aggressively recruited. Continuous learning, performance appraisal, and feedback mechanisms are built into the work schedule and process. These activities occur at every level of the organization. Major milestone meetings are scheduled up to a year in advance and attendance is mandatory. This embedded management process also serves as a way to connect people throughout the organization and for continuous communication "bottom-up and top-down."

Critically important to their enterprise is that everyone in the organization knows exactly what is expected of them, which metrics are being used, and why, and how they are measuring up. People are put at risk and held accountable for certain commitments and they share amply in the rewards for reaching the objectives. High level performance is generously rewarded through pay and promotions. Continuous feedback and learning, and ongoing evaluation create highly motivated people with the tools to meet and exceed expectations. Collegiality, flexibility, the ability to work with and motivate others, and to make good decisions are all highly valued and rewarded. People are regularly moved and promoted and new teams are created to meet new opportunities.

Since GE puts such significant resources into developing the capabilities of its people, it is also keenly aware of the cost of losing those people, whether to competitors or to unrelated industries. Therefore, GE makes what some might consider extraordinary efforts to ensure that the feedback loop runs in all directions and that its people feel like they and their families matter in the organization. Special programs, gifts, dedicated services, and communications all play an important role in building a relationship not just to the worker, but to the person.

No doubt, this is a high intensity environment. The pressure to perform, to dedicate oneself to the organization's values and goals, to meet and exceed objectives is unrelenting. Individuals have to work hard to balance competition and collegiality, and personal and professional obligations. Nevertheless, employee retention is extremely high and people are seldom summarily dismissed. The ongoing evaluative process enables the organization to identify issues or areas in need of improvement early, so that individuals have the opportunity to work on them and improve.

While the goals and some of the values at a global corporation like GE may not align completely with those of an AHC, the need to manage and motivate knowledge workers is highly analogous. The GE example illustrates how it is possible, with the appropriate organizational structures and personnel management policies and processes, to motivate extraordinarily large and diverse organizations of knowledge workers to maintain high levels of performance. It also illustrates how dedicating organizational resources to the development of people can sustain motivation even when policies or processes sometimes fall short.

In the AHC, and in universities more generally, there is nothing like this level of resource commitment or organizational focus for the purpose of supporting faculty and staff in their professional development and in their work. For organizations to attract and retain the best and the brightest in the future, they have no alternative but to adopt many of these proven methods. The example of GE and hundreds of other companies and organizations offers a clear example for AHCs now struggling with the imperatives of the marketplace and with motivating an increasingly unsettled knowledge workforce.

Overcoming cultural barriers

Developing new archetypes

A final critical dimension of the AHC and health professional organization that must be reformed and realigned is the culture of the organization. The

AHC and the medical profession have traditionally been supported by three cultural archetypes. The first is the ideal of the independent and original investigator. For the doctoral degree and for academic and professional advancement, the individual candidate must demonstrate independence of thought and originality of achievement. The training of students and career trajectory of faculty are effectively defined by the requirement to distinguish oneself and one's work from that which preceded it and to show originality relative to the work of one's peers.

The second archetype is the "triple threat" faculty physician. This is a high-energy individual who is a great clinician, a solid, if not brilliant, investigator, and an inspiring teacher and mentor. The triple threat has long served as both an ideal and an idol by which clinical faculty or physician scientists could calibrate their efforts and by which their contributions could be valued and measured for the purposes of career advancement and academic promotion.

The third archetype, less universally admired, but nevertheless widely accepted and cultivated within academia (and academic medicine in particular), has been the strong, independent, charismatic, egocentric, and often authoritarian or highly maverick personality. These characteristics are often associated with legendary figures in the history of medicine akin to Bobby Knight or Woody Hayes of college coaching fame. The indomitable personality is one whose combination of brilliance and independence of thought and eccentric (or worse) behavior is not tolerated or compatible with most organizations or institutions. In academia the combination has been not only tolerated, but often rewarded by a series of increasingly senior and prestigious appointments at a succession of leading universities.

Each of these three academic archetypes, like the organization and management systems they support, is under considerable strain. How these archetypes are addressed will determine a great deal about the viability of the change in the AHC and professional organization. The first archetype, independence and originality, is being tested by both internal and external factors. Internally, as we have described, the methodologies of science, and perhaps of important clinical and educational processes, are converging. Faculty seek out collaborators across the entire spectrum of research, clinical care, and educational programming. Externally, public and private funds are increasingly seeking to maximize return on investment by choosing to support work that can draw on multidisciplinary sources of expertise. More and more progress in science, medicine, and education is occurring as a result of cross-disciplinary and cross-institutional collaboration, whether episodic or long term and continuous. External factors also include market-based pressures that drive the need to reduce costs and create efficiencies in each mission area, including the need to maximize sharing of core facilities, instruments, and other critical resources, as well as knowledge.

Clearly, progress in science, care, and education will continue to require independence and originality. So this underpinning cannot be allowed to crumble; however, it is also clear that teamwork and collaboration are, and increasingly will be, vital to scientific progress. It is therefore necessary to reform the archetype so that it holds up both the development of the independent and original investigator, and the demonstrated ability to work collaboratively.

Internal and external forces are also challenging the second archetype, the triple threat (Pellegrin and Arana, 1998). Increasingly, as people of diverse backgrounds and interests began to fill out medical schools and faculties, the grounds for promotion and advancement broadened and became more flexible. New thinking has challenged the conventional view of scholarship and has contributed to the development of a more sophisticated understanding of the value of several forms of scholarly activity (Angstadt, Nieman, and Morahan, 1998; Boyer, 1990; Nora et al., 2000). At the same time, AHCs and medical schools have developed along a variety of paths, with different emphasis on clinical care, education, or research. The relative value or importance of these characteristics and contributions now vary by institution and by department within institutions. Consideration of academic advancement normally depends upon excellence in at least one mission area and substantial contributions in another.

The external forces threatening the triple threat archetype have been even more daunting than the internal forces. As the market-driven environment imposes itself on the AHC and health care, the necessary focus on faculty productivity and revenue generation has undermined this gold standard. Administrators and faculty alike face the increasing realization that the triple threat no longer serves as a realistic standard by which to measure the value of clinical faculty. For increasing numbers of clinical faculty, clinical productivity, in particular, is becoming a de-facto proxy for the value of their contributions as faculty members.

Nevertheless, the existing departmental structures and their policies largely have yet to incorporate this new reality. Department chairs, deans, and peers continue to send mixed and conflicting messages about standards for faculty performance. Tenure and promotion standards, particularly at the elite, research-centered AHCs, overwhelmingly retain the traditional triple threat as an evaluative gold standard. Yet, specialization in one mission area with substantial expertise and contributions in another is becoming the new real standard. This new model is more compatible with the progress of science and medicine and with the likelihood of ongoing success within academic and professional organizations.

While still representative of the highest attainment in the minds of some, the traditional triple threat is becoming more like an ideal than a real standard for the vast majority of faculty and schools. AHCs and the health professions should cultivate a new triple threat valued and rewarded for:

- Excellence in scholarship and/or achievement in one or more of the core academic mission areas: student-centered education, discovery-centered research, or care-centered research or innovation.
- Excellence in achievement and/or leadership in the core service mission: patient-centered care.
- Excellence in achievement and/or leadership in community, professional, and institutional service to measurably meet societal needs and aspirations for our health care system.

A triple threat built on standards like these would be a worthy successor to the former ideal.

The final archetype, ego-centrism with independence of behavior, is also under severe stress. Internally, deans and senior administrators, not to mention departmental and other affected faculty, increasingly worry about the extent to which intense competition among AHCs to recruit stellar individuals is both costly and, in many cases, extremely disruptive. Recruitment packages can run into millions of dollars in commitments. Recruiting high-profile individuals and providing them with outsized and bountiful resources can be disruptive to departments and even to whole institutions. Very often, appointments of stellar individuals to chairmanships and institute director-ships have been made without regard to the leadership or managerial capa-bilities of the individual. Five years later, the return on this investment can end suddenly as the star is recruited away by a new high bidder. Meanwhile, rising stars within the organization leave, or are recruited away, to pursue other opportunities.

External forces eroding this part of the culture are the same market forces affecting the others. The new environment favors organization and leadership that engenders commonality of purpose and optimal knowledge worker and system performance. Independence and originality of thought, the capacity to create teamwork, inspire loyalty, and manage performance are increasingly prized and rewarded. Ego-centrism, authoritarianism, and independence of behavior are no longer adaptive. They are increasingly counterproductive.

The "Project Professionalism" of the American Board of Internal Medicine (ABIM) is a model of what professional societies can do to promote a new, more adaptive culture for twenty-first century health care. Established in 1992, the Project developed an enhanced definition of professionalism that has been adopted by the ABIM. It identified eight elements of professionalism to be required of candidates seeking specialty certification: altruism, account-ability, excellence, duty, service, honor, integrity, and respect for others. Also identified were seven issues that diminish professionalism, including: abuse of power, arrogance, greed, misrepresentation, impairment, lack of conscien-tiousness, and conflict of interest. Project Professionalism then developed a program that includes guidelines, forms, and other materials by which grad-uate medical education program directors and others learn to mentor and assess residents and candidates for certification. The ABIM project is playing an important role in the formal incorporation of humanistic qualities into the components of clinical competency (American Board of Internal Medicine, 2001).

Leadership development

The General Electric company and many other enterprises, both large and small, have a very different view of leadership development and succession planning. They believe that routinely bringing in new leadership from the outside, as many enterprises do, is often more disruptive than successful.

At GE, leadership development and succession planning are top priorities. The idea of routinely recruiting top leadership from outside the company is an anathema. Rather, they focus on developing that leadership from within. They recruit individuals with high achievement and leadership potential and then invest years of learning and support to help ensure that they develop it. Individuals sought must be strong and able to demonstrate key attributes: independent thought, ability to manage individuals and inspire performance, and a talent for building successful teams. Individuals displaying arrogance, and the penchant for inspiring resentment, mistrust, jealousy, and other de-motivating behaviors are either educated or weeded out. Leaders are cul-tivated throughout the organization and are groomed for what they, their supervisors, and their peers determine together are the appropriate leader-ship positions.

Academic health centers can no longer afford to reward egocentric and authoritarian personalities, who cannot manage people or processes well. The environment and the organization can no longer support this. Academic health centers must build a new cultural archetype that supports stellar, brilliant individuals with strong personalities who can lead change and inspire confidence and performance among knowledge workers and peers. This new cultural archetype can be built by developing a new focus on leadership development and succession planning for key positions throughout the organization, especially department chairs, deans, and other senior administrative and business managers. Recruitment objectives for younger faculty should be revised to include criteria for the identification of potential future leaders. Such internal and occasionally external recruitment policies should be aligned with faculty and staff leadership development programs and integrated into departmental and other administrative unit operations and functions.

External recruitment for high leadership positions need not be discontinued. National and international searches for the best individual or team to fulfill a specific leadership or other significant role can be effective. Academic health centers will, however, likely experience vast improvements in their organizational and leadership capabilities to the extent that such searches increasingly reveal that the best candidates are to be found, because they have been cultivated, within their own institutions.

Recommendations

The Blue Ridge Group offers the following recommendations to AHCs for reshaping their organizational structure and culture in seeking to create value-driven organizations.

Enterprise management

Academic health centers should base their management structures on the "enterprise." Individual components of AHCs that perceive themselves as independent must view themselves as integral to a common enterprise and must commit to accomplishing common goals and objectives.

To make progress in this area, AHCs should develop and implement organizational performance measures for each of their mission areas that address quality, productivity, innovation, and societal value, to measure progress toward organizational objectives, guide decision-making and assure accountability.

Organizational innovation

Academic health centers should develop and implement organizational innovations and programs that enable faculty and staff to achieve societal health care needs and to create a value-driven health care system.

To make progress in this area:

- AHC leadership should adopt the 15 leading chronic conditions identified by the MEPS as "priority conditions" around which to focus organizational reform efforts.
- AHC and other provider health systems should support the development of comprehensive disease and/or demographic centers of care on the model of the NCI Comprehensive Cancer Center designation.
- AHCs should systematically review the roles of existing academic departmental structures and develop new organizational approaches to managing the barriers they pose to clinical, research, and education/training programs.
- AHCs should pursue changes in public and private payment systems that will eliminate payment barriers and disincentives for providers and provider organizations transitioning to practice in such new structures and organizations.
- AHCs should seek federal and other sources of support for needed research and the development of quality and outcomes measures and the application of information technology to quality and outcomes management improvements.
- AHCs should lead efforts to demonstrate the value of organizational restructuring on health care and health status.

Enabling knowledge workers

To enhance value creation, motivate performance, and improve quality and outcomes, AHCs must develop a new understanding of knowledge workers and the types of organizational systems and processes required to manage and lead them. Academic health centers should commit to ongoing leadership, professional, and staff development as an integral part of each mission.

To make progress in this area:
- AHCs should build upon proven leadership and management approaches and human resources development programs, like those of GE, that align with the way highly skilled knowledge workers are properly supported and motivated.
- AHCs should re-evaluate accepted measures of performance and value on an ongoing basis, and identify ways to enable faculty to better manage their roles, responsibilities, and expectations. AHCs must develop more sophisticated measures of value creation to guide the organization, direction, and evaluation of institutional and personnel performance.
- AHCs should ensure that all faculty and staff in management and supervisory positions are provided training and support in the delivery of regular performance feedback and the development and mentoring of professionals.

Academic health centers should develop new and improved human resource capabilities that enable routine performance appraisals, identification of new talent, cultivation of skills, and mentoring of faculty and staff.

To make progress in this area:
- AHCs should experiment with policies that motivate faculty through the distribution of risk and reward.
- AHCs should develop enhanced tools for measuring performance of the system and individuals (i.e., metrics) to promote accountability.
- National organizations, such as the Association of American Medical Colleges (AAMC), Association of Academic Health Centers (AHC), or Institute of Medicine (IOM) should conduct or sponsor studies of enhanced human resources capabilities and infrastructure for AHCs.

Culture recommendation

Academic health centers and health professional organizations should actively work to reform their cultures and archetypes of desirable behavior.

To make progress in this area:
- AHCs should supplement the culture of the independent investigator with a culture that supports a demonstrated ability to establish and be a significant contributor to, or leader of, fruitful and meaningful collaborations and teams.
- AHCs should supplant the traditional ideal of the "triple threat" with one that emphasizes:

- Excellence in scholarship and/or achievement in one or more of the core academic mission areas: student-centered education, discovery-centered research, or care-centered research or innovation.
- Excellence in achievement and/or leadership in the core service mission: patient-centered care.
- Excellence in achievement and/or leadership in community, professional, and institutional service in measurably meeting societal needs and aspirations for our health care system.
- AHCs should replace the archetype of the egocentric, authoritarian, or otherwise organizationally dysfunctional personality and cultivate a new standard that values the stellar, brilliant individual with a strong personality who leads collective change, inspires confidence, and motivates performance among peers, other knowledge workers, and staff.
- AHCs should establish leadership development and succession planning programs that identify and develop the new leaders in health care and biomedical sciences necessary for creation of a health care system for the twenty-first century.
- AHCs and health professional societies should adopt, as a model set of professional standards, the elements of the enhanced definition of professionalism developed by the ABIM through its "Project Professionalism."

Conclusion

A new kind of health system is on the horizon. It is the responsibility of the entire health community to make progress toward the health system of the twenty-first century. Unlocking the promise of the new system will demand new ways of thinking, new modes of working, and new kinds of skills for both professionals and organizations. Optimal performance in the evolving system will require that the external environment supports health care organizations through reimbursement and funding mechanisms that reward quality care and create a national health information infrastructure. In turn, health care organizations must support their staff by creating an organizational culture and structure that enable individual and institutional excellence.

The Institute of Medicine has provided a rallying point for the entire health care system and particularly for AHCs and health professionals as they seek to define a sound way forward. By focusing the public policy spotlight on the inadequacy of existing delivery systems and system goals, and in building on the knowledge, skills, and dedication of the healing professions, the IOM has articulated clear and powerful goals that both health professionals and our public can embrace. It is now up to AHCs and their partners within the health community to take tangible steps towards transforming the vision of a twenty-first century health system into a reality.

The Blue Ridge Group believes that AHCs should begin by assessing their mission, goals, and performance against the goals for the new system. Where gaps exist, there are opportunities for realignment and organizational reforms that seek to truly change organizational performance. Academic health centers should prepare for forthcoming changes by ensuring that their organizational structures foster flexibility and collaboration. Academic health center organizational processes should support faculty and staff through clear expectations and robust human resource functions. Academic health center culture, particularly its archetypes, should be updated to reflect contemporary needs of AHCs and the health community.

As discussed in Chapters 2 and 3, the Blue Ridge Group also believes that AHCs should be leaders in building a value-driven health system for the twenty-first century. This leadership can take a variety of forms: AHCs can lead by example through their organizational change efforts; AHCs can lead by conveying the new vision to audiences throughout the health community; AHCs can help shape the health policy agenda and decisions that will in turn determine how well the external environment supports health organizations and professions in the new system; AHCs can use their research resources to translate the vision into practice by expanding knowledge about what constitutes safe, effective, and efficient care. Equally important, AHCs can help current and future professionals acquire the skills they need to achieve excellent performance consistently.

Absent strong leadership from AHCs and professional societies and the continuing turbulence in health care also threaten the pipeline of bright, idealistic young people willing to choose a career in health care. Nursing and medical technician shortages abound. Academic health centers need to support organizational and cultural changes with comprehensive reforms in the entire spectrum of education of health professionals – a subject that the Blue Ridge Group addressed in *Reforming Medical Education: Urgent Priority for the Academic Health Center in the New Century* (Blue Ridge Academic Health Group, 2003).

The last several decades have been a time of great turbulence and stress for AHCs and health professionals. Now the health community stands at the beginning of a new era, one that could prove to be momentous for the health and history of the nation. It is essential that AHCs not only prepare themselves to succeed in the future environment, but to define it.

REFERENCES

American Board of Internal Medicine (2001). *Project Professionalism*. Philadelphia, PA: American Board of Internal Medicine Publications. Online at www.abim.org.

Angstadt, C. N., Nieman, L. Z. and Morahan, P. S. (1998). Strategies to expand the definition of scholarship for the health professions. *Journal of Allied Health*, **27**(3), 157–61.

Aschenbrener, C. A. (1998). Leadership, culture, and change: critical elements for transformation. In *Mission Management: a New Synthesis*, Volume 2, ed. E. R. Rubin. Washington, DC: Association of Academic Health Centers.

Balas, E. A. (2001). Information systems can prevent errors and improve quality. *Journal of the American Medical Informatics Association*, **8**(4), 398–9.

Blake, D. A. (1996). Whither academic values during the transition from academic medical centers to integrated health delivery systems? *Academic Medicine*, **71**(8), 818–19.

Bloom, S. W. (1998). Structure and ideology in medical education: an analysis of resistance to change. *Journal of Health and Social Behavior*, **29**, 294.

Blue Ridge Academic Health Group (1998). *Academic Health Centers: Getting Down to Business*. Washington, DC: Cap Gemini Ernst & Young US, LLC.

  (2003). *Reforming Medical Education: Urgent Priority for the Academic Health Center in the New Century*. Atlanta, GA: Emory University.

Blumenthal, D. (1997). The future of quality measurement and management in a transforming health care system. *Journal of the American Medical Association*, **278**(19), 1622–5.

Blumenthal, D., Causing, N., Campbell, E. G. and Weissman, J. S. (2001). The relationship of market forces to the satisfaction of faculty at academic health centers. *American Journal of Medicine*, **111**(4), 333–40.

Boyer, L. L. (1990). *Scholarship Reconsidered: Priorities of the Professoriate*. Princeton, NJ: Carnegie Foundation for the Advancement of Teaching.

Bulger, R. J., Osterweis, M. and Rubin, E. eds. (1999). *Mission Management: a New Synthesis*. Washington, DC: Association of Academic Health Centers.

Commonwealth Fund Task Force on Academic Health Centers (2000). *Managing Academic Health Centers: Meeting the Challenges of the New Health Care World*. New York: The Commonwealth Fund. Online at www.cmwf.org.

Drucker, P. F. (1996). *The Executive in Action*. New York: Harper Business Press.

  (1999). *Management Challenges for the 21st Century*. New York: Harper Business Press.

Durkheim, E. (1964). *The Division of Labor in Society*. New York: The Free Press.

  (1966). *Suicide: a Study in Sociology*. New York: The Free Press.

Eisenberg, L. (1999). Whatever happened to the faculty on the way to the Agora? *Archives of Internal Medicine*, **159**(19), 2251–6.

Franzini, L., Low, D. and Proll, M. A. (1997). Using a cost-construction model to assess the cost of educating undergraduate medical students at the University of Texas-Houston Medical School. *Academic Medicine*, **72**(3), 228–37.

Garson, A. (1999). Performance measures and our "art." *Journal of the American College of Cardiology*, **34**, 607–9.

Goodwin, M. C., Gleason, W. M. and Kontos, H. A. (1997). A pilot study of the cost of educating undergraduate medical students at Virginia Commonwealth University. *Academic Medicine*, **72**(2), 211–17.

Hoffman, C., Rice, D. P. and Sung, H. Y. (1996). Persons with chronic conditions: their prevalence and costs. *Journal of the American Medical Association*, **276**(18), 1473–9.

Holmes, E. W., Burks, T. E., Dzau, V., Hindery, M. A., Jones, R. E., Kaye, C. I., Korn, D., Limbird, L. E., Marchase, R. B., Perlmutter, R., Sanfillipo, F. and Strom, B. L. (2000). Measuring contributions to the research mission of medical schools. *Academic Medicine*, **75**(3), 303–13.

Institute of Medicine (2001). *Crossing the Quality Chasm: a New Health System for the 21st Century*. Washington, DC: National Academy Press.

Johns, M. E. and Niparko, J. K. (1996). Averaging excellence out? *Archives of Otolaryngology Head Neck Surgery*, **122**(10), 1839–44.

Jones, R. F. and Korn, D. (1997). On the cost of educating a medical student. *Academic Medicine*, **72**(3), 200–10.

Kataria, S. (1998). The turmoil of academic physicians: what AMCs can do to ease their pain. *Academic Medicine*, **73**(7), 728–30.

Korn, D. (1996). Reengineering academic medical centers: reengineering academic values? *Academic Medicine*, **71**(10), 1033–43.

Ludmerer, K. M. (1999). *Time to Heal: American Medical Education from the Turn of the Century to the Era of Managed Care*. New York: Oxford University Press.

Lynch, J. (2001). *Leveraging Leadership to Drive Growth at GE*. Presentation to the Blue Ridge Academic Health Group.

McKinlay, J. and Arches, J. (1985). Towards the proletarianization of physicians. *International Journal of Health Services*, **15**(2), 161–95.

Medical Education Panel Survey (2000). MEPS HC-0068: 1996. Medical Conditions. Online at http://www.meps.ahrq.gov/catlist.htm.

Nora, L. M., Pomeroy, C., Curry, T. E., Hill, N. S., Tibbs, P. A. and Wilson, E. A. (2000). Revising appointment, promotion, and tenure procedures to incorporate an expanded definition of scholarship: the University of Kentucky College of Medicine experience. *Academic Medicine*, **75**(9), 913–24.

Pellegrin, K. L. and Arana, G. W. (1998). Why the triple threat approach threatens the viability of academic health centers. *Academic Medicine*, **73**(2), 123–5.

Rein, M. F., Randolph, W. J., Short, J. G., Coolidge, K. G., Coates, M. L. and Carey, R. M. (1997). Defining the cost of educating undergraduate medical students at the University of Virginia. *Academic Medicine*, **72**(3), 218–27.

Relman, A. S. (1994). The health care industry: where is it taking us? In *The Nation's Health*, 4th ed. P. R. Lee and C. L. Estes. eds. London: Jones and Bartlett Publishers.

Rouan, G. W. and Wones, R. G. (1999). Rewarding teaching faculty with a reimbursement plan. *Journal of General Internal Medicine*, **6**(14), 327–32.

Stewart, T. A. (1997). *Intellectual Capital: the New Wealth of Organizations*. New York: Doubleday.

Sussman, A. J., Fairchild, D. G., Coblyn, J. and Brennan, T. A. (2001). Primary care compensation at an academic medical center: a model for the mixed-payer environment. *Academic Medicine*, **76**(7), 693–9.

Wagner, E. H. (2000). The role of patient care teams in chronic disease management. *British Medical Journal*, **320**(7234), 569–72.

Weissman, J. S. and MacDonald, E. A. (2001). Current findings on the financial status of academic health centers. Presentation to the Commonwealth Fund Task Force on Academic Health Centers Spring Meeting, April 27.

Appendix

Baylor metrics 2001

Clinical departments

Patient care

1. *Patient care RVUs*: the RVU (relative value unit) describes how much time and effort a physician spends performing a service: a routine clinic visit is approximately 1 RVU whereas heart surgery receives 30 RVUs. This is a measure of how much activity all physicians perform; the higher the number of RVUs, the more outpatient visits and procedures are performed.

2. *Patient care RVUs per private patient care FTE*: this is an efficiency measure, indicating how efficiently physicians spend their time while seeing patients. The number of RVUs is divided by the number of full time equivalents (FTE) devoted to patient care. Each physician spends a certain percentage of their time seeing patients – for example, if he/she spends one day per week out of five, this is 20 percent or 0.2 FTE. If the number of RVUs is divided by the patient care FTE, this normalizes the patient care activity to what a 100 percent physician would spend.

The Medical Group Management Association (MGMA) has benchmark data on private practice physicians throughout the United States. We have chosen this measure as a benchmark for our physicians. For example, if the department of otolaryngology is greater than the 90th percentile for MGMA, this means that Baylor physicians see patients more efficiently than 90 percent of private otolaryngologists.

3. *Patient care expense per RVU*: this is the expense per service. All department expenses related to patient care (e.g., physician salary and fringe, staff, supplies, etc.) divided by RVU. Given the different incomes of physicians, the expense per RVU cannot be meaningfully compared across departments. However, the percentage change from one year to the next in the same department is a measure of change in resource utilization.

158

4. *Patient satisfaction – patient–physician relationship*: an outpatient survey is administered by telephone quarterly. Seven of the questions relate to the physician (for example: competency, caring, enough time spent with the patient). This number is the overall patient assessment of the physician.

5. *Patient satisfaction – process of care*: in the same survey, questions are asked about "process," such as: time to get an appointment, parking, courtesy of the staff, billing. This number is the overall assessment of the process.

Research

6. *Basic science laboratory grant dollars per basic science laboratory*: this is a measure of the efficiency of use of basic science or "bench" laboratory space. The grant dollars are those used to perform basic science – for the most part those investigations requiring animals, genes, chemicals, microscopes, etc. The total grant dollars (direct dollars to the investigator plus the indirect dollars to the institution) are used. The square feet used are those for investigators' basic science laboratories and other shared laboratory support space such as cold rooms. Values more than approximately $350 per square foot indicate crowded laboratories.

7. *Grant and contract dollars per research FTE*: this is a measure of the productivity of researchers. Both basic research (defined above in no. 6) and clinical research (generally research on individual patients such as taking blood pressure, giving drugs, or the support of such research, for example by data collection or computer modeling) are included. The number of grant dollars is divided by the number of FTE devoted to research. Each researcher spends a certain percentage of their time doing research; for example, if he/she spends three days per week out of five, this is 60 percent or 0.6 FTE. If the number of grant dollars is divided by the research FTE, this normalizes the research activity to what a 100 percent researcher would spend. This amount of funding (>$400 000 per research FTE) implies that, on average for the department, each research faculty member holds more than one grant.

Education

8. *Learner evaluation*: periodically (whether after a single lecture, or after a month with a physician, or a year with a mentor), learners (i.e., medical students, graduate students, and residents) are given the opportunity to evaluate their teachers. The evaluation form is similar for each type of learning, and

each asks the overall evaluation of the teacher on a scale of 1 to 7 with 7 being the highest. This metric is the average of every evaluation received by faculty in the department.

Finance

9. *Budget*: each year, each department submits a budget for the upcoming fiscal year. If, at the end of the year, the actual revenue minus expense (overall – all business segments) exceeded the prediction, the goal was exceeded.

10. *Revenue less expense > 0*: if, at the end of the year, the overall revenue less expense was greater than zero (regardless of the prediction), the goal was exceeded.

Basic science departments

Research

1. *NIH grant dollars per tenure track faculty*: for basic scientists, one important measure of the quality of research is whether the National Institutes of Health is funding that grant. Since basic science departments are made up almost exclusively of individuals performing basic science, it is a goal for each tenure-track faculty member to be funded by the National Institutes of Health. While also true in the clinical departments, there are prestigious funding sources for clinical research that might come from other sources, and so this is not a metric for clinical departments. This amount of funding (>$350 000 per faculty member) implies that, on average for the department, each tenure-track investigator holds more than one NIH grant.

2. *Basic science laboratory grant dollars per basic science laboratory square foot*: this is a measure of the efficiency of use of basic science or "bench" laboratory space. The grant dollars are those used to perform basic science – for the most part those investigations requiring animals, genes, chemicals, microscopes, etc. The total grant dollars (direct dollars to the investigator plus the indirect dollars to the institution) are used. The square feet used are those for investigators' basic science laboratories and other shared laboratory support space such as cold rooms. Values more then approximately $350 per square foot indicate crowded laboratories.

3. *Grant and contract dollars per research FTE*: this is a measure of the productivity of researchers. Both basic research and clinical research (generally research on individual patients such as taking blood pressure, giving drugs,

or the support of such research, for example by data collection or computer modeling) are included. The number of grant dollars are divided by the number of FTE devoted to research. Each researcher spends a certain percentage of their time doing research, for example, if he/she spends three days per week out of five, this is 60 percent or 0.6 FTE. If the number of grant dollars is divided by the research FTE, this normalizes the research activity to what a 100 percent researcher would spend. This amount of funding (>$400 000 per research FTE) implies that, on average for the department, each research faculty member holds more than one grant.

4. *Learner evaluation: graduate students and medical students*: periodically (whether after a single lecture, or after a month with a physician, or a year with a mentor), learners (i.e., medical students, graduate students, and residents) are given the opportunity to evaluate their teachers. The evaluation form is similar for each type of learning, and each asks the overall evaluation of the teacher on a scale of 1 to 7 with 7 being the highest. This metric is the average of every evaluation received by faculty in the department. Graduate students rate teachers statistically lower than do medical students, hence the separate metrics.

Finance

5. *Budget*: each year, each department submits a budget for the upcoming fiscal year. If, at the end of the year, the actual revenue minus expense (overall – all business segments) exceeded the prediction, the goal was exceeded.

6. *Revenue less expense > 0*: if, at the end of the year, the overall revenue less expense was greater than zero (regardless of the prediction), the goal was exceeded.

Case study

Organizational evolution of an academic health center enterprise: Oregon Health and Science University

Michael A. Geheb, M.D., Mark L. Penkhus, M.H.A., M.B.A., and Peter O. Kohler, M.D.

Background

Since its inception, and especially over the last 15 years, Oregon Health and Science University has responded to its changing economic and competitive environment. The University of Oregon Medical School, established in 1887, consolidated its clinical functions in 1973 with the merger of the Multnomah County Hospital and the University Hospital and its outpatient clinics. In 1974, the University of Oregon Health Sciences Center, then also including the schools of nursing and dentistry, was independently organized under the State of Oregon Higher Education Authority, and in 1981, was re-named the Oregon Health Sciences University (OHSU). Although OHSU enjoyed greater independence, it remained a state agency still greatly reliant upon state support (28 percent of a $190 million operating budget).

By the mid 1990s, Oregon had become one of the most competitive managed-care marketplaces in the country, and OHSU faced declining state support. As a state agency, OHSU was still unable to set its strategic course and act rapidly, manage its human capital strategically, generate and retain needed revenues for program development, and manage or have access to capital. A deteriorating physical plant was a major impediment to building major academic and clinical programs. At one point, deferred maintenance was estimated to be $400 million with an institutional annual budget of approximately $500 million. OHSU had a bi-modal distribution of clinical services

Michael A. Geheb is Professor of Medicine and Vice President for Institutional Advancement at Oregon Health & Science University. Mark L. Penkhus is Senior Vice President and Chief Development Officer for Sheridan Healthcorp. Peter O. Kohler is President of Oregon Health & Science University.

consisting of some cutting-edge medicine and indigent care, with indigent care predominating. Recruiting and retaining talent was challenging.

Changing the organizational structure

Oregon Health Sciences University's goal was to build nationally recognized educational, research, and clinical programs to benefit the State of Oregon, but remaining part of the State of Oregon Higher Education System would not allow OHSU the flexibility to successfully address the business issues of its environment. Required organizational changes would include committed governance of the enterprise with strategic alignment of its components, management flexibility with effective data-driven decision-making, and access to and focused capital investments. All of these changes were necessary to achieve the strong operating and financial performance critical to accepting the prudent business risk required to implement OHSU's vision.

Two options, becoming a private 501(c)(3) corporation or becoming a non-profit public corporation (a public-private hybrid), were considered. Given key linkages to the State, including a popular employee retirement plan, and liability protection under the Oregon Tort Claims Act, both the State and OHSU preferred to keep OHSU as a public entity, leading to the public benefit corporation being formed in 1995. Under the enabling legislation, OHSU has a board of ten trustees, including the OHSU President (who is responsible for university operations), appointed by the Governor and confirmed by the State Senate. The assets (including schools, research institutes, and hospitals and clinics) are merged and are the property of the OHSU Board (Alexander, Davis, and Kohler, 1997).

Another key organizational step occurred in 2002 with the aggregation of some 30 clinical practice groups into a single 501 (c)(3) corporation, the OHSU Medical Group (OHSUMG), with an elected President (who is responsible for the operations of the clinical practice). While operating as a separate corporation, OHSUMG is controlled by OHSU through its Board composition, and a Memorandum of Understanding (MOU) between OHSU and OHSUMG defines the operating relationship. The Dean of the School of Medicine and the Executive Director of OHSU Hospitals and Clinics sit on the Executive Committee and Board of OHSUMG, as well as the operations oversight group defined in the MOU. With the formation of OHSUMG, clinical department chairs are now jointly evaluated for three sets of responsibilities: clinical service chief of the OHSU hospitals and clinics, academic department chair, and director of the clinical practice within OHSUMG. Evaluations of performance are coordinated by the Dean of the School of Medicine, and reviewed with the Director of the Health System and the President of OHSUMG, these three positions serving as the Compensation Committee of OHSUMG.

Reporting to the OHSU President, the Oregon Health and Science University Foundation – including Doernbecher Children's Hospital Foundation, a 501(c)(3) corporation – is the fund-raising arm for OHSU and is the third structural component of the OHSU enterprise.

Changing the academic operating model

As defined in this chapter, key to OHSU's enterprise management has been the evolution of an academic operating model that recognizes the financial inter-relationships of its mission areas, and that establishes a model of accountability, providing the ability to deal with the cultural issues that often hinder effective management of AHCs (see Table 3.2 in Chapter 3). Given the complexities of AHC funding sources, understanding an institution's "sources" and "uses" of funds and the patterns of cross-subsidization across missions is essential to successful management. In 1999 OHSU began to adapt the "all funds" approach first developed at the University of Alabama at Birmingham (Blue Ridge Group, 1998). This approach defines a common financial language with a single set of rules and accounting standards, distributes financial risk to academic operating units, and is transparent (i.e., uncovers deals) while defining a common set of performance ratios. When combined with nonfinancial "mission metrics," both qualitative and financial aspects of performance by mission can be assessed.

Advances to the model at OHSU include developing a detailed chart of accounts identifying classes of revenue and expense by mission installed on a single financial system (Oracle), used by all OHSU entities (including all schools and research institutes, hospitals, the OHSU Medical Group, and the Oregon Health and Science Foundation). Thus, all fund flows classified by mission across all OHSU entities and their consolidated balances can be tracked. As a result, the deliberate investment of resources with a clear delineation of performance expectations for individual programs can be defined. With clear and common rules, the model allows for decentralization of decision-making and financial risk, giving flexibility to and leaving control at the program level. In theory, creativity and entrepreneurship are enhanced, with better management of the enterprise. Table 4.2 summarizes

Table 4.2 Oregon Health and Science University fiscal year 2002 funds flow analysis

Summary for School of Medicine clinical departments	1999	2000	2001	2002	FY01–02 Variance	Change (%)	2002 Basic Science Mean	2002 Total SoM Mean
Clinical external funds generated / FTE	$ 170 049	$ 181 123	$ 211 535	$ 215 932	$ 4397	2	$ 2527	$ 183 317
Research external funds generated / FTE	$ 80 273	$ 96 643	$ 117 751	$ 114 520	$ (3231)	−3	$ 455 519	$ 167 132
Total external funds generated / FTE	$ 269 024	$ 300 429	$ 356 801	$ 348 800	$ (8001)	−2	$ 489 358	$ 371 754
Total funds generated / FTE	$ 283 703	$ 326 752	$ 377 847	$ 375 403	$ (2444)	−1	$ 492 415	$ 394 787
Institutional investment / FTE	$ 45 739	$ 43 675	$ 46 315	$ 43 234	$ (3081)	−7	$ 101 177	$ 51 258
Total funds invested / FTE	$ 67 457	$ 57 198	$ 64 161	$ 73 718	$ 9557	15	$ 107 849	$ 80 430
Total faculty salaries & benefits / FTE	$ 162 357	$ 179 670	$ 195 936	$ 194 919	$ (1017)	−1	$ 132 067	$ 185 451
Total expenses / FTE	$ 340 438	$ 377 828	$ 430 760	$ 423 543	$ (7217)	−2	$ 567 593	$ 448 864
Department margin / FTE	$ (32 824)	$ (33 871)	$ (32 351)	$ (16 535)	$ 15 816	49	$ (68 648)	$ (23 997)
Department margin	$ (16 636 844)	$ (17 522 484)	$ (16 015 363)	$ (9 476 043)	$ 6 539 319	41	$ (875 148)	$ (539 133)
% Department operating margin	−11.57%	−10.37%	−8.56%	−4.40%	4.16%		−13.94%	−6.08%
Total institutional margin / FTE	$ 10 722	$ 6121	$ 11 248	$ 25 577	$ 14 329	127	$ 32 671	$ 26 353

(cont.)

Table 4.2 (*cont.*)

Summary for School of Medicine clinical departments	1999	2000	2001	2002	FY01–02 Variance	Change (%)	2002 Basic Science Mean	2002 Total SoM Mean
Total institutional margin	$5 434 248	$3 166 777	$5 568 096	$14 658 096	$9 090 000	163	$416 502	$592 058
% Total operating margin	3.05%	1.59%	2.54%	5.69%	3.15%		5.44%	5.55%
Funds generated / total funds invested	$4.21	$5.71	$5.89	$5.09	$(0.80)	−14	$4.57	$4.91
Funds generated / institutional investment	$6.20	$7.48	$8.16	$8.68	$0.52	6	$4.87	$7.70
Total fund balance	$96 820 841	$106 857 496	$106 004 633	$127 624 950	$21 620 317	20	$1 093 403	$4 709 829
Number of FTEs	506.85	517.33	495.05	573.09	78.04	16	13.98	22.47
Number of MDs	399.49	400.75	400.28	455.97	55.69	14	0.78	15.59
Funds generated / total net allocable square feet	$505.25	$594.03	$532.37	$603.85	$71.48	13	$288.92	$421.11
Total net allocable square feet occupied	284 598	284 563	331 786	356 282	24 496	7	21 593	19 834
Faculty compensation								
paid by externally sponsored research		12.29%	11.8%	11.7%	−0.07%		46.47%	16.00%
paid by other research		2.50%	4.3%	4.6%	0.32%		1.78%	4.40%
paid by other		29.70%	27.0%	25.2%	−1.78%		47.23%	26.60%
paid by clinical		55.52%	57.0%	58.6%	1.63%		4.52%	53.00%
Total		100.0%	100.0%	100.0%	0.10%		100.00%	100.0%

RATIO DEFINITION

Clinical external funds generated / FTE

Measures the revenue generated from patient care activities per faculty member. The higher the ratio, the more productive the faculty.

Research external funds generated / FTE

Measures the revenue generated from sponsored project research grants and contracts per faculty member. The higher the ratio, the more productive the faculty.

Total external funds generated / FTE

Measures the revenue generated from external sources via patient care activities and sponsored project research grants as well as via educational and other nonclinical and nonresearch activities.

Total funds generated

Measures the total revenue generated (including grants and contracts, patient care revenue, and other external revenue such as VA contracts as well as internal funds generated such as medical director fees and other clinical service contracts) per faculty member.

Total funds generated / FTE

Measures the total revenue generated (including grants and contracts, patient care revenue and other external revenue such as VA contracts as well as internal funds generated such as medical director fees and other clinical service contracts) per faculty member. The higher the ratio, the more productive the faculty.

Institutional investment / FTE

Measures the income received from the institution directly (e.g. Dean's support and other university commitments) and unreimbursed expenses incurred by the institution on behalf of the department offset by any funds generated by the department that are then retained by the institution (e.g. Dean's tax on clinical revenue & indirect costs retained) per faculty member. The higher the ratio, the greater the institutional investment in the department.

Total funds invested / FTE

Measures the total investment by the institution, department and other outside donors & investors on a per faculty member basis. This includes income received directly from the institution (e.g. Dean's support & other university commitments) and unreimbursed expenses incurred by the institution on behalf of the department offset by any funds generated by the department that are then retained by the institution (ex. clinical revenue & indirect costs retained). It also includes the total revenue received from endowment earnings, interest, or department investment from practice group funds. The higher the ratio, the greater the institutional and departmental support in the department.

(cont.)

Table 4.2 (*Legend cont.*)

Total faculty salaries & benefits / FTE
Measures average expense for a faculty member's salary and benefits.

Total expenses / FTE
Measures the average total expenditures in support of a full-time faculty member.

Department operating margin / FTE
Measures the operating surplus (or deficit) on a per faculty member basis of an academic program before institutional contributions to support the program. (In other words, this measures the operating income or loss if the academic program were to operate on a stand-alone basis.) The higher the deficit, the more institutional support per faculty member that is required for the program to break even financially.

Department operating margin
Measures the operating surplus (or deficit) of a department *before* institutional contributions to support the program.

% Department operating margin
Measures the % profitability (or deficit) position of a department before institutional contributions to support the program. It measures the contribution to the bottom line from every dollar generated by the department and invested in the department by the department only.

Total institutional margin / FTE
Measures the operating surplus (deficit) per faculty member of an academic program considering all sources of funds including institutional funds and all expenses. Since faculties generate the clinical or research activity to generate the funds, this is a measure of the average contribution of each faculty member to the profit or deficit of a department or program. It is the measure of the contribution margin per faculty member.

Total institutional margin
Measures the surplus (or deficit) position of a department or program including all sources and uses of funds as a result of operations.

% Total operating margin
Measures the % profitability (or deficit) position of a department after considering all sources and uses of funds. It measures the contribution to the bottom line from every dollar generated by the department and invested in the department by the department and the institution.

Funds generated / total funds invested

Measures "leverage" of institutional and department funds, looking at the number of times institutional and department funds are multiplied for a given investment in a department or program. The larger the value, the better the "return" on the institutional investment.

Funds generated / institutional investment

Measures "leverage" of institutional funds, looking at the number of times institutional funds are multiplied for a given institutional investment in a department or program. The larger the value, the better the "return" on the institutional investment (excludes departmental investment).

Total fund balance

This balance represents the total fiscal year-end fund balance including all unrestricted and restricted funds held at OHSU, the OHSU Foundation and the OHSU Medical Group.

Number of FTEs

Total number of MD, PhD and other employees defined as faculty in a department or program responsible for generating revenues through patient care, research or other academic activities.

Number of MDs

Total number of MD faculty in a department or program.

Funds generated / total net allocable square feet occupied

Measures the total funds generated for each square foot occupied. The higher the value, the more productive is the use of a department's space. If this ratio is excessively high, it may also represent a need for additional space to enhance a department's or program's growth.

Total net allocable square feet occupied

This is a measurement of the total floor area of rooms, floors and/or buildings, assignable to an operating department (excluding physical plant maintenance and building operation space).

Faculty compensation – paid by

This section demonstrates the composition of funds by mission from which the faculty member's salaries and benefits are paid.

data for the clinical departments of the School of Medicine showing improved productivity and financial performance over the four years. Basic science departments have shown similar improvements in productivity and financial performance.

Developing the OHSU enterprise

Since becoming a public corporation, OHSU has undertaken several steps to enhance its research, education, and clinical care missions. In 1998 OHSU merged with the Oregon Regional Primate Center (now called the Oregon National Primate Research Center) and the Neurological Sciences Institute. In 2001, OHSU merged with the Oregon Graduate Institute (OGI), a research-intensive graduate engineering school, and opened its new Vaccine and Gene Therapy Institute. The execution of these mergers has provided OHSU with specific research and translational capabilities in genomics, computer engineering and information science, and clinical device development. With the OGI merger, OHSU's name was formally changed to the Oregon Health & Science University.

In order to better manage across the continuum of clinical care with its increasing complexity, OHSU is organizing inter- and multidisciplinary clinical programs, recognizing that traditional clinical departmental structures are organized to meet the regulatory and certification requirements for medical education. These centers and institutes are in the School of Medicine with parallel service lines in the clinical system. They include the Casey Eye Institute, the OHSU Cancer Institute (which received NCI designation in 1997), the Center for Women's Health, the Oregon Hearing Research Center, and Doernbecher Children's Hospital's pediatric cardiac center. Other developing programs include clinical neurosciences (including pediatric neuroscience), pediatric surgery, a center for digestive diseases, multidisciplinary critical care, diabetes, orthopedics, and adult cardiac disease. Even given the difficulties in current Medicare reimbursement, the OHSU School of Nursing is developing a Center for Healthy Aging.

Key statistics

As illustrated in Table 4.3, OHSU's operating budget has more than doubled to $1.1 billion since becoming a public benefit corporation (including

Table 4.3 Growth and change at Oregon Health and Science University, 1975–2003

	1975	1985	1990	1995	2000	2003
ECONOMICS AND FUNDING						
Operating budget	$80 million	$190 million	$340 million	$499 million	$882 million	$1.045 billion
State grant	$34 million	$53 million	$65 million	$60 million	$55 million	$48 million
All other revenue	$47 million	$137 million	$275 million	$439 million	$827 million	$997 million
Percent of budget that is state grant	42%	28%	19%	12%	6.4%	4.6%
Percent of budget that is other revenue	58%	72%	81%	88%	93.6%	95.4%
RESEARCH						
Award dollars	$14 million	$18 million	$43 million	$86 million	$168 million	$221 million
Award dollars from out of state	$10.5 million	$13.5 million	$36 million	$74 million	$161 million	$208 million
Percent of award dollars from out of state	75%	77%	83%	86%	96%	94%
Number of awards	a	78	243	362	607	697
Number of inventions	0	2	30	36	32	80
Total companies formed from OHSU technology[d]	1	4	5	15	30	36
HEALTH CARE[b]						
Number of patients	a	69 000	108 000	112 000	153 300	187 800
Patient visits (OHSU hospitals and clinics)	186 969	169 068	247 491	344 408	575 800	631 100
ACADEMICS						
Number of students	1610	1200	1536	1855	1854	2524[c]
Library volumes	137 419	181 343	177 545	216 159	229 796	238 958
Electronic journals	0	0	0	0	439	1349
PHILANTHROPY						
Gift dollars	$3.6 million	$7.5 million	$8 million	$22.5 million	$34 million	$50 million
Number of gifts	a	2201	20438	17 680	28 372	29 211
FACILITIES AND EMPLOYEES						
Number of employees	4300	5200	6500	6600	10 000	11 500
Capital expenditures	a	$5 million	$30 million	$60 million	$79 million	$98 million
Square feet of building space	2.4 million	2.4 million	3.1 million	3.8 million	5 million	5.3 million

[a] Data not available.
[b] More than 40 percent of OHSU's inpatient admissions are low-income (Medicaid or uninsured).
[c] Includes School of Science and Engineering Students. OGI and OHSU merged July 1, 2001.
[d] Cumulative historical number of spin-outs and start-ups.

OHSUMG). State support for operations has continued to decline in dollar amount and will be less than 4 percent of the total operating budget in the fiscal year 2004. Research awards have almost quadrupled to $220 million since 1995. The National Institutes of Health ranks OHSU 29th among 515 competing domestic higher education institutions. Intellectual capital is being captured as is evidenced by the growth of the number of inventions and the total number of companies formed using OHSU technology.

Since 1996, the School of Medicine has increased its research ranking from 52nd to 30th among 122 medical schools funded, with the departments of neurology, ophthalmology, and otolaryngology ranking in the top 10 nationwide. OHSU's School of Nursing has climbed from 21st to 8th in the last five years. OHSU enrolled more than 3500 students and trainees in 2003, and is the principal site in Oregon for graduate health professional training, and after 2001 for graduate engineering training. Clinical growth has also been substantial, with total patient encounters (inpatient and outpatient) tripling since 1995 to greater than 600 000 visits.

Promoting a culture of quality at Oregon Health & Science University

Recent public interest in patient safety and clinical quality provides a unique challenge to and opportunity for AHCs. In 2001, OHSU began re-organizing its clinical operations and clinical education programs to be a leader in patient safety and clinical quality, embracing common quality attributes defined by the Institute of Medicine in *Crossing the Quality Chasm* (IOM, 2001). These defining attributes require that health care should be: safe, effective, patient-centered, timely, efficient, and equitable. At OHSU, these attributes have been refined to five guiding principles: (1) improving the patient experience for all patients; (2) making the hospitals and clinics safe in the delivery of health care; (3) monitoring and improving clinical outcomes; (4) designing better systems to assure timeliness and efficiency; and (5) assuring quality while maintaining fiscal responsibility. OHSU is developing standards of performance for its clinical systems and educational programs to measure success defined by these guiding principles.

To enhance clinical nursing at the OHSU hospitals, especially after a contentious nursing strike, the School of Nursing has been integrated into hospital operations. With the recent definition by the Accreditation Council for Graduate Medical Education (ACGME) of six core competencies for the evaluation of all trainees, physician training is also being reorganized. In addition to a renewed emphasis on professionalism, physician trainees will be explicitly evaluated in evidenced-based practice and how they perform in systems of care. The School of Medicine is revising its evaluation and training of all physician trainees to incorporate OHSU's quality principles into the framework required of the ACGME. The Schools of Medicine and Nursing are working collaboratively with the hospitals and the OHSU Medical Group in defining the OHSU clinical quality program.

Although the benefits of coordinated care are becoming more and more apparent, the training of health professionals is typically isolated by discipline. In addition to being proficient in their respective professions, OHSU intends to train the next generation of health care professionals to be prepared for the kind of collaborative, interdisciplinary care-giving environment they are increasingly likely to find after leaving school. The goal is to create and train health care professionals in a "culture of measurable quality" in which "system" professionalism and competence are as highly valued as individual professionalism and competence. OHSU is building on a good clinical quality record: of reporting University Health System Consortium (UHC) hospitals, OHSU has one of the highest case mix indices and one of the lowest overall mortalities for UHC reporting members.

Information technology is a key to advancing the quality agenda. The IOM has reported, "health care delivery has been relatively untouched by the revolution in information technology that has been transforming nearly every aspect of society" (IOM, 2001). Technology can enhance the patient–practitioner interface, making patient records available at the right time and the right place, and can reduce system errors. OHSU is continuing to develop a lifetime clinical record (LCR), with all lab results, dictated reports and diagnostic imaging now available on a web-based system. OHSU is now completely film-less with all imaging studies being digitally archived. Scanning technology now allows all written records to be stored electronically, making them available on the LCR. At OHSU, technology is making drug delivery safer and is preparing OHSU for computerized physician order entry. Clinical, operating, and financial databases are now being linked. Working with the University HealthSystem Consortium, clinical, operating and financial benchmarking is now being developed, embracing the attributes defined by the IOM.

Conclusion

OHSU has changed substantially over the last 30 years. In 1974 it was highly dependent on state funding and as a state agency did not have the organizational structure or flexibility to deal with an increasingly volatile environment. After becoming a public benefit corporation, committed to its historic public missions, it developed the committed governance and management structure to manage OHSU as an academic health center enterprise. Key to its growth has been the development of an operating model to manage and monitor investments in quality programs associated with outstanding financial performance. Even given the current difficulties in the American and especially the Oregon economy, OHSU has developed an expansive vision enabled by public confidence in its ability to execute that vision. OHSU's organizational structure continues to allow it cope with the instability of public funding, to develop clinical care systems with measurable quality that are patient centered, and to be a catalyst for translational science – from the bench to the bedside – providing business opportunities for the Oregon community.

The challenge for OHSU and other AHCs will be to develop collaborative care models and the human resource systems to support them, the integrated curriculum and training models to educate all health care professionals, and the information technology to enable these models. All of these elements are required to embrace quality improvement principles for health care delivery.

REFERENCES

Alexander, B., Davis, L. and Kohler, P. O. (1997). Changing structure to improve function: one academic health center's experience. *Academic Medicine*, **72**(4), 259–268.

Blue Ridge Academic Health Group (1998). *Academic Health Centers: Getting Down to Business.* Washington, DC: Cap Gemini Ernst & Young US, LLC.

Institute of Medicine (2001). *Crossing the Quality Chasm: a New Health System for the 21st Century.* Washington, DC: National Academy Press.

Commentary

Arthur Garson, Jr., M.D., M.P.H.

Introduction

Individual faculty members, departments, and entire schools have much to gain through the judicious application of measures of performance. Although there are several pitfalls in measurement of academic performance and much more to the achievement of the highest level of academic performance than can necessarily be measured discretely, a well-designed and implemented process to measure performance offers two clear benefits. First, it provides data that support the management of individual departments and the school as an enterprise. For example, one of the major current problems in academic medicine is finding ways to identify, train, and reward excellent teachers. Providing evaluations from students and peers in a consistent way provides needed feedback and can strengthen the effectiveness of individual faculty members.

Second, such a process provides a mechanism for measuring goals related to strategy. After setting a strategic direction for a school, it is absolutely necessary to develop specific timed objectives to determine if that strategy is effective. This is also the case at the department or division level. Each of these units will not have similar objectives and may put emphasis in different areas, but ultimately the summation will need to serve the strategy of the school. Most importantly, the individual faculty members must be able to achieve their goals in academic medicine whether they are in patient care, research, education, or community service. These goals will, of necessity, be the most varied but will summate to the goals of the department. One common theme for each faculty member will be promotion and tenure. Since committees that review faculty members for promotion and tenure are interested to a

Arthur (Tim) Garson is Vice President and Dean of the School of Medicine at the University of Virginia.

certain extent in quantitative data, it becomes helpful to each individual faculty member to develop quantitative goals that can be assessed yearly with a mentor whether it be the department chair, division chief, or other individual.

Learning from experience

In 1995, I led the strategic planning process at Baylor College of Medicine. As part of that process, we decided that an assessment of what the faculty actually did would be an important component of our analysis. We prepared a faculty questionnaire seeking virtually everything that each person did and asked quantitatively how they spent their time in number of hours per year devoted to each of the activities.

When the first set of questionnaires was returned, eight of the Baylor faculty reported working more than three years (per year), 365 days per year, seven days per week. I telephoned one of those faculty members and asked if he would meet with me to discuss his questionnaire response. He told me he did not have the time. I made no more calls. Requesting the number of hours also generated a number of issues including how "on call" hours were handled, since in some specialties, individuals virtually always were required to leave home to see patients (e.g., obstetrics) whereas in others (e.g., pediatric cardiology) a resident and two fellows could handle the majority of the problems with consultation on the telephone. This problem was not limited to the clinical faculty: a scientist wrote on the form that he "thought in the shower" and therefore counted those hours. We learned – the next year, we used percent time.

We did a few things right at the beginning including making the individual faculty data confidential between the faculty member and their immediate supervisor, division chief, or department chair. The dean's office never had access to individual faculty data where the names were associated with the data. This proved to be somewhat comforting to the faculty who feel, appropriately, that their work must be placed in context. The major breakthrough came after the second year in which faculty and departments could compare themselves with their own data from the previous year. National benchmarks are helpful when they are collected in a similar way across schools, but most schools do not collect data the same way (e.g., percent time). In the third year, we simplified the process by collecting fewer data per faculty member and reporting summary data. The most important measures became relative value units (RVUs) per clinical full-time equivalent (FTE), patient satisfaction, grant dollars per research FTE, grant dollars per square foot (at the department level), and evaluation of teaching by students.

In the next year, we abandoned the self-report and the faculty member and his or her immediate supervisor (i.e., division chief or department head) jointly established the assignment of time and effort. We also tied the allocations of faculty time and effort to the budget so that if an individual spent 80 percent of their time on research, whether funded or unfunded, we charged the expense of 80 percent of their salary and fringe to research. Since the faculty time and effort was determined yearly in consultation with the immediate supervisor and since all of the other data could be obtained "noninvasively" from data already being collected at the level of the department or the school, we were able to completely eliminate the faculty questionnaire. The faculty were clearly pleased. In the following year, summary data became available to each division and department monthly on the web. These then became useful management data rather than a yearly event.

Having recently moved to the University of Virginia, I have had the opportunity to consider the process of academic performance measurement and improvement in another setting. At the time of my arrival, the measurement of RVUs per patient care FTE, research grant dollars per square foot, and educational evaluation were already present. Therefore, the "culture of accountability" existed, much to the credit of my predecessors. This allowed for testing the hypotheses of the previous principles. Thus far, we have completed a detailed strategic plan with each team (i.e., patient care, research, education) and identified metrics and benchmarks for those metrics as they relate to the timed objectives produced by the plan. We intend to make the time and effort reporting part of individual faculty goal setting each year and will report these measures monthly. The monthly measures include: RVU per clinical FTE, patient satisfaction (measured quarterly), NIH grant dollars, total grant dollars, grant dollars per square foot, teaching evaluation (aggregated yearly), as well as finance data related to patient care, research, and education.

Major lessons

Our experience with performance measures has been evolutionary with important lessons about the process and the characteristics of ideal metrics emerging along the way. The introduction of performance metrics to an organization must begin with clear articulation of the reason for the measurement (e.g., assessment of individual faculty's goals or relationship to department or school strategic planning). Faculty percent time and effort should be assessed jointly as part of the yearly process of goal setting with immediate supervisor. Data collection should be as noninvasive as possible.

The ideal metric is simple, unambiguous, and helpful to the user. Whether for the individual faculty member, department, or school, the metrics must relate to something they want to accomplish. The metric needs to be understandable and anyone would agree that if it goes up, that is good. The challenge of metrics is to begin with "simple" without going through "complicated." A complex system is not only difficult to administer, but also difficult to justify.

Accurate data are essential for effective metrics. Early in the Baylor process, the consultants that were helping transposed one column and one row in the summary data thereby making the data inaccurate. These data were distributed and nearly destroyed the entire program. The data must be checked, ideally by a subgroup of individual faculty members and chairs, before they are published.

Meaningful metrics are frequently reported (e.g., monthly) with trends and comparison to previous data shown. They are collected in a way that can be applicable for appropriate benchmarking with other institutions and collected across all areas of mission (e.g., patient care, research, education). Further, the best metrics will be unweighted. Some metric systems attempt to weight individual metrics either within or across areas of mission (e.g., a certain number of points for RVUs, compared with a different number of points for research grant and paper). These weighting systems are extremely contentious and may not be as helpful to the individual faculty member as an understanding between the faculty member and the supervisor of what is important to that faculty member.

Finally, we must recognize that everything cannot be a metric. The trick with metrics is to place objective measures in the context of the "art" of what we do. The warmth of the physician, the encouragement of the teacher, the brilliance of the researcher, and the spirit of an organization must also be featured and appreciated. Understanding this balance allows us to be more than automatons and to move our schools forward.

Commentary

Jonathan F. Saxton, J.D. and Michael M. E. Johns, M.D.

The case for changing the traditional culture and organization of the AHC is both strong and urgent. The Institute of Medicine (IOM) made the case best in its report, *Crossing the Quality Chasm: a New Health System for the 21st Century* (IOM, 2001). There it describes an American health system that can provide the best possible care for some people, but one that is in disarray, mired in outdated priorities, practices, and processes, and unable to meet important health care needs of our society. The IOM calls not just for reforming, but for **rebuilding** the health system around the aims of providing health care that is safe, effective, patient centered, timely, efficient, and equitable. What does that have to do with the AHC? It has to do with whether the AHC will lead or follow health care reform in this century.

Academic health centers have provided leadership in the health professions and have been the loci of discovery and progress in the biosciences. Together with their owned and affiliated teaching hospitals, they have also been the primary centers of high-quality, innovative care. This is why the AHC is both deeply implicated in the health care system's dysfunction and absolutely essential to its successful rebuilding.

Medical training and practice in AHCs for half a century have been organized by and for the elite physician scientist, the almost mythic "triple threat," who embodies the model of the supremely capable but autonomous medical professional. This model easily replicated within the university-based academic environment, where clinical departments developed in step with the proliferation of professional subspecialization. Medical education was compartmentalized according to basic science disciplines, followed by clinical (graduate medical education (GME)) training conducted through long-term, intensive immersion and mentoring within specialty "services." Academic

Jonathan F. Saxton is Health Policy Analyst at Emory University. Michael M. E. Johns is Executive Vice President for Health Affairs at Emory University, and Chief Executive Officer, Robert W. Woodruff Health Sciences Center.

health centers trained many of the world's best doctors but primarily in the model of this insular form of medical professionalism. Therefore, while AHCs have been centers of tremendous progress in medicine, that progress has been concentrated in the development of "heroic measures," both personal and technological, designed to intervene in cases of complex and advanced disease and disability. Less well supported have been public health, nursing, and other "allied health" approaches that promote coordinated care, disease prevention, and population health management.

On top of this, the "fee-for-service" insurance and reimbursement system, and the development of the publicly funded Medicare and Medicaid programs ensured that physicians were relatively insulated from conventional market forces. Even community physicians primarily practiced alone or in informal local networks, affiliated (through admitting privileges) with local hospitals.

Only with recent public policy changes ushering in a newly competitive and cost-conscious reimbursement environment has the medical profession and the AHC had to revisit their traditional cultures and organization. Clinical revenues to the AHCs and their parent universities have been put at significant risk in the newly competitive environment for health care. University and AHC leaders now understand that the clinical and educational experience must be adapted to new societal health care priorities. Yet, to change the culture and organization of the AHC is a major challenge for AHC leadership. How can this be accomplished?

This chapter describes the elements of a powerful, value-driven approach that AHC leadership can take to reform the culture and organization of the AHC. A value-driven approach takes a societal view of the changing health care needs and demographics of our society and of the roles and responsibilities of health professionals. It draws upon the most advanced work on organizational theory and on the management of medical and other professionals as knowledge workers. It factors in the imperatives of a competitive marketplace and the need for the redeployment of people and resources. Most importantly perhaps, it builds upon lessons learned to develop new kinds of leaders for a new kind of health system, one that provides incentives to health care providers, payers, individuals, and communities to work together to improve both individual and population health status and to reward innovative and cost-effective improvements in quality health care.

This is a powerful vision and a recipe for change. But can we get there from here? The early signs are that AHCs are moving in that direction, though not without some difficulty. Academic health center schools, hospitals, and clinics remain largely organized along traditional lines. Yet, almost all are now factoring into their planning and operations the demand for patient-centered services that provide better access, a kinder and gentler experience, more comprehensive care management, and the tools by which patients and their families can understand, participate in, and evaluate the quality of the care provided. Innovators are developing new team and inter-professional approaches to care and disease management. Comprehensive cancer centers in select AHCs have long been prime examples of such approaches, but there are also tremendous innovations occurring in areas such as diabetes management, women's health, aging, heart, stroke and vascular disease, disorders of the mind, brain and special senses, transplantation and regeneration, musculoskeletal disorders, and other complex and chronic diseases. In addition, the explosion of new technologies in information management, bioinformatics, genetics, systems biology, and other fields is creating the possibility of a new kind of health care. On the horizon are new capabilities for both individualized and population-wide preventive, pre-emptive, and interventional health strategies. All of these developments and more are being pioneered within AHCs, and while some are still relatively nascent, they represent a vast opportunity for AHCs and their faculties to be leaders in realizing the potential for a new era of health care.

At the Woodruff Health Sciences Center of Emory University, for example, just in the last few years faculty have reached across traditional departmental boundaries to establish comprehensive initatives in the neurosciences, musculoskeletal and spine care, cardiovascular care, and, most recently, bioterrorism research and preparedness. Functionally, we are overcoming the limitations of a fragmented model and are developing comprehensive approaches and cross-professional systems. Additionally, we have established the Woodruff Leadership Academy, a leadership development and training institute that selects, for an intensive six months of seminars and group projects, 20 fellows (faculty and staff) per year nominated from across our system. With our Leadership Academy, the opportunity is to actively cultivate and train leaders within our system who can envision and achieve the promise of patient-centered, value-driven health care.

This is what can differentiate the AHC in this new era. The AHC continues to have the responsibility of bringing scientific expertise together with educational resources and the clinical care enterprise to catalyze progress and innovation in health and healing. But now the AHC must move from being host to heroic individuals and interventions to being institutions that lead the development of comprehensive, patient-centered, and value-driven care.

As with any challenge of this complexity and magnitude, what is required above all else is leadership. Academic health center and other health sector leaders must build upon these nascent initiatives. They must forge the organizational and cultural change that enables AHCs to fulfill their indispensable roles in achieving society's aims for our heath care system. This chapter provides helpful insight and guidance to leaders able and willing to take that responsibility.

REFERENCE

Institute of Medicine (2001). *Crossing the Quality Chasm: a New Health System for the 21st Century*. Washington, DC: National Academy Press.

Commentary

George F. Sheldon, M.D.

Against the background of a changing world, trends, areas, and policies can be identified that require increased or continuing emphasis to change the health care culture to value orientation. Some are already becoming part of the culture of the AHCs; other areas or policies require persuasion or redirection to achieve the goal of a value-driven system.

Rosemary Stephens discussed the future of medicine in the public sphere as expressed through professional organizations in an important article in *The Milbank Quarterly* (Stevens, 2001). Medical organizations were perceived during the 1990s as existing to enhance the well-being of their members rather than the public. She observed that organized medicine is fragmented and that physicians view their specialty societies as their primary professional voice. Fragmentation and lack of leadership of professional organizations led some to predict the end of organized medicine. Another problem is that participation in professional organizations is unattractive to the younger members of the medical profession. They are of a generational orientation that is uninterested in professional societies. The role models and leaders of the current generation have done an inadequate job of emphasizing the importance of participation in professional organizations (Sheldon and Kagarise, 2002).

An important area of cultural change is to convince the generation of physicians in training of the important public role of medical professional organizations. Students and physicians in training are inadequately exposed to the regulatory, educational, advocacy, and research functions of professional organizations. Medicine's public role is overdue for updating to meet today's scientific, economic, and political conditions. The profession, whose voice is through professional organizations, currently lacks clear-cut health policy roles.

George F. Sheldon is Professor of Surgery and Social Medicine and former Chair of Surgery at the University of North Carolina.

Establishing a defined public role through the advocacy positions of professional organizations is a needed cultural change. AHCs should create a culture that encourages participation of students and residents in professional organizations.

One of the problems contributing to the negative public perception of medical societies is the claim to dedication to high quality service, while lacking measurements available to the public to support that position. Stephens notes that lacking public availability of quality measurements, it is understandable that some believe that professional organizations are self-serving and destructive of the public interest.

Happily, a commitment to quality has emerged as a trend of major significance in health care organizations. Two Institute of Medicine (IOM) publications, entitled *To Err is Human*, and *Bridging the Quality Chasm*, list ten expectations for the health care system (IOM, 1999, 2001). The goals of the IOM are ambitious, but have been enthusiastically endorsed by virtually all medical organizations. Some of the goals, such as state-of-the-art health care availability 24 hours a day, are out of reach unless there is a substantial commitment to expand the funding of health care and its workforce. The goal occurs at a time when health care careers are less attractive than previously and shortages are emerging.

In December 2002, the American Hospital Association (AHA), the Federation of American Hospitals, the Association of American Medical Colleges (AAMC), the Joint Commission on Accreditation of Health Care Organizations (JCAHO), the Center for Medicare and Medicaid Services (CMS), the National Quality Forum (NQF), and the Agency for Health Care Research and Quality (AHRQ) launched a public–private initiative designed to provide public information on identified quality indicators. Another positive action was the public advocacy in 1998 of the American Medical Association, the American College of Surgeons, the American College of Physicians, the Academy of Pediatrics, and the Academy of Family Medicine, issuing a public statement calling for universal access to healthcare.

Quality is an essential focus of cultural orientation of AHCs. Commitment to universal access is part of a quality health care system.

A focus on professionalism and its important tenet of professional self-regulation is occurring. Recent emphasis on the importance of professionalism in our evolving health system includes a Presidential Address for the American College of Surgeons, as well as initiatives of the American College of Physicians, American Society of Internal Medicine, the European Society of Internal Medicine, and the Association of American Medical

Colleges (Sheldon, 1998). Peter Drucker predicts that increasing profession-alization of the work force in the knowledge society will be an evolving pos-itive trend. Clark Kerr, past President of the University of California System, predicted a day when the knowledge industry would occupy the same role as the railroad industry did in the nineteenth century. Thorstein Veblin's 60-year-old dream of a professionally run society may be approaching reality. The evolving availability of complex science moved into application through translational research, with examples such as cloning and proteonomics, requires developing standards of professional behavior when new technology raises new ethical questions. This need has been recognized and is well on the way to being effectively included in undergraduate and graduate med-ical education. The six competencies (including professionalism) required for inclusion in the general requirements of the Accreditation Council for Graduate Medical Education (ACGME) and the American Board of Medi-cal Specialties (ABMS) are an important step in the preparation of health providers of the twenty-first century.

Professionalism is a core component of a value oriented culture in AHCs.

Workforce is an area of concern, as it increasingly appears that our AHCs are educating insufficient numbers and the wrong type of physicians. Our medical schools have been operating under three assumptions, which appear to be flawed. New economic trend analysis and marketplace data suggest that a deficit of physicians, a shortage of specialists, and increasing reliance on nonphysician clinicians is occurring (Cooper, 1995). The flawed assump-tions, based on many studies beginning with the Graduate Medical Educa-tion National Advisory Committee (GMENAC) in 1981, are that a significant physician surplus would be present by 2000 and beyond, and the health sys-tem would be loosely modeled on a staff model gate-keeper-controlled health maintenance organization (HMO). The assumptions included the establish-ment of universal health insurance during the last 25 years of the twentieth century, that the health care system would be based on generalists, and that a specialist surplus was likely. Point of service contracts, dissatisfaction with managed care, and the increasing evidence of a specialist shortage demon-strate the difficulty of health workforce planning.

Updating education, undergraduate, graduate, and continuing medical education to the realities of professional skills and behavior in an era of accelerated technological transfer and translational research is a needed cultural change for AHCs. Enhanced sensitivity to workforce needs is an important cultural orientation of AHCs.

The knowledge society favors specialism not generalism. A new concept of generalism is needed which would define generalism as the summation of special knowledge leading to recommendations from a team, rather than a single provider. The conceptual change is the expectation that the generalist concept will be an amalgamation of specialist opinion, rather than expectations that all skills reside in a single generalist or primary care provider. The capacity to summate specialty input to produce a general conclusion requires working within an organization. Prior to 1950, when Peter Drucker identified the profession of management, businesses were not seen as organizations of people, but were viewed merely as product developing and producing entities. Since that time, considerable focus on the dynamics of an organization, and its workforce as professionals has occurred. Such a health care team or organization would include the increasing contributions of nonphysician clinicans (NPC). The need to integrate input from professionals of different background requires the continued evolution of a constructive integrated organization.

The Blue Ridge Group endorses the development of a culture of constructive participation in a broad group culture, to displace the silo orientation sometimes associated with schools of medicine and hospitals. While AHC leadership is sometimes frustrated at the resistance encountered at dispelling parochialism, departments are learning the value of cross-departmental and center collaboration. Currently examples of successful implementation of team focus on disease entities occur in areas where expertise is additive. Cardiology, oncology, critical care, and trauma provide examples where constructive collaboration is well on the way to implementation.

Good models of cross department collaboration exist in AHCs and cultural emphasis should be on highlighting the working models, as examples. Encouraging group working skills is an important cultural change needing continued emphasis.

A common organizational entity within and outside of the AHC is group practice. Group practice is one of the strongest single trends to occur in health care in the past 75 years. It can be considered a maturing of an organization or an industry. In the recent past, the practice of medicine was a cottage industry delivered mostly by general practitioners functioning in solo practice. Since World War II the paradigm has changed with the coalescence of a variety of practice organizations, many stimulated by the successful model of the Mayo Clinic, and similar organizations. Continuity of care is a time-honored concept, valued by patients and emblematic of the physicians' fiduciary responsibility to patients. Unfortunately, it has been eroded significantly to the point that some educators even state that the concept is outmoded. Many if not most primary care practices are available by appointment, and seldom after five o'clock. Emergency rooms have become the primary care provider of after hours of care. Group practice, as it matures as an organizational entity, has the potential to solve the problem of continuity of care and generalism. The cultural change required is to enhance the skills and attitudes for functioning within an organization.

The most important cultural issues to be emphasized by the AHC is the concept of value, cost, and quality. If a healthy society is a stable society, the cultural orientation of AHC should emphasize quality and value, not cost. Addressing these issues in the context of AHC cultural change continues the ancient challenge of physician choices and responsibilities. Tension continues between population-based medicine with its Benthamite concept of the "greatest good to the greatest numbers," and the fiduciary responsibility of a physician to each individual patient as described in the Hippocratic Oath. Health of the public, as well as responsibility to an individual patient, is also a physician responsibility with its focus on public health and prevention. The conflict between these responsibilities is often over resource deployment (e.g., should federal and state resources be used to expand Medicaid coverage or public health initiatives).

The changes required of AHC culture to advance the societal role of 21st century medicine are extensive. A substantial commitment to examine practices and policies of the AHC, teaching hospitals, schools of medicine, and professional organizations is warranted.

REFERENCES

Cooper, R. A. (1995). Perspectives on the physician workforce to the year 2020. *Journal of the American Medical Association*, **274**(19), 1534–43.

Institute of Medicine (1999). *To Err is Human: Building a Safer Health System*. Washington, DC: National Academy Press.

(2001). *Crossing the Quality Chasm: a New Health System for the 21st Century*. Washington, DC: National Academy Press.

Sheldon, G. F. (1998). Professionalism, managed care, and the human rights movement. *Bulletin of the American College of Surgeons*, **83**, 14–33.

Sheldon, G. F. and Kagarise, M. J. (2002). Surgical organizations in the 21st century. *The American Journal of Surgery*, **183**(4), 338–44.

Stevens, R. A. (2001). Public roles for the medical professions in the United States: beyond theories of decline and fall. *The Millbank Quarterly*, **79**(3), 327–53.

5 Managing and leveraging organizational knowledge

Introduction

Enabled by technological developments and accompanied by an economy undergoing fundamental changes, the knowledge age has arrived. Its impact is already evident in the nature, scope, and pace of competition among businesses, work of individuals, and expectations of the public. As this new era unfolds, organizations are assuming new roles, acquiring new capabilities, developing new business models, and interacting with consumers in different ways. Simultaneously, a flood of advances in the ability to preserve health and treat disease is creating exciting prospects and greater challenges for health care organizations and professionals and their patients.

At first glance it might appear that as institutions with a strong tradition of discovering and sharing knowledge, academic health centers (AHCs) would automatically become leaders of the health domain within the emerging knowledge economy. In fact, however, this leadership position is not assured. Academic health centers have been surpassed by other industries in the practices used to manage and leverage knowledge. They face growing competition in the discovery of new knowledge and are being challenged for the role of preferred source of health knowledge. Moreover, they must update their educational models for effectiveness in the digital era. Thus, AHCs need to attend to their organizational knowledge capabilities and to their role in the future health care environment.

Academic health center leaders face the pressing and pivotal question of how to position their organizations for future success. When current medical knowledge is ubiquitous and medical technology widely diffused, what added value can AHCs bring to the patient and student experience? As patients change their approaches to seeking and receiving health care services, how should AHCs adjust the preparation of health professionals? As research becomes more interdisciplinary, inter-institutional, commercialized, and is performed more often by research teams outside academia, how can AHCs remain attractive sites for researchers to ply their talents? As other organizations become more knowledge-focused and capable and technology blurs differences among organizations, what will preclude other organizations from developing innovative ways to provide the services traditionally provided by AHCs? More specifically, which knowledge management practices will contribute the most to AHC performance and to the goal of a value-driven health system? How much should AHCs invest to strengthen their knowledge capabilities?

In light of experience in other industries, the Blue Ridge Group chose to explore the role of knowledge within leading organizations, examine current AHC knowledge practices, and identify ways that AHCs can realign their knowledge capabilities for greater benefit to those they serve. This chapter provides an introduction to knowledge management, shares examples of how a variety of corporations are approaching knowledge management, encourages broader use of knowledge management within AHCs, and explores how knowledge is tied to the leadership role within the health community and is increasingly linked to success in the health care market. The recommendations presented in the chapter advocate action by AHCs in three areas: increased attention and resource allocation to managing their knowledge, preparation of health professionals for the knowledge economy, and participation in the development of a national health information infrastructure. A fourth recommendation encourages other health organizations to support the diffusion of knowledge management within health care.

This chapter builds on three themes of the preceding chapters. First, change is inevitable for AHCs and AHC leaders should seek creative responses to the challenges confronting them. To be successful, the exploitation of internal resources will become as important as seeking increased external resources. Second, information and connectivity technologies play a critical role in improving the performance and strengthening the viability of AHCs. Third, AHCs can demonstrate leadership for the rest of the health care industry by their actions and, in so doing, advance the development of our health system while preserving and expanding their missions of patient care, education, research, and public service.

The chapter also complements the recommendations from the previous chapters. Knowledge management supports and is supported by enterprise-wide management. A knowledge management infrastructure can advance use of organizational performance measures. Moreover, managing knowledge

contributes to the development of a value-driven health system by enabling
the practice of medicine based on evidence, productivity enhancements, and
adoption of innovative practices. Aggressive use of organizational knowledge
and information technology can extend the range of ways that health care professionals and organizations interact with patients, enable patients to assume
more control in managing their health, and support population health management. Developing a knowledge management infrastructure and implementing knowledge management strategies can strengthen organizational
culture by tangibly supporting knowledge workers and in so doing likely
increase productivity and satisfaction within a frequently tumultuous environment. Finally, knowledge management and e-health strategies are com-
plementary, often overlapping, and in some instances inseparable. (See also
Chapter 6.)

The forces shaping health care

Major challenges facing the health care community include providing insurance coverage to the entire population, measurably improving health outcomes, and achieving high-quality services consistently. To accomplish these
objectives, health care organizations and professionals must manage the
health of populations through evidence-based medicine, collaborative care,
and chronic disease management. Simultaneously, they face growing public health challenges, new accreditation requirements, and greater public
scrutiny in their handling of person-specific health information. Underlying all of these challenges is the need to manage and organize cohesively
the ever-growing volume of health-related data and knowledge. Information
systems and processes for managing and communicating knowledge to work
teams and other key stakeholders have become cornerstones for health care
organizations.

In addition to a multitude of developments within health care that are
changing its shape, the health care milieu is also being shaped by a series of
interwoven external forces, including demographic trends, increasing consumerism, advances in telecommunications and computers, and changes in
the nature of economic transactions. As the US population has aged, become
more diverse, and developed new family structures, its needs and desires have
changed. The economic boom of the 1990s and the accompanying increase
in purchasing power of many citizens made them more demanding consumers. Their overall experience, not just the quality or price of a product

or service, is now one of the factors weighed in their consumption decisions (Neuborne, 1999). Thus, health care organizations are striving to replace disjointed service patterns with smooth and convenient patient experiences that are underpinned by well-organized disease management models. Evening and weekend hours for pediatric clinics, physician practices located in grocery stores, drive-up windows for filling prescriptions, and at-home monitoring of chronic conditions are among the approaches health care organizations are using to meet the new needs and demands of patients (Ernst & Young LLP, 1998).

Advances in information technology and communications have changed the nature of work and what is most highly valued in the market (Davis and Meyer, 1998). Telecommunication capabilities make it possible to invest less in physical capital and focus more on intellectual capital. Relationships with many employees are shifting, as they are more likely to be loyal to their work team or profession than to one company. Academic health centers have already experienced this phenomenon with subspecialists in medicine and nursing. In the future, more and more of the workforce will qualify as crucial knowledge workers so that their leaving the organization will add both substantial training and recruiting costs. Thus, there is a greater need to build connections with employees through mentoring, professional development opportunities, or flexible employment models, and to maintain contact after staff leave the organization. Moreover, formal relationships are giving way to evolving roles within economic webs, where competitors may now collaborate and businesses increasingly depend on other businesses for their well-being (Davis and Meyer, 1998). Mergers between organizations present challenges in preserving valuable organizational knowledge, as well as aligning and leveraging the combined knowledge base. Global transactions are now commonplace across most industries and offer new potential markets even for typically local products, but require knowledge of and sensitivity to local cultural and infrastructure concerns.

Not only are businesses responding to consumer demands for higher levels of service, they have begun to customize their services and products. This customization is possible in part because interactions between producers and consumers are increasingly supported by "pervasive connectivity" (Davis and Meyer, 1998). Such connectivity allows greater communication between the customer and producer, and producers use this as an opportunity to learn about customer preferences so that they can anticipate future needs, customize to meet unique needs, and upgrade their offerings through incremental enhancements. For businesses, the ideal interaction with customers involves an exchange of information and emotion (e.g., loyalty, esteem, or engagement), as well as compensation for the goods or service received.

The increased connectivity of the US population has begun to change the nature of patient interactions with health professionals and organizations by offering new tools to patients as well as professionals. An estimated 90 million Americans have used the Internet to seek health information (Madden and Rainie, 2003). The world's largest medical database, MEDLINE, includes references from 4600 medical and scientific journals and over 12 million citations. It handles over 500 million searches per year (National Library of Medicine, 2004). Some physicians have begun to respond to electronic mail both from their patients and the general public (Borowitz and Wyatt, 1998), thereby improving ongoing communication between the patient and physician, in the first case, and providing a service that may or may not result in a referral, in the second. (In both instances, concerns arise about confidentiality, practicing medicine across state lines, and compensation.)

Web sites are a common feature for many hospitals and health systems, but they face stiff competition on the basis of both format and content from a wide variety of independent web sites that provide updates on medical advances and information on specific conditions in user friendly formats. The most well-known sites have been developed and are maintained by firms whose primary function is to serve as managers or brokers of health information and knowledge both for professionals and the general public (e.g., WebMD, Intelihealth, AmericasDoctor) (Miller, 1999). These brokers bring greater interactivity to the use of the Internet for health and offer more options for customizing interactions. Health consumers can obtain virtual consults 24 hours a day, locate physicians in their area, check the compatibility of drugs they are using, learn about clinical trials, participate in specialized support groups, develop personalized health records, and fill drug prescriptions – all via the Internet and without interacting with a traditional health provider organization (National Research Council, 2000a).

In general, however, the health care industry's response to the transform-ing economy is nascent compared to other industries where instantaneous communications and computing capabilities separate selling and the deliv-ery of goods, reduce response time to customers, enable customization, and speed the diffusion of new trends within and across organizations and indus-tries. The banking, travel, and retail industries have already developed the ability to provide services electronically and, in many cases, to improve upon them. They are using the capabilities offered by the Internet and other kinds of information technology to transform how they do business by extending their accessibility, making better use of their organizational information, using encounters with customers to gather new information, and using such information to develop new services.

These developments are influencing the general public's performance expectations for other industries, including health care. If some industries can become more accessible and flexible, provide streamlined services, integrate information, and offer greater value, why not all industries? And, although the pace of development may be mitigated somewhat by concerns about security and privacy, the general direction is irreversible. Ultimately, success will gravitate to those who reliably deliver on these emerging criteria of high performance.

Far more dramatic changes are projected for the not-too-distant future. Ray Kurzweil (who worked on optical character recognition in the 1970s, voice recognition in the 1980s, and print-to-speech reading software in the 1990s) has predicted that by 2009, a $1000 personal computer will be able to perform a trillion calculations per second. At that point, most text will be created using continuous speech recognition; routine business transactions (e.g., purchases, travel reservations) will most often take place between a human and a virtual personality; and intelligent courseware will be a standard means of learning (along with traditional classrooms). According to Kurzweil, things will really start to get interesting around 2029, when a $1000 (in 1999 dollars) unit of computation will have the computing capacity of approximately 1000 brains and direct neural pathways will have been perfected for high-bandwidth connection to the human brain. By that time, automated agents will be learning on their own and significant knowledge will be created by machines with little or no human intervention (Kurzweil, 1999).

Whether or not Kurzweil's predictions are totally on target, the major thrust of his hypotheses is difficult to ignore. Technological advancements will not only continue, but will do so more quickly, with the ultimate impact being unavoidable for our society and economy. Organizations cannot afford to ignore the direction and magnitude of the forthcoming changes.

Knowledge as capital

Competitive success has always been a function of a firm's knowledge about how to optimize its resources. Compared to other assets (i.e., land, capital, and labor), the role of organizational knowledge has grown over time. The current information-based, global economy has transformed this intangible asset into the primary source of wealth for firms and nations. Knowledge and information now are both raw materials and valuable products. Not only has the knowledge intensity of goods and services increased dramatically, but knowledge and information also play a critical role as organizations adapt to their ever-changing environment. The increasing speed of change in markets, staff attrition, growth in the scope of organizations, globalization of markets and firms, growth in networked organizations, and changing consumer expectations all place new demands on organizations that can be offset through management of information and knowledge (Cole, 1998; Stewart, 1997).

Organizational knowledge is typically tacit rather than explicit (Bock, 1998). It appears in unwritten rules, undocumented experiences, and uncaptured expert talent. This important resource tends to be local; taken for granted by those who possess it; not easily codified; and, therefore, often difficult to communicate. As the value of knowledge has grown, the transformation of tacit to explicit knowledge has become one of the most important challenges for organizations. It cannot, however, be met by technology alone. Knowledge transformation and diffusion are most likely to occur in an environment of trust through dialogue and interactive problem solving. Knowledge generally spreads when people gather and share stories or if they make a systematic effort to find it and make it explicit (Nonaka and Takeuchi, 1995).

Once knowledge is captured in a way that allows it to be described, shared, and deployed to do something that could not be done previously, it becomes an organizational asset or intellectual capital (Stewart, 1997). Unlike other assets that are easily accounted for and managed, the value of this asset resides in an organization's people, structures, and relationships. Simply spending more money on experts, information systems, or databases will not, however, increase intellectual capital. These actions must occur within an environment that is shaped by strategies that focus the allocation of organizational knowledge resources on clearly defined goals and that expects and enables colleagues to share and act on information, knowledge, and expertise.

Organizational efforts to develop such strategies and create such an environment are often described as knowledge management. Knowledge management initiatives generally focus on two fundamental objectives: to enable knowledge sharing and to use knowledge to generate value (see Table 5.1). Successful knowledge management initiatives underlie existing business processes; support specific business strategies and objectives; focus on the solution of concrete problems; provide a range of tools that can be skillfully

Table 5.1 Knowledge management goals, strategies, and actions

Goals	Strategies	Actions
Enable knowledge sharing	**Create knowledge management culture** • Make knowledge visible and show role of information within an organization • Instill responsibility for knowledge sharing **Build technical and staffing infrastructure** • Build connections among people as part of the knowledge management infrastructure (both technically and socially) • Assign explicit knowledge roles **Harvest organizational knowledge** • Share expertise and best practices • Capture past experiences and organizational learning • Access valuable knowledge from external sources • Build and mine customer knowledge bases	Demonstrate leadership commitment through vision statement, time on meeting agenda, and investment in knowledge management resources Establish organization-wide knowledge goals Align performance incentives with sharing behaviors Establish ways to recognize outstanding knowledge management practices by staff Appoint a chief knowledge officer Designate knowledge stewards to maintain organizational knowledge bases and provide assistance to staff seeking information or knowledge Rotate staff into and out of specific knowledge management roles Establish networks with common hardware and software platforms Provide electronic access to knowledge bases wherever staff are working Establish electronic connections with customers, suppliers, and other potential partners Develop databases that contain internal and external knowledge (e.g., enter project summary reports into database, document lessons learned, purchase online subscriptions or databases) Distribute knowledge on demand and push knowledge to staff Promote learning opportunities (e.g., mentors, multifunctional project teams, communities of practice, training, technology or best practices fair) Seek to uncover organizational knowledge through knowledge mapping, prototyping, learning history, after-action reviews, and internal benchmarking

(*cont.*)

Table 5.1 (*cont.*)

Goals	Strategies	Actions
Act on organizational knowledge and insights	• Apply organizational knowledge in decisions, processes, and transactions • Embed knowledge in products and services • Create new knowledge through innovation • Use knowledge to strengthen organizational relationships	Try new approaches to stimulate innovation Provide open access to company information Identify or create internal knowledge brokers
Assess value	• Measure knowledge assets and impact of knowledge management	

used by workers; and, most importantly, lead to action as a result of the new knowledge or insight gained.

A growing number of business leaders consider the ability to manage and act on organizational knowledge as essential to the success of firms (Wah, 1999). Increasingly, companies are strengthening and, in some cases, transforming themselves by focusing on, capturing, organizing, communicating, and acting on their organizational knowledge. These companies are succeeding in reducing costs, improving quality, streamlining processes, managing huge organizational changes, creating new products, improving productivity, and retaining critically important knowledge workers (Davenport and Prusak, 1998; McCune, 1999; Stewart, 1997). In essence, these companies are using knowledge to extend capabilities, strengthen relationships, and create value. Along the way, many of them have enhanced their company culture and sense of identity in order to drive substantial changes.

AHCs and knowledge

Although AHCs differ in many ways, knowledge is a core element of these organizations. Each of the AHC missions relies upon communication, application, and analysis of an ever-growing volume of complex information and knowledge. Sharing of information and knowledge among researchers, between clinicians, with patients, from teachers to students, from mentors to residents, and sometimes even across these lines is the cornerstone of daily AHC operations. Academic health centers have been gradually expanding their methods of sharing, developing, and applying knowledge as information technology evolves. To varying degrees and in a variety of ways, AHCs make information and knowledge more accessible for internal and external users, target how knowledge is presented, and insert knowledge into routine processes to improve efficiency or outcomes. Some AHCs are becoming more sophisticated in their use of knowledge as a means of interacting with potential or actual consumers. The emergence of the Internet and the connectivity it offers can be credited for many new knowledge practices (see also Chapter 6).

As primary knowledge repositories for AHCs, health sciences libraries have been at the forefront of acquiring access to and making available the knowledge needed by AHC professionals. The shift from print to digital media is enabling libraries to bring knowledge closer to the actual site of work for more convenient and faster use. In addition, health sciences libraries have used their knowledge resources and staff expertise to support a variety of communities important to, but not physically part of, the AHC. For example, medical student preceptors are often provided access to online knowledge sources. The North Carolina AHEC is building upon this concept by providing preceptors access to a customized library and creating a virtual faculty lounge for them (North Carolina AHEC Program, 1999).

A wide range of information and knowledge needed by AHC staff or their customers is increasingly available online (e.g., institutional policies, medical school applications, residency opportunities, lectures, expertise of faculty within the institution) (Johns Hopkins Medicine, 1999a, 1999b). In some cases, this material is formatted for a specific target audience. For example, as part of an effort to create better patient services, billing, and scheduling, Emory Health System is developing a web site for the general public that offers information on wellness, disease management, clinical trials, and how to access services at Emory (COR Health LLC, 2000; Emory Health System, 2000). In other instances, AHC staff are using information and knowledge that are readily accessible to improve processes (e.g., use standard templates in preparing grant proposals or make online image databases available to assist faculty in preparing lectures) (Johns Hopkins Medicine, 1999c; University of Virginia, 1997). Clinical information systems now include clinical alerts and reminders and real-time access to most current medical knowledge to ensure that complete data are collected, to assist clinicians in making sound decisions, and to minimize adverse events (Bates *et al.*, 1998; Hunt *et al.*, 1998; Sackett and Straus, 1998). Some AHCs (e.g., Vanderbilt University) format clinical protocols for residents to load into Palm Pilots, thereby providing immediate access to important knowledge.

In addition to disseminating knowledge through traditional mechanisms (e.g., classrooms, rounds, publications), AHCs have begun to offer online education opportunities for students, residents, professionals, and patients (Sikorski and Peters, 1998; University of Virginia Health System, 2000a, 2000b). Academic health centers have also begun to repackage the knowledge generated within their institutions for other users to meet specific market needs and to form partnerships that combine knowledge bases or establish more effective knowledge distribution channels. For example, Johns Hopkins publishes the *Johns Hopkins Family Health Book* and Harvard Medical School provides consumer health information to Intelihealth, a consumer health portal managed by Aetna (Intelihealth, 2004; Johns Hopkins, 1999). A consortium of midwest AHCs established a web site to provide specific information resources selected by librarians and information professionals (Health Web, 2000). Another group of AHCs formed WebEBM (now known as Health Gate) to assist clinicians and patients in making informed decisions through the use of evidence-based clinical guidelines (WebEBM, 2000).

Centralized, longitudinal clinical databases derived from clinical records enable AHC faculty to study patients over time or across populations while maintaining patient privacy. Such databases enable a clinical researcher to focus on questions of immediate concern to a particular population and to use the results to inform clinical practices in a fairly short time frame or to compete for extramural research funding (Duke University Medical Center, 2000; University of Virginia Health System, 1999). Through an IAIMS (i.e., Integrated Advanced Information Management System) grant funded by the National Library of Medicine, the University of Chicago is promoting collaborative and translational research by linking basic researchers with clinicians through a series of databases including "individual research interests, gene sequences, genetic maps, antibodies to the proteins encoded by the genes, patient data, and patient slides in the pathology service" (University of Chicago, 1999). Several universities have established technology transfer offices to manage their intellectual property assets (Stanford University, 2000; University of North Carolina-Chapel Hill, 2000). These offices assist faculty in obtaining research support from corporate sponsors, license discoveries developed by faculty and staff, and develop agreements for sending university materials to scientists at other institutions.

Although a wide range of knowledge activities can be found across AHCs, knowledge management activity within and across AHCs is uneven. Despite their wealth of knowledge, large pools of highly educated and motivated professionals, and increasingly robust information technology infrastructures, AHCs underutilize their knowledge. Knowledge enables academic success for AHC professionals, is needed for positive clinical results, and is the basis for ongoing research. It is not, however, a commodity in and of itself. Knowledge is not consistently viewed as a form of capital that ought to be maximized.

The typical AHC organizational structure (i.e., dominated by clinical departments) has been credited with inhibiting the enterprise-wide management of revenues, facilities, and personnel. It also has limited evolution of knowledge management practices within AHCs, which have tended to be localized and often individualized rather than viewed in terms of meeting organizational strategies. Knowledge management within AHCs is often piecemeal and ad hoc, sometimes initiated by the interests of a single faculty member rather than being the result of the decision to respond to a specific organizational need. Typically, knowledge gained during work processes is used for one purpose; rarely is it captured for subsequent application or transferred from one organizational domain to another to improve processes or stimulate new products, as is increasingly practiced in other industries. Just as AHC faculty and staff cross functional lines to perform their work, knowledge resources must be released from rigid organizational structures and made available to all staff who can contribute to or benefit from them.

Academic health centers tend to view organizational knowledge narrowly. In addition to the medical knowledge that is critical for patient care and basic science knowledge that supports research, knowledge exists on a wide range of topics related to patient preferences, suppliers, potential collaborators, work processes, and in-house experts that has only begun to be captured, managed, and leveraged to improve organizational performance. There is a great deal of tacit knowledge within AHC faculty and staff that could advance the strategic objectives of the organization, if it is identified and added to explicit knowledge bases.

As educators, clinicians, and researchers, AHC staff share knowledge on a daily basis with a variety of audiences. Sharing knowledge for purposes of educating students, treating patients, or disseminating research results is, however, very different from sharing knowledge to transform a business. Like other successful businesses, AHCs can find opportunities for innovation throughout their institutions – literally from the ground floor where support services reside, to clinics and patient care units, to classrooms, to research laboratories, to administrative suites. Within each of the missions and the accompanying administrative and support services, there are multiple points for gathering or applying organizational knowledge. At each stage of a work process there may be an opportunity to create greater value simply by making existing knowledge readily available to those who need it.

A knowledge infrastructure

Often the most visible element of an organization's knowledge management initiative is the creation of a knowledge infrastructure or knowledge web. At its most basic level, the knowledge web connects staff with information and knowledge needed for their work and connects them to each other. A knowledge web builds upon and enhances the existing organizational technological infrastructure in at least two ways. First, the technological infrastructure is used to capture and, in some cases, to codify knowledge so that others can access it in the future. By making organizational knowledge readily available, the knowledge web eliminates redundant work steps and enables staff to focus on unique attributes of a task sooner. Second, it goes beyond the support of transactions to support of relationships (among staff, between the organization and staff, and between the organization and its customers or suppliers) that generate value. As an added benefit, establishment of a strong knowledge web prepares the organization for introduction of e-commerce practices into its business.

In addition to a technological infrastructure and the actual content, the knowledge web encompasses processes for gathering, filtering, and disseminating knowledge; policies to guide the organization's development and use of knowledge; and designated staff to manage the knowledge web and support the organization's use of knowledge (Bock, 1998; Davenport and Prusak, 1998). To establish a knowledge infrastructure, an organization must address:

- **Content** to be included, determined in part by focus of the knowledge management effort (e.g., single unit, multiple units, or entire organization) and assessment of the credibility and reliability of data and knowledge sources.

- **Processes** to be used to capture knowledge from professionals without adding substantially to their work, to filter new knowledge to determine usefulness to others, and to classify and code content so that it can be easily accessed by future users.
- **Policies** needed to manage issues surrounding intellectual property and, in the case of health care, to safeguard patient privacy when knowledge resources come from patient data.
- **Resources** needed to support the knowledge infrastructure (e.g., dedicating staff to managing organizational knowledge, expanding existing information technology infrastructure, and ensuring that future information technology investment supports knowledge management objectives).
- **Services** provided by the knowledge infrastructure (e.g., defining shared services, offering integrated services to staff).
- **Relationships** between and **responsibilities** of knowledge management and information technology staff.

Firms may develop a knowledge infrastructure to support a particular kind of knowledge to be managed, to support a particular group of workers, or to resolve a specific organizational need, as has been done by various companies. For example, to maximize the number of problems that can be solved with a single telephone call, technical support representatives at Dell Computer Corporation use a knowledge base that advises them on the kinds of questions to ask callers and guides technicians through problem solving (McCune, 1999). Hewlett Packard has established an electronic network to manage and distribute knowledge in response to customers' demands for rapid service. The system is used by 1900 technical staff members whose job is to keep customers' systems up and running. Once a problem is reported, a description of the problem and its urgency are entered into a database. The database is updated as employees work, so that if the problem is not resolved by the end of shift, it is sent to the next center with full information (Stewart, 1997).

Alternatively, a knowledge web may be designed to provide knowledge resources to the entire organization, as was done by Cap Gemini Ernst & Young LLP (Center for Business Innovation, 1996a). The knowledge web supports 80 000 professionals and has been credited with improving their work experience and contributing to improved staff retention. It includes practice-specific knowledge bases, a catalog, a navigation taxonomy, search engines, a set of templates for use in adding new content, a database describing consultant skills, guidelines for ownership of content, and a standardized technology platform.

A key element of the Cap Gemini Ernst & Young knowledge web is the availability of filtered sets of online material containing essential knowledge that a consultant needs to possess to work in a given area. The knowledge infrastructure includes a chief knowledge officer, a knowledge process committee, knowledge networks for each of the key consulting domains, and three knowledge-focused units. One unit focuses on creating new knowledge, another structures knowledge into methods and automated tools, while the third gathers and stores the firm's acquired knowledge and external knowledge.

A knowledge culture

For a knowledge infrastructure to be effective, the organizational culture must expect and endorse knowledge sharing (McDermott and O'Dell, 2000; O'Dell and Grayson, 1998). Enterprise-wide focus is essential for organizational success, but not easily achieved in environments where units traditionally have been autonomous. Employees may be accustomed to hoarding knowledge in the belief that such behavior protects their power or ensures their value to the organization. Organizations must also overcome broader cultural influences. Contemporary society values individuals with technical expertise and those who create knowledge over those who share knowledge. As a result, staff may be resistant to trying practices developed elsewhere. This situation is exacerbated by lack of awareness of what and how things are done elsewhere in the organization.

Thus, organizations seeking to manage knowledge need to attend to the nontechnical components of the knowledge management infrastructure and begin the gradual process of cultivating an organizational climate for sharing (see Table 5.1). Supporting communities of practice is one way to foster a knowledge-sharing culture. Informal networks known as communities of practice are critical building blocks of a knowledge-based company because they provide the mechanism by which ideas, information, and new practices spread most easily throughout an organization (Senge et al., 1999). Communities of practice or formal work units provide natural boundaries for initiating projects that can then be replicated for similar groups, revised for groups with different needs, or expanded for the entire organization.

Based on research begun in the 1980s, Xerox has emphasized communities of practice in its knowledge management (Murray, 1999). Xerox identified a gap between the knowledge applied in the field by service technicians and information found in manuals. After studying how technicians interact with each other to share knowledge (i.e., tell war stories to teach each other to diagnose and fix machines), the Eureka system was developed to allow technicians to share their stories in the form of electronic tips. Field service representatives create and maintain the knowledge base by contributing tips that are validated by a formal review committee. By using a common documentation method to facilitate lateral communication, the system enables Xerox service teams around the globe to diagnose, solve, and prevent equipment problems. Equally important, other groups within Xerox now access and use the knowledge contained in Eureka to improve their work product. Engineering, manufacturing, and documentation units use the knowledge to improve design, production, user instructions, and technical manuals.

Novartis, a life sciences company created in 1996, has focused on creating a knowledge culture since its inception. Novartis' corporate objectives include the

transmutation of accumulated knowledge into a corporate asset by exploiting the vast amount of knowledge across organizational boundaries; providing easy, rapid access to a global knowledge base; eliminating time and space constraints in communications; and stimulating associates to experience the value of knowledge sharing. (Probst, 1998)

Accordingly, the company designated knowledge managers, established advisory committees and knowledge networks, and created a series of awards for innovative research both within and outside the company. Novartis' knowledge activities include: using its knowledge about consumers to shape its research and development of nonprescription drugs; routinely scouring the work done by small innovative companies who cannot afford to develop their ideas to maximum potential; and developing partnerships to increase its knowledge base on health, safety, and environment issues (Novartis, 1999).

Knowledge management processes

The most tangible results from knowledge management activities often arise from efforts to harvest, transfer, and apply organizational knowledge. Hoffman-LaRoche, a Swiss-based international pharmaceutical company, used a knowledge management initiative to reduce both filing and Food and

Drug Administration approval time for new drugs. Hoffman-LaRoche successfully improved its performance in application preparation and approval time by mapping its existing knowledge and prototyping the application process to determine what knowledge customers need to have and how to create that knowledge. The application for a new indication for one drug resulted in a reduction in filing time from a projected 18 months to 3 months and approval time from a projected 3 years to 9 months, at an estimated savings of $1 million per day (Center for Business Innovation, 1996b).

British Petroleum (BP) seeks to "make the reuse of existing knowledge a routine way of doing business and to create new knowledge to radically improve business performance" (Wah, 1999). British Petroleum's Peer Assist Program has proven to be highly effective in transferring knowledge within the organization (Ernst & Young LLP, 1998). After initial research and data analysis, new project teams identify issues needing clarification. They call on experts within the company to form a group that meets with the project team for one to three days to identify possible solutions to the issues. Invited experts participate willingly, even though the task is in addition to their regular job. They view the invitation as an honor and an opportunity to see what is happening in another part of the company. A project is not complete at BP until those involved have articulated lessons learned, action points for the future, and quantification of key internal measures during completion meetings. Business lessons that emerge from facilitated team sessions are translated into best practices and are added to the corporate knowledge database. In addition, approximately one-quarter of BP business units have knowledge guardians who help their teams harvest newly created knowledge (Wah, 1999).

The World Bank is using knowledge management techniques to streamline its work processes. It has adopted a new approach for responding to technical questions (e.g., education strategy development). Rather than assembling a study team to visit a country and write a report, which usually takes months, a project manager contacts a community of practice within the bank asking for advice. Responses come from bank staff and partners around the world, enabling a report to be produced quickly and added to the bank's knowledge base on development issues. Over 100 communities of practice contribute to the knowledge base, which is envisioned to ultimately be available to anyone via the Internet (World Bank, 2000).

Another class of knowledge management activities focuses on increasing the knowledge of the organization. KPMG LLP, a consulting firm, is using a Web-based curriculum on Internet studies to ensure that all staff in its consulting division, from administrative assistants to senior partners, have the necessary skills to respond to the emergence of the Internet as a major business force. The 50-hour course is offered online, includes a pretest and final exam as well as virtual lectures, and is updated every 90 days. Within three months of its availability online, 95 percent of KPMG's domestic workforce had taken the final test. KPMG has also developed higher-level courses for interested staff (Balu, 2000).

Rising to the challenge

How AHCs respond to the challenges of defining their role, building new capabilities, becoming more responsive, and developing new models for their clinical, educational, and research enterprises will determine their influence in the health system of the twenty-first century – nationally and globally. The Blue Ridge Group believes that AHCs can become leaders within the health community by establishing themselves as premier knowledge managers for all health knowledge domains (such as health maintenance, disease manage-ment, evidence-based medicine, and population health management). Doing so will enable AHCs to evolve from their traditional roots into organizations that are able to respond to contemporary forces and anticipated needs of individual patients, regions, the nation, and beyond.

Pursuing this path will require that AHCs allocate resources to knowl-edge management. Actual investments in the technological infrastructure will depend on the current status of an individual AHC infrastructure, but in virtually all cases, additional attention and investment will be needed to strengthen knowledge management and electronic commerce capabilities (as discussed in Chapter 6). Equally important and perhaps more difficult will be the preparation of staff, not only by building skills to use knowledge management systems, but also for a potentially dramatic transformation of their roles as clinicians, educators, and researchers. Health professionals will increasingly serve as coaches to more of their patients. Instructors may func-tion more as collaborators in the learning process. Researchers may find that some traditional research methodologies are too limited given the new ques-tions they will be seeking to answer and the new capabilities of computers to process increasingly complex problems. From discovery to application to dissemination and all possible combinations of these three activities, net-working will become normative behavior.

Today, all AHC personnel need to be knowledge workers (Drucker, 1988). Faculty and staff need to think in terms of what the organization needs and to define the resources (other than financial) they need from the institution to be effective in their work in a post-Gutenberg world. Academic health centers can use knowledge management activities to promote desired behavior. Moreover, well-designed knowledge management programs can facilitate work processes, enrich work experience, and promote career development of the workforce and thereby increase satisfaction of staff.

A variety of factors may impede knowledge management within AHCs. Academic health center leaders and staff, who already face myriad demands on their time, attention, and financial resources, may underestimate the need to strengthen their knowledge management capabilities and incorporate knowledge management practices into their work processes. Revenue streams for patient care services that depend on externally determined reimbursement mechanisms do not create incentives for health organizations and professionals to pursue nonreimbursable activities such as knowledge management, despite the potential positive impact on patient outcome, organizational efficiency, and ultimately the bottom line. Further, AHCs may not recognize the crucial distinction between explicitly managing their organizational knowledge and developing information systems (see next section). Or, they may possess a false sense of security created by the fact that AHCs have been in the knowledge business since their inception and already have numerous, albeit disjointed, knowledge management activities underway.

Academic health center leaders face substantial challenges in creating an environment in which knowledge and information of all kinds are shared with ease. Such an effort requires decisions and behaviors that will likely conflict with some traditional AHC habits. Previous organizational structures and practices, as well as reimbursement mechanisms, reinforced a tendency to think in terms of departmental needs rather than the whole enterprise and to hold onto information and knowledge rather than to share it. And even if faculty wanted to share information with colleagues, there typically were limited means to do so easily. As a result, sharing information beyond a work unit was not standard practice. There are also knowledge issues that arise because the various business units of the AHC – the medical school, nursing school, hospital, public health school, primary care network, basic science departments, medical libraries, e-health databases, etc. – have different professional and administrative knowledge glossaries, grammars, and standards.

Several knowledge issues of particular concern to AHCs have become more complex as technology and business models have evolved. Libraries face growing challenges in keeping up with the growth in electronic media and the technological infrastructure needed to serve patrons on top of rising subscription costs. Biomedical researchers require increasingly sophisticated capabilities (i.e., access to and expertise in biomedical computer applications) to analyze complex molecular structures and link them to relevant clinical information. Current laws and policies aimed at protecting intellectual property are outmoded in the digital environment and a new policy framework has not yet begun to take shape (National Research Council, 2000b). Managing intellectual property in the AHC environment requires a fine balance between the education of professionals and dissemination of research results to advance health and the protection of intellectual property to maximize potential revenue associated with new discoveries. Moreover, the relationships that AHCs establish to leverage their intellectual capital – through funding or collaboration or for dissemination – require new organizational models and behaviors and raise new conflict of interest issues that need to be managed (Angell, 2000; COR Health LLC, 2000; InteliHealth, 2004).

IT in support of AHC knowledge management

Academic health center leaders and staff may view the presence of an information technology (IT) infrastructure as equivalent to knowledge management. Certainly, mature knowledge management initiatives cannot succeed without a robust IT infrastructure, but knowledge management encompasses much more than technology because knowledge management is ultimately about behaviors and actions. Moreover, not all IT is capable of supporting knowledge management efforts. Ultimately, an organization's knowledge management should inform and drive the IT infrastructure development. To accomplish this objective, some organizations name a chief knowledge officer to oversee knowledge management efforts and to work with the chief information officer. (See Table 5.2 for comparison of chief information officer and chief knowledge officer roles within an AHC.)

Much like their organizational structure, the IT infrastructure of AHCs – including electronic mail, office support software, clinical information systems, online access to health knowledge sources, and a variety of administrative systems – is typically large, complex, fragmented, dominated by the clinical operation, and gradually becoming more integrated.

Table 5.2 Chief information officer role versus chief knowledge officer role

Chief information officer	Chief knowledge officer
Overall responsibility	*Overall responsibility*
Setting strategy for the technical infrastructure design of information systems (IS) to support knowledge management strategy	Identifying knowledge domains and setting strategy for their development. These domains are in clinical, research, and educational knowledge areas
Key relationship is with the chief knowledge officer	Key relationship is with the chief information officer
Specific responsibilities	*Specific responsibilities*
• Fiduciary and management responsibility for the development and ongoing operation of the IS technology network including vendor relationships	• Identification, evaluation, and development of key information databases to be created, acquired, and integrated to establish each domain of knowledge management
• Managing IS professionals with technical expertise	• Managing knowledge management professionals who can organize and assemble content to be deployed using information systems technology
• Developing and maintaining IS policies and standards to ensure ease of use and access, regulatory compliance, and data integrity	• Identifying program needs in knowledge domains and maintenance of relationships with key stakeholders
• Identifying the IS technical needs and maintenance of relationships with key stakeholders	• Identifying and monitoring new knowledge management approaches
• Evaluating new IS technology to support the evolution of knowledge management	• Providing advice on directions and goals of the business processes in each knowledge management domain, including the business processes to support the AHC
• Developing and implementing business processes supported by IS technology, including financial and administrative systems, to support the AHC and its knowledge management domains	
Clinical domain	*Clinical domain*
Stakeholders: groups of patients (populations), individual patients, insurers, referring physicians, AHC physicians, nurses and other care-givers, other employees	Stakeholders: groups of patients (populations), individual patients, insurers, referring physicians, AHC physicians, nurses and other care-givers, other employees
Sample activities:	*Sample activities*:
• Modifying the patient business cycle, including billing and registration, for ease of use	• Standardizing content for medical records, including information to referring physicians and to patients, potentially online
• Developing Web-based strategies to deliver knowledge to patients and referring physicians	• Developing, monitoring, and updating clinical protocols

Table 5.2 (*cont.*)

Chief information officer	Chief knowledge officer
• Providing technical support for laboratory information systems and filmless clinical imaging systems	
Research domain	***Research domain***
Stakeholders: researchers, trainees, and administrators	Stakeholders: researchers, trainees, and administrators
Sample activities:	*Sample activities*:
• Developing databases and sites for dissemination of results	• Establishing standards for scientific databases
• Developing and supporting IS tools for grant management	• Developing knowledge domains for technology transfer
	• Developing standard institutional forms and protocols for submitting grants (both federal and commercial)
Education domain	***Education domain***
Stakeholders: undergraduate and graduate students, including residents, community physicians, nurses, and other practicing health professionals	Stakeholders: undergraduate and graduate students, including residents, community physicians, nurses, and other practicing health professionals
Sample activities:	*Sample activities*:
• Developing and maintaining Web-based application processes for undergraduates, graduates, and postgraduate education	• Developing content for distance and online learning for students, residents, and practicing physicians
• Developing and applying computerized testing technology	• Developing content for secure online testing
• Maintaining online tracking of registration, course billing, and continuing medical education credits	

Academic health centers have advanced their technological platform considerably during the past decade and are continuing to do so by implementing more comprehensive and integrated systems, building institutional web sites and resources, and confronting issues surrounding the control and management of information systems. (See Case Study by Wilkerson and McCoy that accompanies this chapter.) For example, many AHCs are making strides toward achieving the objective of having all relevant patient data available to health professionals during a patient encounter. This represents a threshold improvement for the practice of sound medicine and is not easily achieved in the complex AHC practice environment, as it requires overcoming historical differences in how inpatient and outpatient records were maintained.

Despite the considerable progress achieved, however, significant work remains for information systems to meet the needs of contemporary health care and for individual organizations to implement truly robust systems throughout their organizations. In addition to widely known issues surrounding health care IT (e.g., confidentiality protection, ease of use, standards for data), outstanding needs generate additional requirements for information systems in AHCs (Goldsmith, 2000). For example, one as yet unmet requirement for information systems is the ability to generate three distinct kinds of clinical data sets. In addition to the patient records traditionally maintained by health care organizations to support institutional needs, increasingly patients seek to maintain their own records to aid in the long-term management of their health. The growing emphasis on managing population health requires databases that incorporate health information for the residents of entire regions. Each of these kinds of health records – personal, organizational, and population – impacts research and education, as well as patient care, and is an important element of the health information infrastructure for the country, but until quite recently organizational health records have received the most attention and development (National Committee on Vital and Health Statistics, 1998).

Organizations seeking to manage their knowledge effectively require an even higher level of capabilities from their IT infrastructure. Current information systems within AHCs facilitate communication; collect, organize, and provide access to data; streamline certain work processes (e.g., ordering tests and reporting results); and, in some cases, guide clinical decision-making through alerts or links to knowledge sources. In addition to these functions, a knowledge management infrastructure facilitates connections within communities or practice or work units; provides access to all the kinds of knowledge needed for staff to perform their work; increases organizational knowledge; and promotes the use of knowledge in routine tasks, innovation, and interactions with customers.

Thus, an information system that is part of a knowledge management infrastructure includes standard terminology, directories of available contents, robust search engines, templates for easy collection of knowledge, both global and unit-specific databases and knowledge sources, and prompts or alerts of available knowledge embedded within processes supported by the information system (McCune, 1999). Moreover, the system is supported by staff who focus on the knowledge needs of users. Ideally, such systems provide the knowledge needed by users without them having to think about what they need and how to get it.

A knowledge infrastructure makes needed information and knowledge available automatically as part of the work process, or upon demand to meet specific requests, or via periodic updates that provide a synthesis of developments with easy access to greater detail. Clinicians need immediate, focused access to current and relevant knowledge when making decisions in the course of regular patient care. Clinical alerts (e.g., to prevent adverse reactions) have been shown to be very effective in achieving positive outcomes and are used by many AHCs, but just-in-time knowledge access is not a standard part of each health professional's interaction with their organization's information system (Chueh and Barnett, 1997). Similar opportunities exist to support research and education through just-in-time knowledge strategies as well. For example, AHCs face the ongoing challenges of sharing knowledge among researchers in real time, increasing the efficiency of research, and quickly moving the knowledge created through research into practice and teaching.

A knowledge management system can enable AHCs to optimize resources spent on obtaining access to external knowledge sources as well as the time spent by faculty and staff on keeping up with the knowledge in their field. Individual departments or service centers may provide staff with summaries of seminal journals for their field. Urgent findings can be highlighted in regular bulletins and linked to the records of patients with relevant diagnoses. Costs of subscriptions can then be consolidated and staff can be freed from reviewing every journal to focus on those of particular interest. Summaries of developments across multiple fields can be combined to offer interdisciplinary perspectives on advances in clinical care and research.

An AHC knowledge management system should intersect the clinical arena with the research and education enterprise. If it does not, there is a great likelihood that the information systems for each mission will be designed and implemented so that most of the potential synergy across the missions will be lost. Specific knowledge resources and processes for capturing and formatting organizational knowledge are required to meet the needs of education and research communities of practice. Particular consideration of how to facilitate knowledge transfer across mission domains, organizational units, or specialties is needed. Although a single information system within an AHC is unlikely, consistency among various systems used by staff is desirable and knowledge management practices would be aided by a global index (accessible from each system in use) that identifies how to access various organizational knowledge resources.

Each AHC information system needs to be evaluated in light of the new requirements posed by knowledge management. Does the system reinforce a knowledge management and learning culture? Does the system provide a means of implementing knowledge strategies for patients, referring physicians, students, and staff? Does the system capture the various kinds of information that will form the basis of new organizational knowledge? Does the system offer the potential to create advantage in the market by allowing the institution to provide services or provide them in a way other organizations cannot offer?

Strengthening knowledge management

The Blue Ridge Group believes that knowledge management must become an explicit activity within AHCs and all health care organizations. Strengthening knowledge management capabilities will depend on preparing the workforce, providing the technical infrastructure, and participation by a broad array of actors within the health sector. Thus, the Blue Ridge Group recommends that:

- AHCs should explicitly manage their knowledge as an organizational asset to improve their performance and strengthen their ability to meet both the market and social needs of their immediate community or region and the broader health care community.
- AHCs should help current and future health professionals acquire the skills needed to use existing organizational knowledge, prepare for the new demands associated with their professions in the digital era, and contribute to the new disciplines of knowledge management as they emerge.
- AHCs and other health organizations should vigorously support and participate in efforts to create and maintain a national health information infrastructure (NHII) and a local health information infrastructure (LHII) within their community or region.
- Federal and state governments should help underwrite the creation of a NHII and LHIIs so as to facilitate knowledge management throughout health care and to provide a platform upon which a value-driven health system can be built.

- Federal agencies, philanthropic organizations, and professional organizations should advance understanding of the role of knowledge in the future health system and support activities that will further diffuse successful knowledge management practices in health care.

Each of these recommendations is discussed in the sections that follow.

Managing an AHC asset

The knowledge economy is creating new demands for all organizations. The knowledge age is opening a wide range of possibilities for the future of health and health care (e.g., personalized care made possible through genomic medicine). Meanwhile, health care organizations are grappling with quality concerns, improving the health of the population, and managing costs. The combination of these factors led the Blue Ridge Group to conclude that knowledge management is a critical success factor for AHCs in the twenty-first century. Fortunately, the set of characteristics that define AHCs – multi-mission, large size, complex organizational structure, sophisticated work, highly educated professionals, and a strong tradition of seeking, discovering, and disseminating knowledge – provides the foundation for large gains to be earned through well-conceived knowledge management initiatives.

Such initiatives must be based on clearly defined organizational strategies and support the organizational mission. Thus, a first step for AHCs seeking to expand their knowledge management capacity is to assess their current mission and strategies in the context of the anticipated environment. The multitude of factors to be considered include:

- the impact of the interconnected economy, but not yet fully connected public,
- which parts of the evolving health market (including e-health) it makes sense for an AHC to compete in,
- the extent to and means by which AHCs can advance the health of populations,
- the changing educational environment, as well as the changing base of learners (including health professional students, patients, faculty, and staff),
- the kind of research that will likely be in demand,
- how to build an infrastructure that fosters collaboration across disciplines and across domains,
- how to generate value in each AHC program.

Once an AHC has developed focused organizational strategies for the emerging environment, it can develop corresponding knowledge strategies. An AHC may choose to foster productivity of a particular unit or community of practice, capture existing knowledge for reuse elsewhere in the organization, encourage collaboration among researchers, or embed knowledge in routine encounters with patients and other customers as a means of solidifying market position.

The pace of scientific discovery and the accompanying growth in knowledge about maintaining health and managing diseases, along with the proliferation of users of this knowledge and possible speed of diffusion, present an opportunity for AHCs to reshape their role as educators or disseminators of knowledge. Some AHCs may choose to pursue their role as knowledge managers quite aggressively from the perspective of preparing their patients and citizens to become proficient in using available health knowledge to manage their personal health. Building upon existing community and patient education programs (e.g., mini-med schools) and using existing technological resources (e.g., computer classrooms), these AHCs may develop and offer classes for the general public, selected employers, or targeted patients on how to access health resources on the Internet, assess the quality of those resources, and use it to strengthen their ability to make prudent decisions. By interacting with patients and potential patients in new ways, AHCs may help to solidify local relationships and encourage the emergence of a new kind of community of practice that may benefit the AHC.

Academic health centers can also seek to harvest explicit and tacit knowledge not necessarily captured through traditional means or in traditional places. For example, in addition to the knowledge from the scientific bases, there is knowledge about how the culture of particular groups influences whether or not they will follow treatment protocols, whether an insurer will reimburse for a given treatment, or how to gain authorization for a certain drug expeditiously. These aspects of providing clinical services are not resolved through literature searches, yet can impact the efficiency and effectiveness of services provided as well as patient satisfaction with care.

Patients themselves represent an untapped well of information. Clinicians may find that information shared by patients is nonlinear when juxtaposed against their structured data gathering and evaluation. Those data that are difficult to codify may, however, contain valuable insights for care of that patient or family member, or may point to the need to investigate a broader problem within the population. Academic health centers could explore alternative ways of capturing patient experiences so that patients feel heard, encounters with clinicians are efficient, and potentially useful information is identified and acted upon (possibly by someone other than the primary clinician). Patients are unlikely to know what information is most useful to clinicians, or know what has been captured from previous visits, and would likely benefit from education on how to have effective interactions with clinicians. Patient encounters can shed light not only on immediate health needs, but also on broader health needs and service preferences if such information is captured and shared within the organization.

If AHCs follow a path similar to that of organizations with robust knowledge management programs, knowledge management practices and infrastructure will become a visible and integral part of daily operations. Academic health centers can improve their ability to share and act on knowledge within and external to the organization by building facile enterprise-wide knowledge webs to support the various communities of practice that exist within AHCs or in which AHCs participate (including patients, localities, and surrounding regions). Knowledge management initiatives, however, need not and probably should not begin with organization-wide implementation. A phased implementation is more likely to yield desired results and complement availability of organizational resources. For example, an AHC can initiate limited scope, high-impact knowledge projects or build upon existing knowledge activity in the near term to strengthen their knowledge management skills, while concurrently developing a comprehensive knowledge management infrastructure.

A variety of activities are appropriate for the first phase of an AHC knowledge management program. Academic health centers can begin by identifying their existing knowledge management activities and assessing their value and potential to serve as organizational models. Units displaying clear evidence of explicit knowledge management or early adopters of IT are strong candidates for participation in larger pilot projects. Pilot projects should be designed to provide specific knowledge management capabilities to a defined community of practice. Pilot projects and ongoing programs should both have a clear strategy and be evaluated to determine if objectives are met and to identify those factors that contributed to or hindered successful knowledge management within that organization. Highlighting early projects can introduce other staff to the concepts and benefits of knowledge management, as well as reinforce the organization's commitment to the endeavor.

Once pilot projects are underway, an AHC can attend to the design of its knowledge web (i.e., goals, policies, content, processes, staff, and technological infrastructure). This design process should incorporate lessons learned from the pilot or previous knowledge management experiences, build on work accomplished or underway within information technology units and the library (including information technology and resources already in place), and focus on meeting the current and projected needs of the communities of practice. In addition, AHCs should assign responsibility for leading knowledge management efforts within the organization to "knowledge officers" and introduce performance expectations that address knowledge management behaviors by staff. Subsequent phases will likely involve expansion of pilot programs and development of the knowledge web with sustainable budgets so that the AHC as a learning organization can continue its progression.

By already serving as a steward of some AHC knowledge, providing integrated services to multiple audiences, and adapting to an increasingly technology-intensive environment, the health sciences library is well positioned to play an active role in AHC knowledge management development. (See Commentary by Watson and Fuller that accompanies this chapter.) Library staff can contribute to the development of the technological infrastructure and consideration of how to manage the organizational knowledge that resides outside standard knowledge bases. Aided by IAIMS funding from the National Library of Medicine, some health sciences libraries have already sought such a role (IAIMS Consortium, 2000).

Preparing AHC professionals

Academic health centers face substantial education and training challenges as they increase their knowledge focus and as health professionals grapple with their evolving roles. These issues impact both the educational and operational domains of AHCs, require both immediate and longer-term responses, affect current and future health professionals alike, and can be addressed through a combination of traditional and innovative approaches. The content and methodologies used in the education of health professionals will shift perceptibly as health professionals will be expected to possess competency in patient-centered care, interdisciplinary teams, evidenced-based practices, quality improvement, and informatics (Association of American Medical Colleges, 2000; Blue Ridge Academic Health Group, 2003; Institute of Medicine, 2003a). A primary objective is to lessen the distance and discomfort between human (carbon-based) and computer (silicon-based) knowledge so that accessing, processing, and applying the growing knowledge base becomes second-nature for all professionals, whether or not they are already accustomed to information technology and inclined toward ongoing knowledge synthesis.

From the perspective of transitioning an AHC into a knowledge-managed organization, the most pressing need is to ensure that staff and students alike understand that the application of relevant knowledge resources is an integral part of health care processes. This requires proficiency in the use of information systems in general and the organization's information systems specifically. It also requires that health professionals and students develop, expand, or reinforce a consistent habit of incorporating available knowledge into their work processes.

Subsequently, AHCs can focus attention on developing more subtle but equally important skills. Data management, identifying gaps in knowledge, developing strategies to fill gaps, and capturing new knowledge that emerges from organizational experience are capabilities that all health professionals need to master. Traditional classroom and training experiences, collaboratories (see below), online tutorials, new curriculum content, updated incentives, individual and work unit role models, information systems, processes, and policies can all be used to promote knowledge management learning.

Defining professionalism in, and preparing students and professionals for, a changing environment presents a complex set of questions for AHCs. What are proper roles and professional values? What proficiencies are required? And how does one demonstrate accountability in the knowledge-based, consumer-focused health economy? These questions are particularly germane as the care system shifts from one designed for and oriented to the deliverer to one designed for and oriented to the user. A critical challenge facing AHCs is to mobilize human adaptability to achieve better performance while remaining connected to and guided by the set of essential values and virtues that have traditionally shaped health professionals. Faculty and staff need to be supported during these anticipated transitions since all are at varying starting points.

A shift in the balance of power can be expected and will be a particularly important cultural change. Hierarchical practices will be replaced by collaborative models. Academic health centers need to create an environment where new behaviors and models can be developed and assessed so that health professionals can determine which approaches are most effective. This will likely result in new roles being created and new kinds of interactions emerging. Explicit boundary-spanning roles, such as clinician-executives, clinician-educators, and clinician-researchers, need to become more prevalent as a means of maintaining balance among the AHC missions of research, service, and teaching (Levinson and Rubenstein, 1999). Such individuals equipped with computer-based data repositories and support programs can assure that knowledge flows across boundaries and that the databases used by learners contain sufficient common language across domains to carry messages clearly. In time, new models of professional development may be appropriate, including knowledge managers as a specific discipline within library science or as part of the role of the clinician-educator or clinician-manager.

Learning and practice will be more interdisciplinary and will engage people working in teams or *collaboratories* (Detmer, 1997; Duderstadt, 2000). These deliberately formed educational teams include representatives of various disciplines and various roles (e.g., faculty, residents, students) and come together to address timely and often real problems. The goal of such a model is more effective knowledge transfer. Collaboratories seek to move beyond simple mastery of knowledge through memory and study to real-time learning that develops problem-solving skills, and provide opportunities to actually implement strategies. As an added benefit, the organization can capture and apply the output. New models for care, education, and research are likely to emerge from communities of practice provided with such stimulating environments.

A national health information infrastructure

Just as health care organizations need a robust information infrastructure to facilitate communication, support data capture and management, and enable knowledge development and dissemination, the health sector as a whole needs an information infrastructure to support its various domains. A national health information infrastructure (NHII) is increasingly viewed as pivotal to improving patient safety and health care quality, strengthening the public health infrastructure, and expediting the creation and dissemination of new knowledge (Detmer, 2003; Institute of Medicine, 2003b; National Committee on Vital and Health Statistics, 2001). The NHII is "the set of technologies, standards, applications, systems, values, and laws that support all facets of individual health, health care, and public health" (NHII, 2003). It will be "a comprehensive knowledge-based network of interoperable systems of clinical, public health, and personal health information" that improves decision-making by making health information available when and where it is needed and supporting the generation of new knowledge (NHII, 2003).

Much of the work in creating and managing the NHII will be done at the local or regional level. Local health information infrastructures (LHIIs) are telecommunications systems that provide the knowledge management, data processing, and communications capabilities needed to improve the health of a region. Data and communication standards will allow LHIIs to form a national network so that data can be compared across communities and new knowledge and practices can be communicated efficiently among regions.

At present, the NHII is primarily a conceptual framework with prototypes of its various components scattered across the country. Substantial attention, investment, and collaboration are needed to create the environment in which the NHII can flourish. Standards must be embraced, legal impediments removed, and incentives for IT investment and data management established (Detmer, 2003; National Committee on Vital and Health Statistics, 2001). Momentum for NHII development is building however. Since the National Committee on Vital and Health Statistics released *Information for Health* in late 2001, the federal government has begun to focus more resources and attention on the NHII.

In September 2002, the Department of Health and Human Services (DHHS) named a senior advisor to oversee the NHII initiative within the Office of Assistant Secretary for Planning and Evaluation. The federal budget for fiscal year (FY) 2004 included $50 million for demonstration projects related to the NHII and $10 million for the development of clinical terminology, messaging standards, and other tools needed to accelerate use of information technology. These same levels were proposed for the FY 2005 budget. The federal government has taken several important steps to accelerate the use of standards, including the adoption of five key health information standards for all future health information systems used by federal agencies and making a previously proprietary common medical language (i.e., SNOMED) available to the US health care community free of charge. These actions are important steps towards building a NHII and they must be continued and expanded upon. Specifically, DHHS should appoint an assistant secretary for the NHII in the office of the secretary of DHHS and direct additional funding to NHII development.

The private sector is also active in NHII development as demonstrated by the formation of several coalitions focused specifically on promoting the NHII and working to eliminate barriers to its development. The *eHealth Initiative* was launched in spring 2001. This national advocacy and trade organization represents stakeholders in the health care technology community and seeks to "drive improvement in the quality, safety and efficiency of healthcare through information and information technology" (eHealth Initiative, 2003). Among the eHealth Initiative projects underway is Connecting Communities for

Better Health. This $3.9 million program is funded by the Health Resources and Services Administration to provide seed funding and support to multi-stakeholder collaboratives within communities who are using information exchange and other IT tools to improve health care quality and efficiency (eHealth Initiative, 2003).

In spring 2002, the National Alliance for Health Information Technology, a coalition to develop voluntary IT standards for health care, was established (National Alliance for Health Information Technology, 2003). The Markle Foundation established and funded a public-private sector collaborative, Connecting for Health, in fall 2002 to address the challenges of mobilizing health information to "improve quality, conduct timely research, empower patients to become full participants in their care and bolster the public health infrastructure" (Connecting for Health, 2004). In January 2004, Connecting for Health launched its second phase of activities aimed at advancing the NHII and announced the addition of the Robert Wood Johnson Foundation as funding partner. The 2003 Institute of Medicine report on how to improve patient safety information outlines a work plan for implementing health data standards that are the "building blocks" of the NHII (Institute of Medicine, 2003b).

Academic health centers have a vested interest in seeing the NHII evolve in a timely and coherent manner and they have much to contribute to its evolution. First, AHCs and their professional organizations have considerable influence locally, regionally, and nationally that can be used to bring attention to the need for the NHII as a means of enabling knowledge management and improving health. They can help to educate the public and policy-makers on the need for substantial NHII investment to strengthen the US health system and call on the DHHS to increase the budget, visibility, and staffing for the NHII initiative.

Second, AHCs can stay informed of NHII developments and ensure that their institutional information systems keep up with NHII progress. Third, AHCs can develop training programs that will prepare all health professionals to be able to use the NHII and increase the number or size of programs that train professionals capable of building the NHII. Fourth, AHCs can participate in NHII research and development through collaborative projects in their regions (e.g., local health information infrastructures), by assessing the effectiveness of NHII projects and technologies, or by exploring how the NHII can be made most useful for health care organizations, professionals, and individual patients through its use in their own institutions. Finally, AHCs will play an ongoing role in developing the knowledge that will be made available through the NHII to support evidence-based decision-making in the health sector.

Looking even more broadly, AHCs can also contribute to and benefit from the evolution of a global health information infrastructure. By partnering with international organizations, AHCs can help to make existing knowledge more readily available to health professionals elsewhere and identify new teaching and research opportunities for their faculty. Shared knowledge may provide the foundation for collaborative relationships and structures that extend the influence of an AHC in its efforts to advance health (Michigan State University, 1999).

Partners in knowledge

For knowledge management to become an integral part of the future health system in the United States, a variety of public and private organizations must continue, expand, or initiate programs that promote both the cultural and technological requirements needed for effective knowledge management within health care organizations. The federal government bears significant responsibility for creating a knowledge management culture in the health sector and can do so through its policies and funding. The NHII initiative within the DHHS constitutes a critical step in this direction.

In addition, the National Library of Medicine (NLM) has played and continues to play a vital role in developing the knowledge management capabilities of the US health system. The NLM has built the world's largest database of peer-reviewed articles (i.e., MEDLINE); offers free access to a central repository of journal articles (i.e., PubMed Central); and developed an information resource for the public that includes access to consumer health information, clearinghouses, health organizations, and clinical trials (i.e., MEDLINE*plus*). It also developed and provides access to a database of three-dimensional images of the entire human body (i.e., the Visible Human Project) and provides access to all known DNA sequences (i.e., GenBank) and the assembled Human Genome data. In addition to providing access to medical knowledge resources, NLM conducts research on improving health care information dissemination and use as well as in computational biology and dissemination of biomedical information. Further, NLM's extramural grant programs support research in medical informatics, health information science, and biotechnology information as well as network planning and development within institutions. The Integrated Advanced Information Management Systems (IAIMS) program has supported AHCs in building information networks and organizational mechanisms for information management since 1984. The IAIMS grant program has recently been revised to reflect the current information environment facing AHCs and offers a wider range of funding mechanisms for applicant organizations (Florance and Masys, 2002).

In the private sector, AHC professional associations (i.e., the Association of American Medical Colleges, Association of Academic Health Centers, and the University HealthSystem Consortium) already support and practice knowledge management by pooling and making available AHC information to their constituents, as well as by bringing AHCs together to share knowledge and collaborate on specific initiatives. For example, AAMC maintains a web site on research compliance with links to institutions with model policies, guidelines, and training materials (AAMC, 2002a). The Health Education Assets Library (HEAL) is a national digital library created by a consortium of medical schools and funded by the National Science Foundation that provides free multimedia resources for health sciences education (HEAL, 2003).

These organizations, along with the American Medical Informatics Association (AMIA) and specialty societies, can play advocacy and educational roles as well. They can consistently articulate the need for a robust NHII to improve health in the United State to their members and policy-makers. For example, the AAMC report *Better Health 2010* describes how medical schools and teaching hospitals can "make optimal use of information technology and the Internet to improve the health of people and communities" (AAMC, 2002b). They can also develop educational programs to assist their members to develop and refine knowledge management skills. Further, these organizations can participate in shaping and developing the NHII. Many AMIA members have been and continue to be active in projects that support the NHII (e.g., standards and open source development in support of the NHII) (AMIA, 2003).

The accomplishments to date in both public and private sectors should be applauded. A significant challenge remains however. The current environment does not provide sufficient incentives for health care organizations to invest in the IT that will provide the backbone for knowledge management practices. Current reimbursement mechanisms for health care services do not reward, and in some instances penalize, health care organizations that improve their performance through IT investment (Detmer, 2003). Federal agencies, accreditation organizations, third-party payers, and the business community must create incentives that reward organizations and individuals for investing IT and using knowledge management practices to improve the quality of their services. The work of the Leapfrog Group (described in the Commentary by Galvin accompanying Chapter 2) provides an excellent model of how this objective can be achieved.

Conclusion

Increasing connectivity resulting from advances in computing and communications technology, accompanied by an increasingly consumer-driven market, is changing the speed and nature of economic interactions, as well as creating a new source of value for individuals and organizations. Organizations are changing what they do, how they do it, and how quickly they do it. At the same time, the health care sector continues to face a set of challenges that impact the nation's health, such as lack of universal coverage, the need to create safer care systems, and a gap between available and applied medical knowledge (Haynes, Hayward, and Lomas, 1995; Institute of Medicine, 1999, 2001, 2003a). Information systems and knowledge management are linked to the resolution of many of the issues facing health care organizations and will likely account for dramatic changes in health care in the next decade.

The Blue Ridge Academic Health Group is convinced that AHCs must confront the forthcoming changes directly and deliberately define their role within a health care industry that is experiencing constant change, amidst an economy that is simultaneously undergoing transformation. Despite an already full agenda and, in some cases, serious financial concerns, AHCs need to anticipate and manage their forthcoming organizational metamorphosis. To do so, AHCs will need to acquire the organizational capabilities to function effectively in an environment that is increasingly knowledge-driven, connected, fluid, dependent on more players, and much more responsive to consumers.

Academic health centers can and should expand their knowledge management capacity to convert a potential threat into an unprecedented opportunity and solidly advance their organizations. Incorporating knowledge management practices into work processes and routinely acting on insights gained from organizational knowledge will benefit each mission area, each organizational unit, and potentially each patient and staff member. Sound knowledge management is essential to AHCs as they strive to become value-driven organizations where:

- Patients feel connected and view the institution as a resource not just when they are sick, but as they manage their health on a daily basis.
- The surrounding community can visibly see how the AHC is contributing to monitoring and improving the population's health.
- The faculty and residents are supported in their clinical care decisions through comprehensive, validated, targeted information and knowledge – including clinical, financial, and administrative data.
- The education process is streamlined, interactive, customized, multidisciplinary, reflective of the current practice environment, and flexible to meet the needs of students.
- Researchers rely on institutional knowledge systems to develop proposals, manage research grants, and disseminate findings, as well as to build communities of collaborators where data are shared, combined in new ways, analyzed, and used to create new knowledge.
- The influence and revenue-generating opportunities extend beyond its immediate area.
- Collaboration and innovation are evident throughout the organization.
- Staff share a common understanding of the institution's goals and each individual decision is understood as an opportunity to support those goals.

Academic health centers (individually and as a group) possess phenomenal energy and intellectual assets with which to transform their organizations in response to changing societal needs and expectations and emerging technology. Academic health centers can use all their various kinds of knowledge to innovate their roles in the health system and can use the organizational processes to fulfill those roles. They can also identify new resources and form new collaborative relationships that will enable them to increase the visibility of knowledge management as a standard practice for effective health care, education, and research. Moreover, they can promote the development and use of a national information infrastructure as a means of advancing health. Academic health centers are well positioned to be leaders of the health community throughout the knowledge age. They must, however, take full advantage of their organizational knowledge to do so.

REFERENCES

American Medical Informatics Association (2003). *Open Source in Support of the NHII.* Bethesda, MD: AMIA. Online at http://aspe.hhs.gov/sp/nhii/documents.

Association of American Medical Colleges (AAMC) (2000). Delphi study makes prediction for the future. *AAMC Reporter*, **9**(5), 2000.

(2002a). *AAMC Research Compliance Resources*. Washington, DC: Association of American Medical Colleges. Online at www.aamc.org/research/dbr/compliance/startcom.htm.

(2002b). *Better Health 2010: a Report by the AAMC's Better Health 2010 Advisory Board*, ed. V. Florance. Washington, DC: Association of American Medical Colleges. Online at www.aamc.org/betterhealth.

Angell, M. (2000). Is academic medicine for sale? *New England Journal of Medicine*, **342**(20), 508–10.

Balu, R. (2000). KPMG faces the Internet test. *Fast Company*, March, pp. 50–2.

Bates, D. W., Leape, L. L., Cullen, D. J., Laird, N., Peterson, L. A., Teich, J. M., Burdick, E., Hickey, M., Kleefield, S., Shea, B., Vander Vliet, M. and Seger, D. L. (1998). Effect of computerized physician order entry and a team intervention on prevention of serious medication errors. *Journal of the American Medical Association*, **280**(15), 1311–16.

Blue Ridge Academic Health Group (2003). *Reforming Medical Education: Urgent Priority for the Academic Health Center in the New Century*. Atlanta, GA: Emory University.

Bock, F. (1998). The intelligent organization. In *Prism*. Cambridge, MA: Arthur D. Little.

Borowitz, S. M. and Wyatt, J. C. (1998). The origin, content, and workload of e-mail consultations. *Journal of the American Medical Association*, **280**(15), 1331–4.

Center for Business Innovation (1996a). *Case Study: Knowledge Management at Ernst & Young*. Washington, DC: Ernst & Young LLP.

(1996b). *Case Study: Knowledge Management at Hoffman-LaRoche*. Washington, DC: Ernst & Young LLP.

Chueh, H. and Barnett, G. O. (1997). "Just-in-time" clinical information. *Academic Medicine*, **72**, 512–17.

Cole, R. E. (1998). Introduction: knowledge and the firm. *California Management Review*, **40**(3), 15–21.

Connecting for Health (2004). *Press Release: Connecting for Health Announces Commitment to Create Incremental Roadmap for Achieving Electronic Connectivity in Health Care*. Online at http://www.connectingforhealth.org.

COR Health LLC (2000). Research drives Emory site design, structure, and strategy. *Internet Healthcare Strategies*, **2**(4), 5–8.

Davenport, T. H. and Prusak, L. (1998). *Working Knowledge: How Organizations Manage What They Know*. Boston, MA: Harvard Business School Press.

Davis, S. and Meyer, C. (1998). *Blur: the Speed of Change in the Connected Economy*. Reading, MA: Addison-Wesley.

Detmer, D. E. (1997). Knowledge: a mountain or a stream? *Science*, **275**, March 28. Online at http://www.sciencemag.org.

(2003). Building the national health information infrastructure for personal health, health care services, and research. *BMC Medical Informatics and Decision Making*, **3**(1), 1.

Drucker, P. F. (1988). The coming of the new organization. *Harvard Business Review*, January-February **66**(1), 45–9.

Duderstadt, J. J. (2000). *A University for the 21st Century*. Ann Arbor, MI: University of Michigan Press.

Duke University Medical Center (2000). *Heart Center First*. Online at http://heartcenter.mc.duke.edu/heartcenternsf/webpagesfirsts.

eHealth Initiative (2003). *Who we are*. Online at http://www.ehealthinitiative.org.

Emory Health System (2000). *Emory Health Connection*. Online at http://www.emory.org/healthconnection.

Ernst & Young LLP (1998). *Lessons Learned* Business Case Studies. Washington, DC: Ernst & Young LLP.

Florance, V. and Masys, D. (2002). *Next Generation IAIMS: Binding Knowledge to Effective Action*. Washington, DC: Association of American Medical Colleges. Online at http://www.aamc.org/programs/betterhealth/iaimsinside.pdf.

Goldsmith, J. (2000). How will the Internet change our health system? *Health Affairs*, **19**(1), 148–56.

Haynes, R. B., Hayward, R. S. A. and Lomas, J. (1995). Bridges between health care research evidence and clinical practice. *Journal of the American Medical Informatics Association*, **2**, 342–50.

Health Education Assets Library (HEAL) (2003). *Heal History*. Online at www.health central.org.

Health Web (2000). *Health Web*. Online at http://healthweb.org/index.html.

Hunt, D. L., Haynes, R. B., Hanna, S. E. and Smith, K. (1998). Effects of computer-based clinical decision support on physician performance and patient outcomes: a systematic review. *Journal of the American Medical Association*, **280**(15), 1339–46.

IAIMS Consortium (2000). *IAIMS Grant Recipients*. Online at http://www.urmc.rochester.edu/iaims/consortium/recipients.html.

Institute of Medicine (1999). *To Err is Human*. Washington, DC: National Academy Press.

   (2001). *Crossing the Quality Chasm: a New Health System for the 21st Century*. Washington, DC: National Academy Press.

   (2003a). *Health Professions Education: a Bridge to Quality*. Washington, DC: National Academy Press.

   (2003b). *Patient Safety: Achieving a New Standard*. Washington, DC: National Academy Press.

InteliHealth (2004). *The Harvard Medical School – InteliHealth Partnership*. Online at http://www.intelihealth.com.

Johns Hopkins (1999). *Johns Hopkins Family Health Book*. New York: Harper Collins.

Johns Hopkins Medicine (1999a). *Education and Training Opportunities*. Online at http://infonet.welch.jhu.edu/education.

   (1999b). *Healthcare Information*. Online at http://infonet.welch.jhu.edu/clinical.

   (1999c). *Research*. Online at http://infonet.welch.jhu.edu/research.

Kurzweil, R (1999). *The Age of Spiritual Machines*. New York: Viking.

Levinson, W. and Rubenstein, A. (1999). Mission critical: integrating clinician-educators into academic medical centers. *New England Journal of Medicine*, **341**, 840–44.

Madden, M. and Rainie, L. (2003). *America's Online Pursuits: the Changing Picture of Who's Online and What They Do*. Washington, DC: Pew Internet & American Life Project. Online at www.pewinternet.org.

McCune, J. C. (1999). Thirst for knowledge. *Management Review*, **88**(4), 10–12.

McDermott, R. and O'Dell, C. (2000). *Overcoming the Cultural Barriers to Sharing Knowledge*. Online at http://www.apqc.org/free/articles.km/0200.

Michigan State University (1999). *The Institute of International Health*. Online at http://www.msu.edu/unit/iih.

Miller, L. (1999). Guidelines: libraries offer cures for web confusion. *USA Today* July 14, 5D.

Murray, G. (1999). *Connecting Communities: the Power of Sharing Knowledge*. White Paper, International Data Corporation. Online at www.computerworld.com.

National Alliance for Health Information Technology (2003). *About Us*. Online at http://www.hospitalconnect.com/nahit/about.html.

National Committee on Vital and Health Statistics (NCVHS) (1998). *Assuring a Health Dimension for the National Health Information Infrastructure*. Online at http://ncvhs.hhs.gov/hii-nii.htm.

   (2001). *Information for Health: a Strategy for Building the National Health Information Infrastructure*. Washington, DC: US Department of Health and Human Services. Online at http://www.ncvhs.hhs.gov/nhiilayo.pdf.

National Health Information Infrastructure (NHII) (2003). *Frequently Asked Questions About the NHII*. Washington, DC: US Department of Health and Human Services. Online at http://aspe.hhs.gov/nhii/FAQ.html.

National Library of Medicine (2004). *Fact Sheet: the National Library of Medicine*. Bethesda, MD: National Library of Medicine. Online at http://www.nlm.nih.gov/pubs/factsheets.nlm.html.

National Research Council (2000a). *Networking Health: Prescriptions for the Internet*. Washington, DC: National Academy Press.

   (2000b). *The Digital Dilemma: Intellectual Property in the Information Age*. Washington, DC: National Academy Press.

Neuborne, E. (1999). It's showtime. *Business Week*, June 7.

Nonaka, I. and Takeuchi, H. (1995). *The Knowledge-Creating Company*. New York: Oxford University Press.

North Carolina AHEC Program (1999). *AHEC Digital Library and Resource System, Business Plan*. Online at www.hsl.unc.edu/ahec/adlrs/bizplan.htm.

Novartis (1999). *Our Commitment to Life Sciences and Our Research and Development Strategy*. Online at www.novartis.com.

O'Dell, C. and Grayson, C. J. (1998). If only we knew what we know: identification and transfer of internal best practices. *California Management Review*, **40**(3), 90–111.

Probst, G. J. B. (1998). Practical knowledge management: a model that works. In: *Prism*. Cambridge, MA: Arthur D. Little.

Sackett, D. L. and Straus, S. E. (1998). Finding and applying evidence during clinical rounds: the "evidence cart." *Journal of the American Medical Association*, **280**(15), 1336–8.

Senge, P., Kleiner, A., Roberts, C., Ross, R., Roth, G. and Smith, B. (1999). *The Dance of Change: the Challenges of Sustaining Momentum in Learning Organizations*. New York: Doubleday.

Sikorski, R. and Peters, R. (1998). Tools for change: CME on the Internet. *Journal of the American Medical Association*, **280**(11), 1013–14.

Stanford University (2000). *Office of Technological Licensing*. Online at http://otl.stanford.edu/about/what.html.

Stewart, T. (1997). *Intellectual Capital: the New Wealth of Organizations*. New York: Doubleday.

University of Chicago (1999). *Welcome to UC-IAIMS!* Online at http://www.uciaims.uchicago.edu/interface/welcome.htm.

University of North Carolina-Chapel Hill (2000). *Office of Technology Development*. Online at http://research.unc.edu/otd/services/services.html.

University of Virginia (1997). UVA faculty share teaching images on the web. *Inside Information.* Online at http://www.med.virginia.edu/hslibrary/newsletter/1997/imagedb.html.

University of Virginia Health System (1999). *Clinical Data Repository.* Online at http://www.med.virginia.edu/achs/health_informatics/cdr/generalinfo.html.

(2000a). *Educational Materials for Healthcare Professionals.* Online at http://hsc.virginia.edu/medicine/clinical/pediatrics/CMC/edmaterials.html.

(2000b). *Multimedia Tutorials for Children and Parents.* Online at http://hsc.virginia.edu/medicine/clinical/pediatrics/CMC/tutorial.html.

Wah, L. (1999). Behind the buzz. *Management Review,* **88**(4), 16–26.

WebEBM (2000). *Evidence-Based Medicine.* Online at http//www.webebm.com.

World Bank (2000). *Education Strategy: Examples of Knowledge Sharing.* Online at http://www.worldbank.org/ks/hatml/examples_education.html.

Case study

Whose knowledge is it anyway? David Geffen School of Medicine, University of California, Los Angeles

LuAnn Wilkerson, Ed.D. and J. Michael McCoy, M.D.

Part I: the website proliferation saga

As the Internet expanded its influence in the late 1990s, websites proliferated at the University of California, Los Angeles (UCLA) medical center and medical school with many individuals and academic groups establishing a homepage, each one offering a distinct entry into different segments of the institution. With this proliferation of unconnected sites, faculty and staff users began to complain to the chief information officer (CIO) about how difficult it was to find the information or resources that they needed to get their work done. After hearing Sherrilynne Fuller from the University of Washington speak about the effectiveness of creating an internal, or intranet, web site that would provide a collection of tools to support the practice and research needs of faculty and staff, a "what do you need to do today" view of on-line resources, the CIO decided to build a similar portal. The CIO envisioned the portal as the entrance to two separate web sites: an *intranet* site for faculty physicians and staff for patient care purposes and an *extranet* to provide the information resources that would be useful to patients and the communities served by UCLA.

The intranet proved easier to accomplish since the CIO already controlled many of the resources for patient care. Five years earlier, a massive effort to centralize email had created a unified system for the enterprise and the new web page would provide a place to enter the email system for everyone in the institution. Other services such as digital paging, faculty directories, and links to departmental websites that were beginning to emerge could also be directly accessed from this page. He explored what medical center admissions

LuAnn Wilkerson is Senior Associate Dean for Medical Education and Director of the Center for Educational Development and Research in the David Geffen School of Medicine at UCLA. J. Michael McCoy is Chief Information Officer, UCLA Healthcare, Senior Associate Director, UCLA Medical Center, and Associate Dean, David Geffen School of Medicine at UCLA.

and billing, the biomedical library, and the medical school wanted to add to the site to support patient care. The resulting page was rolled out almost overnight with the purpose of providing one-stop shopping for physicians in the enterprise. By 1996, the site included links to Health Topics, News, For Health Care Providers, General Information, the Biomedical Library, the Health Network, and the School of Medicine.

The needs of the students, teachers, and researchers in the institution were much harder to meet and the culture of going it alone was well established. Given the difficulty experienced by the medical school staff in accessing the medical center server to install new web materials for education and research as they were developed, in 1998 the medical school decided to establish its own website separate from that of the medical center. The plan for a coalition of websites began to unravel quickly. The office of medical student affairs created a new site for admissions information, applications, and financial aid. The dean of research set up a site for locating specific investigators and research tools. The library expanded its online presence as part of a system-wide initiative with a growing resource of digital texts, journals, and databases. The University mandated a common "look and feel" and created yet another health care homepage that could be entered from the front door of the University.

Part II: developing a front door

By 1999, there were two homepages – an intranet for the medical center and a public site for the medical school – with no one willing or able to coordinate the continuing growth of departmental and individual faculty websites. In addition, the patients who found their way to either of these UCLA medical sites did not find information relevant to getting health care services or learning more about their disease.

The situation came to a head in late 2001 when the installation of new workstations in the medical center and clinics led to a debate over which site to use as the homepage – the medical center or the medical school. Marketing, focused on the need to better connect the medical center services and patients, pushed an expensive, flashy proposal by an external consulting firm to replace the clunky intranet. The CIO, determined to keep the management of knowledge resources for patient care, research, and education paramount in the new product, insisted that an internal task force of marketing, research, education, and technology staff be appointed to plan and develop a fully integrated and consistent website traversing the entire depth of the healthcare enterprise. After a grueling six months of struggle over the goal of this new product, the task force recommended that the Medical Sciences (i.e., medical center and medical school) site use a database for information architecture with all content owned and updated by individual departments and programs and displayed in a single institutional website under one of three major categories: Patient Care, Education, and Research. Rather than commit to the Mayo Medical Center approach of building a patient education presence, the task force recommended using *MedLine Plus* delivered within the institutional template for easy movement between this National Library of Medicine resource and local resources. The task force recommended identifying incentives for conversion to the new site by individual programs and departments rather than requiring participation (e.g, individual ownership of information, an authoring environment and template to make site creation and maintenance easier, improved searching, and the use of medical center promotional dollars to benefit all constituencies). Eighteen months after the initial commitment to solve this knowledge management problem by the director of the medical center, a new prototype was distributed widely for comment and critique. Two months later, conversion began in earnest. A pilot period in which the old and new sites were both maintained resulted in a full transition within six months, bringing the entire process from initial problem definition to resolution within two years. One final step is underway to migrate resources for providers located on the existing intranet to the new portal.

Commentary

Linda Watson, M.L.S and Sherrilynne Fuller, Ph.D.

Introduction

Interwoven throughout this chapter is recognition of the critical roles that libraries and information technology play in the knowledge work of an AHC (i.e., research, education, patient care, and community service). The chapter emphasizes that defining the knowledge assets of an enterprise as complex as an AHC goes far beyond the more commonly understood "knowledge-based information" such as that represented in books and journals and more recently in databases of gene sequences. The expanded definition includes organizational knowledge that is embedded in the daily routines of employees, the patient and transactional data collected, the processes, and communication that takes place across the enterprise and beyond, including population-based data. Most importantly, at its core, the knowledge assets of the enterprise must be made available in increasingly interdisciplinary ways throughout the enterprise and beyond – wherever decisions are being made. This commentary recognizes that within the familiar idea of libraries as knowledge repositories, the environment is changing considerably, and with it, the role of the librarian. We urge AHCs to leverage the expertise of librarians to address the task of managing broader organizational knowledge and communications and, indeed, play a role in transforming the role of the AHC in the knowledge economy.

Linda Watson is Associate Dean at University of Virginia School of Medicine and Director of the Claude Moore Health Sciences Library, University of Virginia. Sherrilynne Fuller is Professor of Biomedical and Health Informatics at the University of Washington School of Medicine and Director of Health Sciences Libraries at the University of Washington Health Sciences Center.

Knowledge repositories

Libraries have been the time-honored repository for access to recorded knowledge such as that found in printed books, journals, and other published information, and collectively have served as a world archive, a somewhat passive role that required users to come to a physical location. With the advent of increased information in electronic form, whether derived from a print version or "born digital," the landscape has become more complex with distributed access to resources the norm. Technology has greatly facilitated access to information, but at the same time has created significant challenges in accessing, managing, and preserving these vital resources. The scholarly communication system is under serious stress fueled by rising journal costs as well as shifting application and interpretations of copyright law in the digital age.

In 1995, Nina Matheson, one of the visionaries of medical librarianship, observed that one of the grand challenges facing society was

the creation of digital knowledge management systems that can acquire, conserve, organize, retrieve, display, and distribute what is known today in a manner that informs and educates, facilitates the discovery and creation of new knowledge, and contributes to the health and welfare of the planet. (Matheson, 1995)

She envisioned a future in which all scholarly scientific knowledge was accessible in the public domain, with ownership (and the corresponding responsibility for quality, access, integrity, and preservation of the knowledge) shifting to the creators or their institutions. She also envisioned that an effective system of the future be built and maintained through the collaboration of librarians, computer scientists, and subject experts. We are no closer now to achieving that vision than we were in 1995.

Are AHCs willing to assume the role as stewards of their own scientific knowledge, rather than relinquishing that role to commercial journal and textbook publishers as in the current system of scholarly communication and in the process gain increased visibility and recognition for their value to science and society? Eight years after Matheson's vision, a movement is growing among research libraries to foster the development of institutional repositories – digital collections of an institution's intellectual output (Crow, 2002). Such a repository could include articles, data sets, images, video, courseware, and websites. One could further imagine content from clinical care – best practices, clinical pathways, and other significant efforts to be shared with the world. The library, with its expertise in classification of knowledge and cataloging of resources, could create metadata for consistent and flexible retrieval and use. Connections could readily be made between research results reported by faculty, facilitating interdisciplinary work, both within the institution and externally (Fuller *et al.*, 2002). The library could be the agent that coordinates the process, sets up the technology for submission and preservation, and builds partnerships with groups of faculty to ensure continuity of the system. The DSpace Federation, for example, is a group of universities using digital repository software developed at Massachusetts Institute of Technology to capture, store, index, preserve, and redistribute the intellectual output of a university's research faculty in digital formats.

Consider linking this publicly available repository with a parallel internal repository to which is added more proprietary information, and which also links to the AHC's Electronic Medical Record (EMR). The library would work with the technology teams developing the EMR to assure transparent navigation from the EMR environment to the knowledge resource environment through various vocabulary and coding systems (Tarczy-Hornoch *et al.*, 1997). The teams would also create or apply technologies to permit data mining and analysis. From reports of fledging attempts to build repositories, however, it has been clear that this is no small undertaking and the process has to be driven by faculty who are willing to submit their works and publish in this way. It is not at all evident that medical faculty or their AHCs are ready for this investment. But should they be encouraged in this direction?

This is not a new concept. Since 1984, the National Library of Medicine (NLM) through its IAIMS program has offered grants to help organizations create institution-wide information management policies and build institution-wide computer networks that link and relate library systems with individual and institutional databases and information files, within and external to the institution, for patient care, research, education, and administration. In a review of IAIMS that took place from 1998 to 2000, the following observation was made:

The information "space" in which decisions are made and learning takes place is fed by hundreds of thousands of information sources of varying quality. The markers of quality and authority upon which people traditionally base their information choices in the print world (e.g., peer-reviewed journal, scientifically sound experimental method, physician-dictated notes in a patient record) are more difficult to discern and confirm. Many kinds of information can be presented to the decision-maker or learner or patient at the same time. How best to draw from the common information space the right subset of information and present it in the way most effective for a given problem and person is a fundamental challenge for academic health sciences centers in the coming decade. (Florance and Masys, 2002)

The librarian's role

The key is getting the right information to the right person at the right time to make a decision or take an action. It will take time until systems are conceived and developed that can accomplish this consistently. In the meantime, AHCs that want to leverage the tacit knowledge residing in the expertise and know-how of their clinicians, researchers and employees, should more fully leverage the knowledge of their librarians towards that end (Association of Academic Health Sciences Libraries, 2003). With the advent of do-it-yourself searching, and the ubiquitous Google approach to finding floods of information on the Internet, requests for expert searching by librarians have plummeted. But at what cost in quality of information received and time expended to get it? Recent reports have pointed to the importance of medical librarian expertise in reducing medical errors (Homan, 2002; McLellan, 2001). The medical library profession has begun to explore a redefinition of service roles in order to bring their expertise closer to the point of care or to the research bench (Davidoff and Florance, 2000; Shipman et al., 2002). Some envision a hybrid professional with formal training in both information management and the discipline being served, an "in-context" professional who is an integral part of the patient care or research team and is the human focal point for knowledge management. This would require not only an investment in training, but also an institutional investment in employing enough of these professionals to effectively serve the most critical information needs (Florance, Guise, and Ketchell, 2002).

   In the absence of sufficient numbers to provide every health professional with a "personal knowledge manager" librarians have traditionally been at the forefront of teaching next-generation health professionals about how to manage information and knowledge, and are also increasingly working with patients, families, and the general public. In the past that teaching was often done on an elective basis with students introduced during ori-entations at the beginning of medical school and later as they participated in problem-based elective courses. Increasingly, however, librarians are now teaching core courses, along with medical faculty, focused on course-integrated information retrieval, evaluation, and management. Termed "information literacy," these skills are critical for teaching students to rapidly locate and critically evaluate core information in support of the practice of evidence-based medicine (Burrows *et al.*, 2003; Sackett, 2000). Skill in identifying, assessing, and managing information for better decision-making is a critical underpinning to life-long learning so essential for keeping up with the changes in science and healthcare. AHCs should require that information mastery and critical thinking be considered core competencies and that training and tools be provided for all students and practitioners across the continuum of learning, from undergraduate to graduate to continuing education.

Managing the knowledge of the organization

Organizational knowledge consists of all the procedural, research data, institutional practices, business practices, clinical data as well as the published contributions of faculty, staff, and students. Increasingly there is a demand for information that cross-cuts all of these types of knowledge and, in fact, organizes it in new ways to answer challenging management questions. The Health Insurance Portability and Accountability Act requirements, human subjects review procedures, research policies, and procedures to name just a few are causing substantial changes in the way that we look at the design of information systems and services. No longer will data and information existing in database "silos" support the critical information challenges facing AHCs, as they must become more and more interdisciplinary in their education, teaching, and, most importantly, research. Librarians have shown that they can play a critical role in transforming these information systems and resources because they are viewed as neutral entities in the organization with a broad mission to support the research, education, clinical, and service missions of the AHC.

At the University of Virginia, the health system website began under the direction of the health sciences library with a focus on the academic mission. When organizational strategy began to envision more integration with the clinical mission, it moved to a home within health systems computing. The health system webmaster, however, is a librarian who has brought her organizational and knowledge management skills to bear on the design and development of the site. This has recently extended to an intranet site with the goal to better manage the organization's internal knowledge.

At the University of Washington (UW), IAIMS planning and implementation were co-led by the Library Director and the Medical Director for the Harborview Medical Center. The IAIMS process resulted in a transformation of the library as well as the information systems of the institution itself. New roles emerged for librarians, including being members of the clinical information systems development team; leader of the development of an academic program in biomedical and health informatics; educator of health sciences students and faculty; and developer of integrated tools and web resources in clinical care, bioinformatics, education, and community services (Fuller *et al.*, 1995, 2000). A key lesson learned from the IAIMS processes at UW and other IAIMS institutions is that the major challenges of such systems are not technical but social and cultural. Time and again IAIMS processes have shown that librarians possess critical organizational and leadership skills in creating processes for moving complex information systems developments forward.

Conclusion

Dr William Stead has very eloquently described the challenge and reward of placing the library at the center of knowledge management for the enterprise:

The changing economic environment in which our biomedical enterprises operate presents unparalleled opportunities to the profession of medical librarianship. Evidence-based medicine, patient empowerment, asynchronous learning networks, and research collaboratories each involve a new type of shared information, or access to information in new ways or by different people. These tasks are ones with which librarianship is directly involved. Librarians are therefore placed perfectly to provide new products and services. To position the library at the epicenter of the networked biomedical enterprise we must meet three challenges. We must align the library's business strategy with that of the larger enterprise. We must provide services in ways that will scale-up to enable new business strategies. We must measure the effectiveness of services in ways that document their role in supporting the enterprise. (Stead, 1998)

The challenge for AHCs is to invest fully in and leverage the assets of the Health Sciences Library to transform knowledge management throughout the organization. Thus AHCs should:

- Become stewards of the scientific knowledge production process and re-assert their rights to utilize that knowledge in the best interests of society.
- Invest in integrated interdisciplinary knowledge systems to include organizational knowledge, scientific research findings, and clinical information systems to support the production of new knowledge.
- Utilize the knowledge and skills of librarians in managing knowledge as an organizational asset and teaching critical knowledge management skills.

REFERENCES

Association of Academic Health Sciences Libraries (2003). *Building on Success: Charting the Future of Knowledge Management within the Academic Health Center.* Seattle, WA: The Association of Academic Health Sciences Libraries. Online at http://www.aahsl.org/new/display_page.cfm?file_id=170.

Burrows, S., Moore, K., Arriaga, J., Paulaitis, G. and Lemkau, H. L. (2003). Developing an "evidence-based medicine and use of the biomedical literature" component as a longitudinal theme of an outcomes-based medical school curriculum: year 1. *Journal of the Medical Library Association,* **91**(1), 34–41.

Crow, R. (2002). *The Case for Institutional Repositories: a SPARC Position Paper.* Washington, DC: The Scholarly Publishing & Academic Resources Coalition. Online at http://www.arl.org/sparc/IR/ir.html.

Davidoff, F. and Florance, V. (2000). The informationist: a new health profession? [editorial]. *Annals of Internal Medicine,* **32**(12), 996–8.

Florance, V. and Masys, D. (2002). *Next-Generation IAIMS: Binding Knowledge to Effective Action.* Washington, DC: Association of American Medical Colleges. Online at http://www.aamc.org/programs/betterhealth/iaimsinside.pdf.

Florance, V., Guise, N. B. and Ketchell, D. S. (2002). Information in context: integrating information specialists into practice settings. *Journal of the Medical Library Association,* **90**(1), 49–58.

Fuller, S., Kalet, I. and Tarczy-Hornoch, P. (2000). Biomedical and health informatics research and education at the University of Washington. In *Yearbook of Medical Informatics,* pp. 107–13. Stuttgart, Germany: Schattauer.

Fuller, S., Braude, R. M., Florance, V. and Frisse, M. E. (1995). Managing information in the academic medical center: building an integrated information environment. *Academic Medicine,* **70**(10), 887–91.

Fuller, S., Revere, D., Soderland, S., Bugni, P., Kadiyska, Y., Reber, L., Fuller, H. and Martin, G. (2002). Modeling a concept-based information system to promote scientific discovery: the Telemakus System. In *Proceedings of the Annual Symposium of the American Medical Informatics Association,* p. 1023. Bethesda, MD: American Medical Informatics Association.

Homan, J. M. (2002). The role of medical librarians in reducing medical errors. *Health Leaders Online,* September 16. Online at http://www.healthleaders.com/news/print.php?contentid=38058.

Matheson, N. W. (1995). Things to come: postmodern digital knowledge management and medical informatics. *Journal of the American Medical Informatics Association*, **2**(2), 73–8.

McLellan, F. (2001). 1966 and all that – when is a literature search done? *Lancet*, **358**, 646.

Sackett, D. L. (2000). *Evidence-based Medicine: How to Practice and Teach EBM*. New York: Churchill Livingstone.

Shipman, J. P., Cunningham, D. J., Holst, R. and Watson, L. (2002). The Informationist Conference: report. *Journal of the Medical Library Association*, **90**(4), 458–64.

Stead, W. (1998). Positioning the library at the epicenter of the networked biomedical enterprise. *Bulletin of the Medical Library Association*, **86**(1), 26–30.

Tarczy-Hornoch, P., Kwan-Gett, T. S., Fouche, L., Hoath, J., Fuller, S., Ibrahim, K. N., Ketchell, D. S. and LoGerfo, J. P. (1997). Meeting clinician information needs by integrating access to the medical record and knowledge resources via the WEB. *Journal of the American Medical Informatics Association. Symposium Supplement. Proceedings of the 1997 AMIA Annual Fall Symposium*, pp. 809–813.

6   e-Health challenges and opportunities

Introduction

The advent of the Internet has been almost universally heralded. It has been compared to most of the important technological milestones in human history, from the capture of fire to the development of electricity, the steam engine, and the telephone. The Internet's dynamic, even explosive, growth is often described using biological metaphors (e.g., "a squirming, protoplasmic nexus of informational activity") that suggest the development of a nascent hypertrophic organism of uncertain but highly promising ontogeny (Valovic, 2000, p. 24).

Indeed, the Internet, as a technology platform, is having a significant, even revolutionary, impact on communications, on the flow of and access to information, on the speed and efficiency of many types of transactions, and on connectivity between and among an ever-growing mass of electronically networked individuals, organizations, and systems. It is affecting everything from the behavior of individuals to the conduct of commerce. "The Net" has spawned whole industries and transformed others. It has created new categories of jobs and career paths, while making others obsolete. It has affected many aspects of our culture, from language, to customs, to the meaning of symbols. Its ubiquity crosses national borders and political boundaries. It has created untold thousands of virtual or cyber communities and has forever transformed many real communities. It sparked "irrationally exuberant" activity in the nation's stock market, catalyzing the creation (and then subsequently destruction) of new wealth.

Novel applications of Internet-based technologies are found or created almost daily. And several public and private initiatives, including the government sponsored Next Generation Initiative (NGI) and the private-sector sponsored Internet 2 Consortium, are currently working to develop vastly enhanced networking technologies, applications, and new Internet platforms for a variety of commercial, governmental, research, and communications applications (National Research Council, 2000).

This nascent technology, perhaps somewhat like a developing nervous system, is vectoring in multiple directions, creating new connections through multiple signaling pathways, and triggering adaptive (including protective and competitive) responses of many kinds. It is impossible to predict at this stage what this evolving system will eventually look like, how it will function, or even whether it will proliferate into an "Internet-work" of Internet platforms. It is quite possible that the Internet's proliferation will be such that it will never be completely comprehensible; that what we now call the Internet will give way to simply ubiquitous connectivity among increasingly intelligent agents endowed with a combination of continuous, at will, and/or contingent, "with permission" data sharing. In any case, it is relatively certain that the Internet as a technology platform will continue for the foreseeable future to grow and to spawn unprecedented and increasingly ubiquitous connectivity among networked users and systems.

Yet relative to other industries, health care organizations including AHCs have been slow to adopt Internet technologies and capabilities and push the boundaries of e-health. Most health care policy-makers and leaders recognize that the Internet and its related technologies hold great promise for enhancing health care, health sciences research and training, and drug and device development. But few AHCs or other health care organizations have aggressively pursued the development of Internet-based resources or technologies to support their core missions, competencies, or competitiveness in the short term (i.e., three to five years).

The Blue Ridge Group believes that e-health capabilities are essential for twenty-first century health care organizations and that AHCs have much to contribute as centers for innovation, collaboration, and nationwide advocacy in the development of Internet-based capabilities in the health sector. Further, the Internet and the evolving domain of e-health will be pivotal to the development of a value-driven health system and value-driven health organizations (see Chapter 2). The Internet is playing a major role in the standardization of health industry data, connectivity, and communications, and is highlighting the need for industry-wide rationalization of provider and payer systems. It is providing a platform that fosters collaboration in the creation of new knowledge and increases the efficiency of knowledge dissemination. It is empowering providers and patients in the care process through access to new health and care-related information and technologies and is supporting the growth of self-care, remote care, and customized care capabilities. It offers as yet untapped capabilities for increasing the speed of and reducing the costs of administrative functions (e.g., assessing eligibility). And it offers a mechanism for capturing and sharing performance data that can be used to guide health care decisions and in so doing support urgently needed efficiencies in the health sector.

This chapter surveys the status and trajectory of Internet technologies, resources, and commerce in the health care sector. It explores how AHCs can leverage the Internet to strengthen their knowledge management capabilities, find efficient ways provide their current services, develop new services for their customers, and become value-driven organizations. The chapter presents a series of findings, recommendations, and implementation guidelines for leaders and policy-makers seeking to understand and prioritize the evaluation, adoption, development, or enhancement of Internet-based health care, research, and training resources with a five to ten year horizon.

Connectivity for e-Health

Development and adoption of common standards are vital to the growth and maturation of most modern industries. The Internet has emerged as a major driver for and enabler of standards in the health sector. It is a common platform upon which an important array of new communications and connectivity technologies must be developed and deployed. With it, health care organizations can standardize data utilization and transmission, integrate disparate clinical and administrative systems, improve access to medical knowledge, open new research frontiers in bioinformatics, pharmacogenomics, and other emerging fields, and if the architecture can be sorted out, allow creative new combinations to emerge. In aggregate and over time these capabilities will enable the standardization of health and illness care (e.g., elimination of inappropriate practice variation) with accompanying quality improvement and cost savings.

The web has become the preferred connectivity technology because of the early and virtually universal acceptance and use of standard underlying software languages. Hypertext Markup Language (HTML), with Extensive Markup Language (XML), and other emerging standards allow web sites to be linked and their contents to be transmitted to one another through a relatively simple and easy to use web browser. Browsers can be employed on everything from dedicated terminals, to desktop and portable computers, to cell phones and other devices, thus enabling unprecedented and relatively inexpensive communication among users, systems, and sites. Also important to the power of the Internet as a common platform is the increasing use of sophisticated database coding. For instance, object-oriented, relational databases enable the discrete labeling and identification of every element in a database. This labeling enables the data to be utilized, analyzed, and manipulated with almost unlimited flexibility and power.

Connectivity challenges

It has long been recognized that facile communication and data transmittal are essential to improving the quality and efficiency of health care. Yet data sharing and processing are among the most daunting issues in the health care industry. Health care is in a pre-industrial era in terms of its integration and commitment to common standards and strategies. Health-related standards such as HL-7, SNOMED-CT, LOINC, and others under development will allow biomedical transactions to flow upon the "highways" offered by the Internet. The progress achieved to date, however, is the result of a long and arduous process and much work remains to be done.

Many record keeping and clinical assessment and reporting systems, including relatively sophisticated computer and software systems, proliferated over the course of the twentieth century. But most developed as proprietary systems and were designed to address local and/or payer specific recording and reporting needs and not to facilitate communication with other systems. With an estimated 30 billion eligibility, claim, laboratory, and referral transactions per year alone, the health care industry is notorious for the difficulties encountered in deriving and sharing data among payers, providers, laboratories, and patients.

The sheer volume of transactions creates one hurdle. A second major hurdle in the implementation of standardized health-related data systems is the diversity and complexity of the records that are created and utilized in support of the care process. The entire spectrum includes medical histories, diagnoses, examination notes, treatment records, prescriptions, test and lab results, regulatory compliance reports, insurance eligibility, billing and collection functions, scheduling, referral data, hospitalization records, and so forth. (In addition, outside the traditional clinical setting, workplace-related health and risk management initiatives also generate health-related data.) Today many of these records are generated at dedicated-computer-aided patient intake stations, some on paper forms. Some records are jotted down by hand by the health care professional, and some are transmitted by facsimile or dedicated electronic pipeline from provider to payer. The average medical center or health care system uses at least six different clinical and administrative systems. The complexity of the record creation and record keeping functions, and the multiple administrative and delivery situations that give rise to them, have so far defied standardization.

Farthest along in electronic transmission are insurance-related transactions. Two-thirds of health claims are processed electronically; the majority of these are pharmaceutical claims. Eighty-seven percent of hospital claims are submitted electronically. However, many of these are transferred in tape media, and the vast majority flow through dedicated, proprietary lines from legacy systems that are extremely expensive to maintain and cumbersome to operate. Heretofore, even with electronic submission, relatively few claims have been adjudicated electronically, creating industry-wide problems with the management of billions of denied and delayed claims (Goldsmith, 2000).

This situation should improve as the Center for Medicare and Medicaid Services (CMS) moves closer to its objective of eliminating paper reimbursement claims, except for limited circumstances, and the practices and standards that health care providers adopt to meet CMS requirements spill over to how they submit claims to other payers (CMS, 2004). The administrative simplification sections of the Health Insurance Portability and Accountability Act of 1996 (HIPAA, P.L. 104–191) constitute the US government's first step in setting transmission standards for health data and has already yielded significant progress on this front. (Other recent steps are highlighted in the discussion of a national health information infrastructure in Chapter 5.)

A third hurdle in achieving ubiquitous connectivity is the requirement that personal health data are protected by systems and practices that protect the privacy of patient data to the extent humanly possible. The HIPAA included provisions to establish federal privacy standards and thus provide the foundation for the health sector to start addressing this hurdle. In response to HIPAA, the Department of Health and Human Services (DHHS) has established regulations for obtaining, holding, transmitting, authenticating, and utilizing sensitive health data (US DHHS, 2003). Each "organized health care arrangement" must establish administrative, physical, and technical safeguards to ensure the confidentiality, integrity, and availability of all electronic, protected health information (US DHHS, 2003). Among the required safeguards are: an organizational risk analysis and sanction policy; reporting of suspecting security incidents; data backup, disaster recovery, and emergency mode operation plan; unique user identification; automatic logoff; and audit controls. These requirements encompass basic practices advocated by industry experts, make the burden of protecting health information explicit, and introduce penalties for negligence. But they are adding substantial costs and administrative burdens to health care institutions as well.

The final hurdle in data processing is that not all health system stakeholders have equal incentives to adopt common data processing standards or efficient connectivity systems. Payers often derive financial benefit from delays in making payments caused by the complexities and inefficiencies in claims authorization and processing. Providers have many barriers and very few incentives to establish electronic connectivity to patients that can alter work flows and increase workloads without commensurate remuneration, proper staffing, and new mechanisms for risk management. Those organizations who have made the most progress have made the commitment to information technology (IT) systems and only later have reaped impressive benefits. While HIPAA is designed to address structural impediments to efficient and secure electronic processing, unequal and often "perverse" incentives are rife in the health system and should not be underestimated (Kleinke, 2000). The federal government and private sector are exploring various options to remove or address these barriers (e.g., financial bonuses, low-cost capital, or requirements for Medicare participation) to reverse this trend (Institute of Medicine, 2003).

Opportunities

The Internet is spawning a universe of devices and capabilities designed for use in the recording, processing, analysis, reporting, and transmission of data in almost every conceivable environment for health care practice, administration, research, and teaching. New software is increasingly enabling the conversion of pre-existing or legacy content into the newer standardized code, while more and more original content is being entered and created online or in digital formats easily migrated online. This mass migration towards web-based information technologies and systems is driven by the possibility of significant cost savings and productivity gains, with vastly more effective and efficient record keeping, including data mining, transmission, and communication among providers, payers, and patients, and the streamlining or improvement of many other elements of the administration and management of care.

The web has enabled new capabilities for extending connectivity and care into the home and ever more remote environments. Already, the wired world of the Internet is rapidly being augmented, and in many areas virtually replaced, by wireless technologies that provide sophisticated mobile capabilities suitable to the full spectrum of care, teaching, and other nonstatic and remote environments. Increasingly intelligent systems and devices are aiding all decision-makers, from the patient to the provider to the payer to the researcher, by enabling the conversion of complex data into accessible information and knowledge. As sufficient connectivity bandwidth becomes more available, the goal of universal connectivity moves closer to realization.

While the web provides a common standardization platform, there are many vendors and technologies providing a variety of pathways for system migration, from the incremental to the global. Appropriate decision-making concerning the financing, adoption, and deployment of these new technologies requires health care organizations to acquire the knowledge or expert assistance necessary for organizational planning and prioritizing. Evaluation, planning, and implementation capabilities for web-based operational and administrative systems must be a core competency of all health care organizations, and especially AHCs with their tripartite missions of care, research, and education. Further, institutional systems and strategies must be implemented in the context of broader industry developments, particularly the emerging national health information infrastructure (NHII) described in Chapter 5. Thus, individual organizations need to track and participate in NHII progress.

Connectivity recommendations

- AHC and other health care organizations should be engaged in ongoing, governing board- and leadership-level evaluation of operational and administrative capabilities and opportunities presented by new web-based technologies to enhance, revise, or redesign current service and business processes and patient care capabilities. AHCs and other health care organizations should pursue opportunities for cost savings, operational improvement, and process reform in the areas of administration, human resources, claims processing, customer relations, and marketing. They should also seek to improve capabilities in evaluating the efficacy and efficiency of care and in communicating and sharing data with patients and third-party payers.
- In the short or near term, health care, research, and training organizations should prioritize the development of Internet-based capabilities that strengthen local or regional market position, and assure services that are reliable, scalable, customer-friendly, and flexible.

- AHCs should collaborate with local health information infrastructure (LHII) initiatives that create a network beneath the entire local care system so that population as well as individual strategies are achievable.
- AHC leadership should explore opportunities across and among academic centers for shared investment in, or outsourcing of, web-based operational and administrative systems.

Health care delivery and the Internet

The complexity and diversity of health care practices have hindered the development and adoption of a broadly accepted or indispensable model for care delivery and management. The Internet offers a common platform upon which care delivery, management, and payment can be coordinated and united through shared data and connectivity among providers, payers, pharmacies, patients, and other authorized parties.

Online practice management should enable the realization of significant efficiencies and cost savings in the utilization and transmission of care-related data. Providers and provider organizations will realize new levels of administrative effectiveness in the management of medical records and patient flow. Patients and their care givers (e.g., families, neighbors, children in distant states) should reach new levels of satisfaction with easier and more reliable scheduling, billing, and medical record keeping, and with enhanced connectivity for the purposes of communicating with or accessing resources and information from providers and payers. (See Case study on PatientSite.) Providers and payers will achieve new levels of accuracy and timeliness in the processing of eligibility and insurance claims. Perhaps the greatest impact of the Internet on health care delivery is that it is empowering clinicians and patients alike through the health information it makes available and the self-care, remote care, and customized care it supports. Each of these advancements will contribute to the development of a value-driven health system by enabling the most effective and efficient use of resources.

Empowering health care providers

With the exception of seeking information, physicians as a group have been slow to adopt Internet-based technologies in their clinical practice or to adapt clinical practice to new Internet-based or enhanced technologies. A recent survey of physicians found that the majority of respondents used the Internet to find journal articles, drug information, and health news (85, 68 and 67 percent respectively) and many used the Internet for online continuing medical education (CME), treatment updates, and practice guidelines (43, 41, and 41 percent respectively). However, physicians have significant concerns that communicating with patients via email or storing electronic medical records on the Internet will increase the risk of violations to patient privacy (WebSurveyResearch, 2001). Limited utilization of the Internet for care-related activities other than seeking information can also be attributed to the lack of demonstrated utility and value of Internet technologies to the care process and the cost of investing in and maintaining the technology. Until very recently, only a few Internet or web technologies were capable of providing physicians with new capabilities, efficiencies, practical benefits, or cost savings in the actual provision of care that would justify their adoption. Internet technologies have begun to yield noticeable benefits in three key areas – automation of routine tasks, clinical decision support, and remote care monitoring.

Several vendors (e.g., *Allscripts*) have pioneered the development of portable or hand-held wireless electronic prescription capabilities that enable physicians to create electronic prescriptions in the exam room. Prescriptions can then be sent electronically to the local retail, mail order, or Internet pharmacies, printed in the office, or for the most commonly prescribed medications, dispensed in the physician's office. On a separate track into the physician's workflow, other vendors (e.g., *Mdeverywhere*) have developed wireless charge capture devices for use by physicians at the point of care.

Clinical decision support has become technically feasible as both search engines and clinical practice guidelines have become increasingly sophisticated. Decision support in medicine requires an extremely complex set of capabilities, including computer terminals or appliances that are easy to use, portable, and can access and quickly and reliably display data and patient records in real time. Also required are extensive and sophisticated databases that include up-to-date research and clinical findings and protocols. Rendering all of this information available and useful to diagnosis and treatment requires search engines and software that can process and analyze the data in ways that are useful to the clinician in the clinical setting.

SKOLARMD is a search engine designed for use by physicians and other providers to conduct rapid searches across multiple medical references (skolar.com). Users can access the most up-to-date medical information and clinical decision support at the point of care. SKOLARMD also promotes the concept of physician-initiated in-context learning, providing the opportunity to earn continuing medical education credits in a "learning while doing" model. *Clineguide* is a point of care clinical decision support system that can be integrated with an electronic medical record system or function as a stand alone resource (clineguide.com). It can be customized by adding local formulary, alerts, and guidelines and has provided patient- and disease-specific care recommendations. Even more general search engines such as Google may provide utility in plucking out specific medical information in a timely fashion, so a range of options and capabilities are available.

E-disease management (i.e., application of web-based technology to manage care and support for patients with chronic illness) is a growing domain of Internet applications (LeGrow and Metzger, 2001). These programs or modules are available for care generally as well as a wide range of specific illnesses (e.g., cancer, diabetes, hemophilia, lupus, and Parkinson's) and may be organized to provide support in the clinician practice site, to the patient with linkage to the physician, to the patient with linkage to a case manager, or to the patient through self-directed tools without electronic linkage to others involved in care. Robust e-disease management programs offer the following features:

- Patients can enter health and other information in stages rather than all at once.
- The program stratifies patients into risk bands and notifies providers of high-risk patients.
- Medical devices enable automatic data entry.
- Patients can reach a provider in real time.
- Reminders can be sent by email reminder.
- Support groups are available.
- E-commerce functions provide access to medical supplies.

Internet-based or enhanced telemedicine capabilities are poised to move from the status of esoteric technologies of marginal utility, to mainstream care management tools. Already, many pathology and radiology practices routinely employ the Internet to transmit images and data. Various telemedicine systems are employed to connect providers to patients in homes, assisted living and skilled nursing facilities, and correctional institutions. (See Case Study on IDEATel.)

Home health care is beginning to emerge as a market with increasingly sophisticated and practical technologies of interest to payers, providers, and patients. Remote monitoring and other connectivity products have the potential to reach millions of patients, especially those with chronic diseases and conditions who represent the highest cost cohort in the health care system. *American TeleCare* (americantelecare.com), *Medtronic* (medtronic.com), *BabyCareLink* (babycarelink.com), and several other companies have developed and are refining systems that connect the home and other remote locations to the provider. Terminals enable audio, visual, and digital communication, as well as the reading, monitoring, and transmission of health metrics such as blood pressure, blood oxygen levels, weight, heart rate, and glucose levels. Regular, ongoing monitoring of these and other metrics, along with visual and voice communications, should allow providers to better manage patients' health, increase patient compliance, and help prevent both over- and under-utilization of care. Some early models have been successful but are quite expensive. Unit cost is expected to drop as standards emerge and greater competition develops.

While these and other initiatives are pioneering new ground in e-health care, there are significant technical, operational, legal, privacy and security, reimbursement, and quality assurance issues with which both vendors and e-care utilizers must contend. Migration of clinical decision support and other clinical functions online can be accomplished only with operational accommodations in all clinical settings. Hospitals, physicians, other providers, administrators, and staff must be open to incorporating new capabilities, learning new skills, adjusting patient flow, and helping to test and refine new technologies.

Electronically enhanced or extended care creates legal issues and responsibilities in the areas of professional licensing, provider, vendor, and payer liabilities, privacy, reimbursement, ethics, and other areas (Silverman, 2000). Remote consultation technologies enabling new diagnostic and treatment options, and practice innovations of many kinds will all require payment adjustments and accommodations by both public and private payers. New technologies will require and enable unprecedented quality and safety assessment and assurance measures for use by providers, payers, employers, regulators, and patients alike.

Health care recommendations

- AHCs should institutionalize and formalize the capacity to support the development and implementation of Internet-based technologies that can enhance and extend care. AHCs can conduct trials and demonstration projects encompassing their regions in concert with other regional providers and expand their research agendas to facilitate exploration of the question: how is health care going to be transformed because of new Internet capabilities?

- As an important basis from which to expand and assert AHC leadership in Internet health care innovation, AHCs should embrace health informatics as a full-fledged professional specialty in medicine, nursing, and public health.

- AHCs should create high-level working groups to identify and support, on an ongoing basis, the evaluation, development, and testing of Internet-based clinical capabilities within and between their centers. Clinicians, departments, and/or clinical delivery services that are willing and positioned to participate should be identified and enlisted in these efforts. Appropriate IT, legal, and administrative resources must be committed to these efforts.

- AHCs should begin by identifying processes that need to be fixed or strengthened within the overall clinical and business strategy. AHC leaders should not allow strategy to be controlled or driven by technology. AHCs are most likely to make progress in this arena by focusing on basic and incremental steps while working with new technologies to improve quality, cost, and delivery of care.

Empowering patients

From the point of view of the patient and the public, there has been remarkable development of Internet-based health care resources. The Internet is providing access to health information in unprecedented volume, depth, and breadth. But beyond simply providing information, hundreds of online commercial and noncommercial initiatives are deploying new capabilities for health care services that enable individuals to engage more effectively in managing their health, insurance coverage, and care. As these capabilities become more broadly and equally accessible, patients and health consumers are increasingly empowered to participate in managing their care.

The first stage of patient and public access to health information came with the explosive growth of consumer-focused health information portals. Among the early leaders with a strong academic pedigree were *Intelihealth* (originally a joint venture of Johns Hopkins Medical School and Aetna US Health Care and now a partnership between Harvard Medical School and Aetna), *Mayoclinic.com*, and *HIVInSite* (developed by the Center for HIV Information at the University of California San Francisco). More commercially oriented portals such as *HealthCentral, HealthGate,* and *OnHealth* also emerged. These site portals provided a broad range of easily navigable resources and information but their current status reflects the high level of transition within the online health information domain. *Health-Central* is still functioning as a consumer health portal, but *HealthGate* now offers its services to hospitals, and *OnHealth* has been assumed by *WebMD.*

In the late 1990s *WebMD* came to epitomize the commercial health care portal. Through a series of major strategic alliances and acquisitions, *WebMD* achieved an unparalleled size, scope, and market presence across almost the entire spectrum of e-health services and capabilities. Although *WebMD* has undergone some retrenchment, it remains a strong e-health presence. *WebMDHealth* is a major source of health information for consumers and providers; *WebMD Practice Services* provide physician practice management software; *WebMD Envoy* provides transaction processing and reimbursement cycle management.

Also sponsoring major web-based health information portals are many governmental agencies (e.g., health.nih.gov, clinicaltrials.gov, and healthfinder.gov), professional associations (e.g., the American Academy of Family Medicine, familydoctor.org; Pharmaceutical Research and Manufacturers Association of America, helpingpatients.org), health maintenance and other provider and payer organizations (e.g., Kaiser Permanente, Kaiser-permanent.org), philanthropic and policy organizations (e.g., the Nemours Foundation, kidshealth.org; the World Health Organization, who.int), and university medical centers. *HealthWise,* a nonprofit health promotion organization and publisher of popular self-care guides, has become a leading vendor of online consumer-oriented, evidence-based, self-care guidelines and information, which can be licensed by managed care organizations, health plans, hospitals, and employers for use with their members and employees.

A different model, and equally important to the diffusion of better health knowledge and the empowerment of patients and the public, has been the development of online communities of interest centered around diseases and conditions or cohorts. Online communities have a wide variety of sponsors, from individuals to dedicated, disease-specific advocacy organizations, to the major health portals. These online communities have played very important roles in the evolution of expectations for health knowledge acquisition and interactivity both between providers and patients and among patients and others with shared disease or other health-related experiences and interests. In addition, there are thousands of informal networks of individuals who share experiences, anecdotes, gossip, rumors, facts, and information of all kinds in web site chat rooms and forums. Many health care organizations and providers are well aware of the importance and power of such informal networks in affecting patient and public perceptions and steering patients towards particular therapies, practitioners, or institutions.

Yet research shows that consumers want even more. In most other service and consumer industries, the level of informational access that has been achieved in health care has been supplemented with important follow-on transactional capabilities that enable levels of service and commerce that have so far not developed in health care. As a result, health portals continue to move towards consumer customization and the integration of health-related products, services, interactivity, and information. Consumers increasingly can go online with any of the major portals not just to find information, but to purchase health products and pharmaceuticals, maintain personal and family health data, track and assess personal health status, join discussion forums, and identify and communicate with health care professionals, insurance companies, health plans, or employee benefits managers.

Beansprout.com is an example of the trend towards integrating both health and related services to particular cohorts of consumers. *Beansprout* targets parents of young children with an online service that connects parents, pediatricians, child care professionals, and dedicated childcare resources. The American Association of Retired Persons (AARP) sponsors a web site providing comprehensive coverage of issues of importance to senior citizens, including a health site, aarp.org/health. Seniors can find a wide range of articles, books, research, and legislative advocacy materials on health care, fitness, nutrition and wellness, care giving, health insurance, Medicare, Medicaid, managed care, long-term care, and other issues.

One of the greatest challenges for patients and the health-interested public (and for health professionals as well depending on the topic) is evaluating the quality of health information they find on the Internet (Greenberg, D'Andrea, and Lorence, 2003). There is reason to be concerned. A 2001 RAND study found that information on health web sites is often incomplete, out of date, or difficult for the average consumer to understand (RAND, 2001). Approximately 6 percent of the 66 million American Internet users search for health information each day, but almost 70 percent of those consumers do not discuss the information they find with a health professional (Fox and Fallows, 2003; Madden and Rainie, 2003). Putting up a website is relatively easy; the genuine challenge is maintaining it with evidence-based timely information.

There are a variety of efforts underway to improve this situation. The National Cancer Institute and American Association of Retired Persons web sites include articles describing how consumers can evaluate health information on the Internet. The US government's *healthfinder* Website does not accept paid advertising, content, or links in any form and evaluates the reliability of information before including it in the site's health library. *Quackwatch.com*, a nonprofit organization with a Web site run by a physician, provides guidance on health information and care. Its purpose is to identify and debunk health-related frauds, myths, fads, and fallacies. This site works with volunteers to investigate questionable claims for medical procedures, cures, products, and outcomes as well as misleading or illegal marketing of health products. Patients and those interested in health can receive regular email updates on various issues and concerns, submit questions, or report questionable claims and practices.

The Consumer and Patient Health Information Section of the Medical Library Association evaluates web sites based on credibility, sponsorship/authorship, content, audience, disclosure, purpose, links, design, interactivity, and disclaimers, and identifies the ten most useful health web sites (www.mlanet.org/resources/medspeak/topten.html). In 2000, the nonprofit Health Internet Ethics (or Hi-Ethics) issued a set of 14 principles to guide Internet health services and information. These principles are applied by URAC, an independent, nonprofit accreditation organization, in its health web sites accreditation program. Consumer WebWatch, a grant-funded project of the nonprofit publishers Consumers Union, seeks to investigate, inform, and improve the quality of information (including health information) available on the web through research, promotion of web publishing guidelines, and web site ratings. In December 2003 Consumer Web Watch and URAC outlined a national agenda for improving online health searches in the United States (Greenberg, D'Andrea, and Lorence, 2003).

These efforts extend beyond the United States. The Health on the Internet (HON) Foundation was founded in 1995 to promote the effective and reliable use of new technologies for telemedicine in healthcare around the world. Among HON's accomplishments are the creation of two widely used medical search tools (i.e., MedHunt© and HONselect©) and the HON Code of Conduct for the provision of authoritative, trustworthy web-based information. The European Union is now actively exploring how to develop a framework that ensures "the ongoing availability of timely, high-quality, accessible, understandable, reliable and relevant information for patients and their carers" (Detmer *et al.*, 2003).

The World Health Organization (WHO) is pursuing a novel course to enhance the credibility of health information offered worldwide. The WHO applied to the Internet Corporation for Assigned Names and Numbers (ICANN) to become the registrar of a new top level domain (TLD) – health. Within the ICANN framework, new top level domains may be restricted or unrestricted. A restricted TLD empowers the sponsoring organization to set policy on how the TLD is allocated and used, including who may apply for a registration within the domain, and what uses may be made of those registrations. As registrar of the health domain, the WHO would have the ability to require domain name holders to adhere to a common set of standards for online health content and services. Though not yet successful, this effort illuminates the importance of establishing worldwide standards of care and suggests that WHO is seeking to increase the importance and use of IT in its operations and culture.

Efforts such as these to promote standardization and evaluation of care are controversial and complex, but inevitable. There are many unresolved difficulties in defining, tracking, measuring, and assessing health claims and information, professional competence, patient compliance, and clinical outcomes. Nevertheless, the objective of defining, measuring, and enforcing standards in all of these areas has long been embraced. Professional societies, national and state regulatory and accrediting bodies, and, not uncommonly, the courts all have had a role in developing, promulgating, evaluating, and enforcing professional ethics, truth in advertising, product safety, and practice standards. Individuals and communities too have always formed opinions and points of view about practitioners, institutions, products, and information. That the Internet is now serving as a platform for the migration and further development of this process online should not be surprising. The vast data generation and handling technologies coming online guarantee that there will be unprecedented, ongoing development of resources to assess quality, safety, performance, outcomes, and other health care metrics.

Patient empowerment recommendations

- AHCs should take a leadership role in identifying, making available, and assuring quality health care information for their patients and the public over the Internet.
- AHCs should create or seek partnerships in a web site or sites that provide their patients and public with relevant, reliable, timely, and trustworthy health information and educational materials, particularly for their

localities where good sources of support may not be widely known. AHCs not yet ready or able to create their own sites can often partner in the editorial and quality control of e-health content for web sites otherwise available to patients and the public.

The Internet and evolution of health insurance

Many payers are leveraging the Internet to provide new levels of information, service, and choice to consumers and patients. Increasingly payers allow members, employers, and providers to conduct online transactions and have begun to implement electronic disease management capabilities (First Consulting Group, 2000; LeGrow and Metzger, 2001). Along with greater information and choice, insurers have begun to introduce new coverage models that require and enable consumers to assume increased responsibility for managing the costs and administration of their care (Gabel, Lo Sasso, and Rice, 2002; Galvin and Milstein, 2002; Goldsmith, 2000; Iglehart, 2002).

Blue Cross/Blue Shield of California subscribers can check health benefits information, research providers' backgrounds, compare hospitals, find treatment options, choose care providers, and provide quality assurance and customer satisfaction feedback (www.mylifepath.com). At the same site, subscribers can view the full range of consumer health news and information. Blue Cross/Blue Shield of South Carolina provides online access to a variety of information and functions for members, employers, providers, and brokers. Members can use the online *My Insurance Manager* to check claims status, inpatient and outpatient eligibility and authorization status, the status of bills, and how much they have paid towards their deductible (southcarolinablues.com). Companies such as Highmark Blue Cross/Blue Shield of Pennsylvania (highmark.com) and *eHealthInsurance* (ehealthinsurance.com) are selling health insurance online directly to consumers and small employers, thereby removing the middle man/insurance brokers (many of whom are scrambling to web-enable their businesses).

By moving these capabilities online, insurers can use the Internet platform to further customize information, services, and functions while collecting, tracking, and analyzing extraordinary new data resources by which they can reduce costs and manage care. They can customize and deliver interactive disease management resources to high-risk subscribers, track variability in patient risk and cost in delivery systems, and promote informed choice concerning invasive versus noninvasive or alternative therapies. By linking patients with their physicians, either with automatic alerts or manual

querying, they can head off emergency room visits and other costly inefficiencies or mistakes. And of course in connecting directly with providers and
employers, payers can accelerate claims and eligibility review, instantaneously
make payments, and automatically bill patients' credit cards for any required
co-payments.

By employing an Internet platform, insurers have an opportunity to introduce improved efficiencies and new levels of customer satisfaction. Based
on estimates from other industries, e-enabling administrative and transaction processes could yield cost savings in the billions of dollars. For instance,
the retail banking industry put the costs for manual teller transactions at
$1.07 per transaction. Moving transactions to the Internet reduced these
costs to $0.10 or less. Traditional paper systems for claims processing cost
an average of $7 per claim to submit. The same claims submitted over the
Internet cost $0.30. Potential savings from electronic management and trans-
actions for the health insurance industry have been estimated to be $18 billion
(Darlington, 1998). The arcane aspects of healthcare financing in the United
States might offer resistance to realizing these savings but in time reductions
are certain to occur.

Beyond seeking efficiencies in administration of current plans, insurers and
employers are looking for ways to "reconcile the strong demand for medical
services with the means to pay for them" through consumer-driven health
plans (Iglehart, 2002). There are two basic approaches to consumer-driven
health plans (Gabel, Lo Sasso, and Rice, 2002). First, consumers may be given
a health reimbursement account from which to draw to pay for health care
purchases. Once the account is depleted, enrollees pay out of pocket until the
annual deductible is met. At that time, the plan becomes a traditional major
medical plan. Second, employees may design their own network and benefit
packages and thus their premiums for their individual plan. The employer
provides a fixed (or defined) contribution for health expenses; employees pay
costs incurred above the defined contribution. In addition, tiered benefits,
in which employees face different cost-sharing requirements for different
preferred providers or prescription drug choices, are a common feature of
consumer-driven health plans. Tiered benefits represent a particular challenge
for AHCs that may be excluded from preferred lists developed solely on the
basis of cost.

An estimated 1.5 million Americans were enrolled in consumer-driven
health plans in 2002 (Gabel, Lo Sasso, and Rice, 2002). Start up companies
were first in this market but several large insurers have developed consumer-
driven health plans and a recent survey found that health insurers consider
consumer-driven health plans to be an essential component of their business

strategy. These plans rely heavily on web-based information tools to provide individual subscribers with information on individual spending, costs of various treatments, wellness, and provider quality ratings. Some of the plans have subscribers choose plan benefits, cost-sharing requirements, and primary and specialist physicians on the web.

Consumer-driven health plans present a significant opportunity for insurers to recast their businesses, for employers to reduce their benefits costs, and for employees to achieve new levels of health market choice, but they also present a series of challenges and questions (Gabel, Lo Sasso, and Rice, 2002). First, is there adequate performance information available to support consumers in their selection of providers and are consumers capable of using that information effectively? Second, will consumer-driven health plans lower health care costs or simply shift costs from employers to employees? Third, will consumer-driven health plans appeal to consumers, and, if so, will they further fragment employer risk pools? At this early stage, the only certainty surrounding consumer-driven health plans is that they present many research opportunities.

Recommendations

- AHCs and other provider organizations should explore opportunities to vastly improve relationships with payers through online transaction and information processing.
- AHCs should seek to work closely with employers and insurers to ensure that consumer-driven health plans rely on sound quality, outcomes, and other metrics of care necessary to informed consumer choice of plan and provider.

Research and the Internet

Background and challenges

Through the first seven decades of the twentieth century, basic biomedical (including behavioral) and clinical research were almost exclusively the province of AHCs and their affiliated hospitals, a few private hospitals and treatment centers, and philanthropically supported care and research centers. The pharmaceutical industry also conducted and sponsored basic and clinical research, but focused primarily on applying discoveries to the drug development and marketing process. Over the century, standards for the conduct and reporting of research were developed through the auspices of the National Institutes of Health (NIH), the National Science Foundation (NSF), and other federal agencies, professional societies and associations, and private foundations, all of whom have cooperated to ensure the quality and integrity of the research enterprise. As popular trust in and support for biomedical research grew, so did federal dollars allocated to the NIH, NSF, the Department of Defense, and other agencies to support sponsored research.

Beginning in the late 1970s, the explosive emergence and growth of the biotechnology industry signaled the maturation of biomedical science to the point where it could generate and support a national and international marketplace with a constant and widening spectrum of new products. As the biotechnology and pharmaceutical industries captured unprecedented financing and found or created huge new markets, competitors increasingly looked for ways to accelerate, lower the costs, and improve the efficiency of the drug and device development process. The traditional university-centered biomedical and clinical research enterprise came under intense pressure to provide better administrative support and vastly improved efficiency and industrial responsiveness for their clinical trials and technology transfer capabilities. Most AHCs have not been able to achieve the levels of operational effectiveness and productivity in clinical research desired by industry.

Into this competitive fissure grew a new industry of contract research organizations (CROs) competing to provide the biotechnology and pharmaceutical industries with efficient and effective drug and device development services. Many in the biotech and pharmaceutical industries also added new research and development capabilities, and all hired leading scientists and some of the most promising younger scientists away from traditional academic careers. As universities have struggled to improve industry-sponsored development and clinical research services, the new CRO and biotechnology industries have proven effective competitors. While universities conduct the vast majority of sponsored basic research, it is estimated that universities now conduct only about 30 percent of industry-sponsored clinical research, down from 70 percent two decades ago (Rich, 2000). The rapid development and consolidation of the highly competitive and well capitalized biotechnology, pharmaceutical, and CRO industries continue to put a premium on improving the efficiency and efficacy of drug and device development.

While academic researchers and physicians continue in their vital role at the leading edge of discovery, research and clinical innovation, the pharmaceutical industry is assuming unprecedented leadership in defining and driving the future of treatments for disease and disability. Research and development spending by the pharmaceutical industry, which reached $26.4 billion in the year 2000, is now 50 percent higher than the $17.8 billion sponsored research budget of the NIH (Drews, 1996). Pharmaceutical industry spending will accelerate clinical research and drug and device development over the next ten years. The industry has approximately 500 biological targets for drug development. With advances in molecular biology and the successful mapping of the human genome, within a few years there will be up to 10 000 such targets, vastly expanding the universe of treatable conditions and the efficacy of treatments. The industry is targeting currently untreatable conditions, especially cancer, and lifestyle drugs, such as Viagra®.

The roles that AHCs will play and the extent of their participation in the surge of pharmaceuticals development are a matter of some uncertainty. Academic health centers have lost significant ground in their traditional role of conducting clinical trials to test the efficacy of therapeutics. As suggested above, AHCs have been only partially and inconsistently successful in improving their capacities to reliably conduct efficient and effective clinical studies. Most centers are plagued by administrative difficulties, especially in recruiting and retaining sufficient trials participants, in records management, and in timely management of human subjects and other regulatory requirements. Nevertheless, AHCs remain a compelling locus for such studies, if they can solve the critical administrative and process issues. Academic health center faculties are well suited to the complex challenges of arbitrating and translating information to and from clinical practice.

Opportunities

The Internet is proving to be a very compelling and promising medium through which to expand and further enhance biomedical research and the drug and device development process. In basic research, the Internet has been widely employed by researchers to increase the speed and efficiency of the transfer and sharing of information. Collaborators are more easily and quickly sharing data, feedback, and results. Peer review panels now save weeks or more in the manuscript review process by being able to post reviews and otherwise streamline study section administrative processes online. Bioinformatics appears poised to assume a larger role in academic medicine, nursing, and public health. Significant programs now exist at Boston University, Northeastern University, Stanford University School of Medicine, University of California at Santa Cruz, Harvard, Duke, and Washington University in St. Louis, among others.

The Internet is also serving as an excellent platform for databases that allow researchers virtually unlimited access. Major online databases include the National Library of Medicine's MEDLINE, an index of the entire biomedical serial literature since 1966; PubMed, a search engine hosted by the National Center for Biotechnology Information; GENBANK, the major database of DNA sequences, hosted by the National Institutes of Health; and OMIM, Online Mendelian Inheritance in Man, hosted by the National Center for Biotechnology Information (NCBI). Many other important databases are available online, both free and by subscription. These online resources have become basic tool sets and forums for collaboration in biomedical research and for rapid growth in the field of bioinformatics.

Yet, the research community has struggled with the implications of this efficient new medium. For instance, in 1999 Harold Varmus and colleagues at NIH proposed the creation of an Internet repository, E-Biomed, for the posting and disclosure of both peer- and nonpeer reviewed research results and papers (Varmus, 1999). The proposal envisioned an international repository where researchers worldwide could share results and discoveries with unprecedented speed, receive feedback, respond to queries and criticisms, and in many other ways open up, accelerate, and improve the research publication, review, and dissemination process. While well received by many researchers, the proposal was met with a torrent of criticism from many others and from journal publishers, professional societies, and other quarters. Much of the criticism stemmed from the fear of the damage such speedy dissemination could do to the integrity of the research review process and to public trust in the research enterprise. PubMed Central, a free access digital archive of life sciences journal articles operated by NCBI, emerged from these deliberations, but the concept as initially conceived has not been implemented.

Other models of open access are emerging as well. BioMed Central is an online commercial publishing house that provides free access to peer-reviewed biomedical research. Authors who publish original research articles in journals published by BioMed Central retain copyright over their work, but agree to allow free and unrestricted noncommercial use of the work by others. The Public Library of Science (PLoS) is a nonprofit organization of scientists and physicians seeking to make the world's scientific and medical literature a public resource by developing a new business model for scientific publishing. PloS published its first journal, *PloS Biology*, online and in print in October 2003.

The Internet is being used to achieve new levels of collaboration and efficiency in clinical trials. Online participant recruitment, electronic data capture, and multicenter collaboration have already been explored by several organizations (Bunn, 2003; Farup, 2003; Formica *et al.*, 2004; McAlindon *et al.*, 2003). An evaluation of a randomized placebo controlled trial found that costs per participant were $1000 less than traditional trials, adherence and retention rates were satisfactory, and participants responded favorably to the online trial experience (McAlindon *et al.*, 2003). The Internet provides a robust platform for addressing and managing virtually all aspects of clinical trials, including:

- recruitment of physicians and patients,
- feasibility assessments,
- study design and protocols,
- data collection, processing, and management,
- labs and clinical supplies ordering and tracking,
- real time information on status of trial and access to educational materials, news, and study documents,
- clinical monitoring and audits,
- ethics, human subjects, and regulatory requirements,
- adverse event reporting,
- online training.

The development of this level of comprehensive online capability may be beyond the reach of many AHCs. But AHCs can partner with other organizations having such capabilities if AHCs acquire or create appropriate electronic or Internet-based administrative and data management capabilities.

Research recommendations

- AHCs should aggressively pursue opportunities for the development or acquisition of online clinical trials design and management.
- AHC faculty must become thought leaders and innovators in the new environment.
- AHC leadership should seek strategic partnerships for online connectivity and collaboration with contract research and pharmaceutical organizations.

Health professions education and the Internet

Challenges

One of the most daunting ongoing challenges in medical education is the amount of information, skills, and knowledge that must be assimilated by medical students and other health professions students. The quantity of scientific and clinical knowledge has grown tremendously over the last century. Nearly 10 000 randomized clinical trials results are now published annually, providing an ever-growing base of evidence for clinical practice and professional education (Chassin, 1998). The rate of growth of biomedical knowledge is increasing due to advances in technology, the growth of the research enterprise, and the opening of whole new areas of inquiry, especially in genomics, structural biology, and many other emerging fields. Some fields are advancing so quickly that it is difficult to keep published texts, and even journals, up to date.

Accompanying the increase in the amount and complexity of medical information that must be assimilated is the pedagogical challenge of finding the best methods to facilitate the learning process. Schools that traditionally imparted basic science and skills information to individuals through large lecture classes increasingly have moved to adopt group seminar formats that allow a focus on individual and group problem solving. Pedagogical approaches also have changed in the clinical setting, which has been made more challenging because of managed care and changed reimbursement scales. With hospitalization rates and lengths of stay falling, medical educators have been hard-pressed to provide students with the patient exposure necessary to ensure thorough clinical training. Many schools have experimented with substituting volunteer and paid actors for real patients in order to present medical students with live subjects from whom they can learn and practice the many skills involved in taking histories and diagnosing health problems.

Increasingly, students are expected to utilize expert information, technology, and decision support systems. There are experiments in training students to learn and share skills and expertise in teams, including teams where more responsibility is allocated to skilled and advanced nurses, physician assistants, and other allied health professionals. Biostatistics, epidemiology, behavioral modification, health services research, and bioinformatics are all gaining a more prominent role in health professions education.

Opportunities

The advent of the Internet and growth of the World Wide Web are transforming medical and health professions education. A broad range of medical and public health information is widely available online, increasing the student's access to new and existing knowledge. Among the resources readily obtainable from public and commercial sources are professional journals, reports, and presentations (sometimes live) from professional and scientific meetings, a full range of major medical reference works, and databases. In addition, health professions students have access to search engines that enable extensive and sophisticated information searches, to continuing medical education courses and materials, as well as to supplies, devices, and equipment they might require.

Medical, dental, pharmacy, and nursing school educational resources increasingly are being moved online. Health sciences libraries are migrating publications, catalogs, and most other library resources and services online. Many schools have moved significant elements of their curricula online for ready access by students and faculty. Additionally, thousands of web sites are maintained by medical students, organizations and schools, pre-med preparation companies, medical textbook publishers, and many others with information on virtually any medical-school-related subject or topic.

The University of Pennsylvania School of Medicine and Tufts University Health Sciences Center provide two notable examples of using electronic connectivity to strengthen an AHC's education mission. Building around a dynamically populated database, Virtual Curriculum 2000® currently allows students to access all their lectures (audio and video), images, and slides on demand, seven days a week, 24 hours a day anywhere in the world, within two hours of any session via the Internet. As of late 2003, the system included 4000 hours of digitized web-based lectures synchronized with slides and indexed by key words, and 350 000 digitized slides and images. It also allows students to provide feedback on curriculum blocks and provides an electronic bulletin board for each course to facilitate communication between students and faculty.

Launched in 1995, the Tufts online Health Sciences Database is an online curriculum resource that combines the capability of a digital library with a course delivery system and a curriculum management system. The Database contains an image database (e.g., micro slides), course syllabi (including some textbooks), video clips, lecture slides with audio, and self-assessment quizzes to monitor progress. More than 70 percent of the first and second year curriculum was online in 2001. An object-oriented database provides flexible, expandable, and integrated content that can be utilized, searched, updated, and customized. The Database provides students with integrated course materials that can be accessed and utilized in a variety of formats. Faculty and students can build on and refine course materials. All users can share materials with one another and with users outside the institution.

Advances are also being made in continuing medical education (CME) and schools of public health and nursing. Many medical schools now offer online courses where physicians can earn CME credits. The private sector is playing strongly in this field. CMEWeb.com, for instance, now provides more than 1500 hours of online accredited continuing medical education testing and processing. The Rollins School of Public Health of Emory University, for instance, has developed eLearn, a suite of programs to deliver electronic materials via the web. The school offers a Career MPH degree, a 42 credit-hour program in which students participate in both traditional face-to-face classroom sessions and on the web. The eLearn system enables students and faculty to interact via chat rooms, an electronic whiteboard, and Internet video conferencing. The program is designed to allow working professionals to complete an MPH degree in approximately two and a half years.

Nursing schools long have been innovators in distance learning. Many are rapidly adding innovative and extensive online learning programs. At Duke University School of Nursing (DUSON), for instance, nurse practitioner and clinical nurse specialist students can participate in web-based courses and programs, including MSN degrees in Nursing Informatics, Health Systems and Leadership Outcomes, and Clinical Research Management. The DUSON is also one of a growing number of schools with an informatics program, emphasizing clinical informatics tools for the improvement of patient health outcomes.

As medical and other health professional schools migrate their curriculum online, the opportunities for sharing and cross-fertilization in the elaboration of pedagogical tools and biomedical knowledge and skills will increase exponentially. Towards that end, Johns Hopkins Medicine and leading professional medical societies founded MedBiquitous to create standards that support online professional medical education (www.medbiq.org). Most expert observers see these developments as only the very beginning of capabilities that will likely revolutionize education and training in the health professions over the next two decades. The better_health@here.now project of the Association of American Medical Colleges (AAMC) concluded that medical education in the year 2010 will be suffused and enhanced by a host of new Internet-based technologies and capabilities (AAMC, 2002). Among the projections for the future:

- A set of refereed multimedia cases that cover core medical concepts will be used for instruction at most medical schools.
- Lecture time will be replaced by small group sessions that build on independent study of web-accessed information and resources.

- Intelligent information systems will provide learning materials that continuously adapt to learners' needs and accomplishments.
- Procedure skills will be taught first on a digital simulator.
- Patient simulations (i.e., virtual patients) will be core experiences in widespread use for the evaluation of clinical skills and medical decision making.
- Continuing education will be personalized, delivered by online modules based on physician performance needs with his or her own patients.

Internet-enabled enhancements to health professions education will drive educators to rethink and even re-conceptualize traditional pedagogical methods (Blue Ridge Group, 2003). Internet-based curricula will soon be capable of providing customized elements of the basic curriculum that are directed and updated by intelligent online teaching systems; in fact, most nonexperiential learning is likely to be accomplished over the Internet. The implications for faculties and students are just beginning to emerge. Will the educational model move from the traditional focus on memory to process-based learning? Will faculties be reduced in size or will faculty size remain stable with curricula leveraging online learning to enable faculties to spend more time providing individualized clinical mentoring and counseling, critically assessing and guiding the development of professional values and ethics? Will the criteria by which students are selected change to focus differently on certain character traits, intelligence, adaptability, communication skills, leadership attributes, ability to interface both with technologies and between digital and biological systems?

What will constitute a school under these circumstances? What would it mean to matriculate? If much of the basic curriculum can be conducted interactively online, will hospitals or health plans or other organizations stake a claim to the necessary hands-on health professions training? If curricular material can be packaged into intelligent learning systems, will commercial companies, such as the Kaplan test preparation organization or privately owned for-profit professional schools, became leaders in the development of such systems, with a legitimate claim of being able to provide or halt the training? Could any or all of this apply to residency and other advanced training?

The Blue Ridge Group believes that the optimal scenario is that new Internet-based capabilities will serve to strengthen the existing system of health professions education, enriching the curriculum and enabling more individually, culturally, and technically nuanced training of a diverse cohort of students. Faculty can be freed of more mundane and repetitive tasks and have more time for trainee contact and mentoring, and to pursue unprecedented opportunities for curricular and pedagogical innovation.

Education recommendations

- AHCs should actively investigate the opportunities and challenges for the development of online curricular and pedagogical resources for students and faculty.
- Medical and other health professions schools should prioritize strategic evaluation and planning designed to maximize the impact of online curricula and resources for health professions training.
- Medical schools should work closely with the Association of American Medical Colleges (AAMC), the Liaison Committee on Medical Education (LCME), the Liaison Committee on Graduate Medical Education (LCGME), specialty boards, specialty societies, and other relevant health professional education associations to maximize the utility of curricular innovation and to ensure the integrity and quality of online educational resources and programs.

Conclusion

The Internet is rapidly becoming a major force in the transformation of health care. It enables the standardization of health industry data and allows connectivity for transactions and communications. Perhaps more than any single technological advance, it holds the potential to be THE disruptive technology that will allow health care to cross the quality, efficiency, and safety chasm, and become a genuine industry rather than being a massive, disjointed enterprise committed to piecework with only marginal performance accountability (Christensen, Bohmer, and Kenagy, 2000). The Internet empowers providers and patients in the care process and is likely to contribute significantly to the evolution of health insurance products that provide choice for consumers but also require responsible decisions from them.

For AHCs, the Internet and Internet-based technologies serve many functions and can be employed to support core missions in research, education, and patient care. In turn, AHCs and their faculties are well positioned to play critical roles in shaping and enhancing online health resources and capabilities. The Internet is spawning many of the tools and technologies necessary to the establishment of a value-driven health care system. Academic health centers and other health care organizations are well advised to take full advantage of this extraordinary opportunity.

REFERENCES

Association of American Medical Colleges (AAMC) (2002). *Better Health 2010: a Report by the AAMC's better health 2010 Advisory Board.* Washington, DC: AAMC. Online at www.aamc.org/betterhealth.

Blue Ridge Academic Health Group (2003). *Reforming Medical Education: Urgent Priority for the Academic Health Center in the New Century.* Atlanta, GA: Emory University.

Bunn, G. (2003). *Achieving Success with eDC.* Research Triangle Park, NC: Quintiles Transnational. Online at www.quintiles.com/performance/presentations.htm.

Center for Medicare and Medicaid Services (2004). *Medicare EDI (Electronic Data Interchange).* Online at http://www.cms.hhs.gov/providers/edi/.

Chassin, H. R. (1998). Is health care ready for six sigma quality? *Milbant Quarterly*, **76**(4), 565–91.

Christensen, C. M., Bohmer, R. and Kenagy, J. (2000). Will disruptive innovations cure health care? *Harvard Business Review*, Sept-Oct, 102–12.

Darlington, L. (1998). Banking without boundaries: how the banking industry is transforming itself for the digital age. In *Blueprint to the Digital Economy: Creating Wealth in the Era of E-Business*, ed. D. Tapscott, A. Lowy, and D. Ticoll. New York: McGraw Hill.

Detmer, D. E., Singleton, P. D., MacLeod, A., Taylor, M. and Ridgwell, J. (2003). *The Informed Patient: Study Report.* Cambridge, UK: University of Cambridge.

Drews, J. (1996). Genomic sciences and the medicine of tomorrow: commentary on drug development. *Nature Biotechnology*, **14**(11), 1516–18.

Farup, P. G. (2003). Treatment of *Heliocobacter pylori* infection – results and experiences with an Internet-based collaboration trial. *Tidsskr Nor Laegeforen*, **123**(22), 3214–17.

First Consulting Group (2000). *Survey: Health Plans on the Road to e-Health.* Online at www.fcg.com.

Formica, M., Kabbara, K., Clark, R. and McAlindon, T. (2004). Can clinical trials requiring frequent participant contact be conducted over the Internet? Results from an online randomized controlled trial evaluating a topical ointment for herpes labialis. *Journal of Medical Internet Research* **6**(1), e6.

Fox, S. and Fallows, D. (2003). *Internet Health Resources.* Washington, DC: Pew Internet & American Life Project. Online at http://www.pewinternet.org.

Gabel, J. R., Lo Sasso, A. T. and Rice, T. (2002). Consumer-driven health plans: are they more than talk now? *Health Affairs Web Exclusive*, Nov 20, W395–W407. Online at www.healthaffairs.org.

Galvin, R. and Milstein, A. (2002). Large employers' new strategies in health care. *New England Journal of Medicine*, **347**(12), 939–42.

Goldsmith, J. (2000). The Internet and managed care: a new wave of innovation. *Health Affairs*, **19**(6), 42–56.

Greenberg, L., D'Andrea, G. and Lorence, D. (2003). *Setting the Public Agenda for Online Health: a White Paper and Action Agenda.* Washington, DC: URAC. Online at www.urac.org.

Iglehart, J. K. (2002). Changing health insurance trends. *New England Journal of Medicine*, **347**(12), 956–62.

Institute of Medicine (2003). *Letter Report: Key Capabilities of an Electronic Health Record System*. Washington, DC: National Academy Press. Online at www.nap.edu.

Kleinke, J. D. (2000). Vaporware.com: the failed promise of the health care Internet. *Health Affairs*, **19**(6), 57–71.

LeGrow, G. and Metzger, J. (2001). *E-disease management*. Online at www.fcg.com.

Madden, M. and Rainie, L. (2003). *America's Online Pursuits: the Changing Picture of Who's Online and What They Do*. Washington, DC: Pew Internet and American Life Project. Online at www.pewinternet.org.

McAlindon, T., Formica, M., Kabbara, K., LaValley, M. and Lehmer, M. (2003). Conducting clinical trials over the Internet: feasibility study. *British Medical Journal*, **327**, 484–7.

National Research Council (2000). *Networking Health: Prescriptions for the Internet*. Washington, DC: National Academy Press.

RAND (2001). *Proceed with Caution: a Report on the Quality of Health Information on the Internet*. Oakland, CA: California Health Care Foundation. Online at www.chcf.org.

Rich, R. (2000). Personal communication.

Silverman, R. D. (2000). Regulating medical practice in the cyber age: issues and challenges for state medical boards. *American Journal of Law and Medicine*, **26**, 255–76.

US Department of Health and Human Services (2003). *Federal Register 45 CFR Parts 160, 162, and 164 Health Insurance Reform: Security Standards; Final Rule*. February 20.

Valovic, T. S. (2000). *Digital Mythologies: the Hidden Complexities of the Internet*. New Brunswick, NJ: Rutgers University Press.

Varmus, H. (1999). *E-BIOMED: a Proposal for Electronic Publications in the Biomedical Sciences*. Bethesda, MD: National Institutes of Health. Online at http://www.nih.gov/about/director/ebiomed/ebi.htm.

WebSurveyResearch (2001). *Physicians on the Web*. Online at www.websurvey.research.com.

Case study

Informatics for Diabetes Education and Telemedicine (IDEATel)

Steven Shea, M.D., Justin Starren, M.D., Ph.D., and
Ruth S. Weinstock, M.D., Ph.D.

Two AHCs – Columbia University Medical Center, which comprises Columbia University Health Sciences and NewYork–Presbyterian Hospital, and State University of New York (SUNY) Upstate Medical University at Syracuse – working in partnership have responded to the opportunity to implement a large-scale trial of home telemedicine. The Informatics for Diabetes Education and Telemedicine (IDEATel) Project is a randomized trial of home telemedicine versus usual care. The project has enrolled a total of 1665 Medicare beneficiaries with diabetes who live in federally designated medically underserved areas in New York City and rural upstate New York (Shea *et al.*, 2002). Technical implementation has required large-scale systems integration efforts (Starren *et al.*, 2002). The Centers for Medicare and Medicaid Services (CMS) funded the trial. The motivating policy issue for IDEATel is the need for data to inform decisions about whether and how to reimburse electronically delivered health care services.

A "digital divide" separates the approximately 80 percent of US citizens who have access to computers and the World Wide Web and the skills to use web-based resources from the approximately 20 percent who do not. The IDEATel project is targeted at older people living in federally designated medically underserved areas in New York State, most of whom are unmistakably on the far side of the digital divide. One of the aims of IDEATel is to demonstrate that with adequate resources it is feasible to bridge the physical, educational, social, and cultural obstacles to computer use in the context of health care.

Steven Shea is Professor of Medicine and Epidemiology (in Biomedical Informatics) and Chief, Division of General Medicine at Columbia University. Justin Starren is Assistant Professor of Biomedical Informatics and Radiology at Columbia University, College of Physicians and Surgeons. Ruth S. Weinstock is Professor of Medicine and Chief, Endrocrinology, Diabetes and Metabolism at SUNY Upstate Medical University and Department of Veterans Affairs Medical Center at Syracuse.

Both the clinical and technical aspects of the project have produced new ideas about ways in which AHCs can innovate and contribute to value creation in the health care system. The electronic integration of primary care and specialty care providers in diabetes management suggests that teamwork and communication among providers can be enhanced using new technologies. The clinical network suggests that electronic integration of health care delivery services may be possible without institutional mergers. For example, the project created a virtual interinstitutional electronic medical record that includes a unified approach to identification of individual patients. The computer network integration component provided an opportunity for both participating AHCs to test HIPAA (i.e., Health Insurance Portability and Accountability Act of 1996) compliance strategies (Association of American Medical Colleges, 2002). At Columbia University Medical Center this experience led to a design for an integrated systems architecture to automate many of the requirements of HIPAA for the conduct of clinical research and for institution-wide health care data security.

We draw two conclusions. First, the innovative aspects of the project could not have been accomplished without pre-existing experience in clinical diabetes care, medical informatics, and clinical research at the collaborating AHCs. Second, the most relevant lesson from planning and implementing IDEATel is the need to think at the systems level in terms of electronic data interchange to support distributed but integrated clinical care for large numbers of patients over a widely dispersed geographic area. These are not new insights, but they reinforce the strategic importance for AHCs of building local excellence in areas of innovation and at the same time participating in collaborative opportunities on a larger scale.

REFERENCES

Association of American Medical Colleges (2002). *Memorandum #2–29: Final Revisions to HIPAA Privacy Regulations.* August 23.

Shea, S., Starren, J., Weinstock, R. S., Knudson, P. E., Teresi, J., Holmes, D., Field, L., Goland, R., Tuck, C., Hripcsak, G., Capps, L. and Liss, D. (2002). Columbia University's Informatics for Diabetes Education and Telemedicine (IDEATel) Project: rationale and design. *Journal of the American Medical Informatics Association*, **9**(1), 49–62.

Starren, J., Hripcsak, G., Sengupta, S., Abbruscato, C. R., Knudson, P. E., Weinstock, R. W. and Shea, S. (2002). Columbia University's Informatics for Diabetes Education and Telemedicine (IDEATel) Project: technical implementation. *Journal of the American Medical Informatics Association*, **9**(1), 25–36.

Case study

PatientSite: CareGroup HealthCare System

Alice Lee, David Delaney, M.D., and Jim Brophy

Project description

PatientSite is a user-friendly, personalized messaging system, allowing secure communication among patients, clinicians, and office staff via a secure web site. Through PatientSite, patients can request prescription renewals, appointments, and referrals. Patients can also securely view their own electronic medical record. Providers are able to prescribe educational materials. Finally, patients can maintain a personal health record.

Business objective

Focus groups and national surveys had shown us that many of our patients were using the Internet, wanted improved connectivity with their providers, demanded greater convenience when interacting with their physicians' practices, and wished to better manage their health online. Creating a forum to achieve this functionality would increase patient/provider satisfaction, improve customer loyalty, and make our organization a market leader. After exploring possible ideas with our users, we created a secure web site that provided a messaging infrastructure. Then, we combined this infrastructure with technology that allowed us to web-expose heterogeneous clinical system information, thereby capitalizing on our clinical information systems. The resultant product featured:

- Secure messaging.
- Automated routing of patient messages.

Alice Lee is Vice President of Clinical Systems at CareGroup HealthCare System. David Delaney is Technical Director, Web Applications at CareGroup HealthCare System. Jim Brophy is PatientSite Project Leader at CareGroup HealthCare System.

- A site for patients to maintain links to health information.
- A mechanism for physicians to prescribe health information to their patients.
- Ability to request prescription renewals, appointments, and referrals.
- Ability to archive messages.
- A secure mechanism for patients to view their clinical records.

Constituents served

The primary goal of the project has been a coordinated deployment of the PatientSite web-based application to all interested clinical health care system affiliates and their patients. Its purpose is to provide patients with convenience and communication tools, and to enhance the quality of service and satisfaction. Second, we wanted to provide clinicians with an application that allows them to better manage the health of their patients. Finally, we wanted to provide practice staff with an application that supports patient-care management by streamlining various processes within their practices. For example, requests for prescription renewals are sent only to those individuals within the practice who are responsible for handling this task. The same applies to appointment and referral requests.

Key obstacles and solutions

The initial barrier was related to concerns about the security of this communication method. Although these concerns may have merit in the context of conventional electronic mail, PatientSite utilizes advanced web security to ensure the privacy of users.

One of the biggest obstacles to overcome is the reluctance to add yet one more method of communication to the provider and practice staff. PatientSite has a feature that was proactively designed to address this challenge: a new message notification function. When a PatientSite message is received, the recipient is notified through their regular email account that they have a PatientSite message waiting for them. The user simply has to click on a link and log into the site to retrieve their message. This process eliminates the need for a user to continually check for new messages in their PatientSite account. A second concern has been message routing within the practice. PatientSite can be set up to mirror workflow by routing specific types of messages to the appropriate person(s) within the practice.

Providers who are contemplating using the system within their practice worry that patients will overuse the system. In actual fact, statistics collected to date have been fairly constant and indicate reasonable use. Every 100 patients registered on the system send about 45 clinical messages per month. These 100 patients generate an average of two to four prescription renewal requests, referral requests, and appointment requests per month.

Direct patient access to medical records is a new idea, and one that feels uncomfortable to many physicians. To accommodate physician concerns, we incorporated the following protocols into PatientSite:

- HIV results are not available through PatientSite.
- Test results can be viewed on PatientSite as soon as the results are finalized, but we embargo pathology results and radiology results to allow physicians a chance to review them.
- Patient access to various aspects of their record is currently controlled by physician preference, however for patients who are cared for by multiple physicians the most permissive setting applies.

Conclusion

PatientSite is a pioneering e-health system, created by an integrated health delivery network that provides a platform for secure clinical communication, customer convenience transactions, patient education, and web-exposure of the clinical record. It provides value to the patients/consumers, to providers of healthcare, and to practices.

Commentary

John Glaser, Ph.D. and Cynthia Bero, M.P.H.

In the last ten years, the world has seen the dramatic and tumultuous introduction of the Internet and the World Wide Web. This period of time saw a tidal wave of unwarranted optimism about the revolutionary nature of the Internet. Industries were going to be transformed. An old economy was to be replaced by a new economy. Fortunes were to be made in cyberspace. A new vocabulary, including terms such as "dis-intermediation," "B2B," "B2C," and "Internet Time," entered the management discourse. This period of time has also seen a tidal wave of unwarranted pessimism about the Internet. The NASDAQ fell dramatically from a peak of nearly 5000. Hundreds of dot coms are no more.

History has shown us that it is usually quite difficult to accurately predict the future that results from the implementation of significant technologies. The second- and third-order effects of profound technologies such as the automobile, the internal combustion engine, and flight were difficult to imagine accurately when the technology was first introduced. In the early 1900s, few people understood that the automobile would lead to suburbs, exodus from the inner city in some cities, and the modern vacation industry (Malone and Rocart, 1991). Flight is an excellent example of the conflicting optimism and pessimism that confronts the discussion of a profound technology early in its life. Many a science fiction writer in the early 1900s thought that our cities would have "airline taxis" cruising the streets several hundred feet in the air. Others, watching pilots get lost or planes crashing with great regularity, thought that the airplane would go nowhere. Similarly, the full impact of the Internet on health care is difficult to see with great clarity.

While it is impossible to see into the future, the Internet is here and our world is changing. More than two-thirds of adults who use the Internet seek health information (Fox and Fallows, 2003). Physicians report that more than

John Glaser is Vice President and Chief Information Officer at Partners HealthCare System. Cynthia Bero is Chief Information Officer at Partners Community HealthCare Inc.

one-third of the patients arrive for visits with information downloaded from the Internet (Pew Internet & American Life Project, 2002). In November 2002, consumers spent nearly $6.2 billion online, an increase of 22 percent over the same period in the previous year (Ewalt, 2002).

While the impact of the Internet on health care is still in its early stages, what have we learned?

Knowledge of how to apply the Internet and leverage the strategies of an organization is still very immature. Many assumptions about the impact of the Internet have proven to be naive. It is difficult to disintermediate individuals and organizations that actually provide value. It can be very hard to connect thousands of suppliers to thousands of hospitals. While hundreds of millions of people use the Internet as a source of health information, a recent VHA survey (VHA, 2002) found that 72 percent of respondents prefer their physician as the primary source of health information with only 4 percent preferring the Internet. There is still significant room for experimentation and learning.

The Internet remains a profound technology. The use of the Internet enables organizations to extend their systems into the home and across the globe with an ease that has the historical equivalent of the radio. The Internet offers the potential to intelligently connect computers, appliances, and people in a fashion whose nearest analog is electricity. The Internet has the potential to deliver an "experience" that is richer – more customized and more interactive – than the previous leap in a rich experience, the television.

The diversity of applications of the Internet is broad. Perhaps this is not surprising since there are very diverse industries, organizations, and activities involved in information distribution and service delivery and that can benefit greatly from extending their processes to customers and other organizations. A health care organization will find a very wide range of possible Internet opportunities, some more potent than others, but a wide range nonetheless.

Those Internet efforts that have been successful have focused on the core sources of IT advantage – leveraging processes, obtaining critical organizational data, and product and service differentiation and creation. Amazon.com has arguably revolutionized the retail industry by making the process of buying a book more convenient. Moreover, Amazon uses data about prior purchases to suggest books (and other merchandise). Amazon enables book readers to leave their critiques of books for other readers, providing a differentiation of the book purchasing experience. Travel reservation web sites are intended to ease the process of arranging travel or a vacation. The consumer conducting the transaction reduces the cost, to the airline or hotel, of the transaction. Data entered by the traveler enables the site to be tailored to them and provides valuable information to the service provider.

The boundaries between "Internet-based" applications and "regular" applications have become blurry. Internet applications often extend regular applications and regular applications are often critical to effective Internet applications. For example, a web site to order children's toys needs a regular materials management application to handle toy inventory and logistics. The use of a web-based application to provide access to clinical data to a referring physician needs a hospital information system to serve the data. Rarely does one find a "pure" web-based application that has no need for a "regular" application in order to be effective. And one finds that most, but not all, regular applications can be made more potent by extending them through web technologies.

Internet technology has become the underpinning of virtually all information technology. Increasingly, all information systems are moving to an Internet foundation. Clinical information systems have a browser interface as the default user interaction. Systems communicate with each other using Internet-based network protocols. Applications are being developed using a web services architecture approach.

The effectiveness of Internet applications is highly dependent upon the thoughtfulness of an organization's strategy and the intelligence of its approach to leveraging core activities. For a while, the Internet jargon of "New Economy," "Internet Time," "B2B," and "B2C" implied that traditional management thinking and strategy prowess were irrelevant. A new way of thinking was necessary if one was going to thrive in "Cyber-space." But positive operating margins, knowing your customer, thinking long and hard about how to improve a process, skillful organizational change, and execution matter as much in the new economy as they did in the old economy.

Effective application of Internet and web applications is hard work. The Internet has not removed many of the challenges associated with the implementation of information systems in health care. While the Internet may facilitate physician use of a computerized medical record, the size of the investment, the lack of financial incentives, and the significant work flow changes remain as significant issues. The Internet may technically enable consumers and patients to receive remote care but the reimbursement model has not moved much beyond payment for face-to-face encounters. Internet-based purchasing collaboratives have not been able to achieve greater savings than can already be found in group purchasing organizations. Lou Gerstner, former chief executive officer of IBM, summarized this well:

I think for a lot of people, the 'e' in e-business came to
stand for 'easy.' Easy money. Easy success. Easy life.
When you strip it down to bare metal, e-business is just business.
And real business is serious work. (Gerstner, 2002, p. 175)

So what should the leadership of AHCs do about the Internet?

- **Maintain a sober but interested outlook on the role of the Internet**. The wild and wooly first years of the Internet should not lead to dismissal of the relevance of the Internet or the uncritical embracing of it. The technology is immature and there is much to be learned. But the technology is profound.
- **Continue to experiment with the application of Internet technologies and learn from the experiments of others**. There are success stories – eBay, extension of data access to community physicians, and teleradiology. There will be more success stories in the intermediate future (e.g., reimbursement for e-visits).
- **Do not separate the Internet discussion from the "normal" information technology discussion**. The boundaries between the two are virtually gone. The information technology strategy discussion should be very well integrated into the overall strategy discussion.
- **Remember that the impact of the Internet is likely to be more evolutionary than revolutionary in health care**. Nonetheless, fossils illustrate that evolution has resulted in victims.

REFERENCES

Ewalt, D. (2002). Cash registers ring with the jingle of online sales. *Information Week*, Dec, **23**: 17.

Fox, S. and Fallows, D. (2003). *Internet Health Resources*. Washington, DC: Pew Internet & American Life Project. Online at http://www.pewinternet.org.

Gerstner, L. (2002). *Who Says Elephants Can't Dance? Inside IBM's Historic Turnaround*. New York: HarperCollins.

Malone, T. and Rockart, J. (1991). Computers, networks and the corporation. *Scientific American*, **265**(3), 128–36.

Pew Internet and American Life Project (2002). *Search Engines: a Pew Internet Project Data Memo*.

VHA. (2002). *Consumers Look at Clinical Quality; Beyond Bricks and Mortar*. Irving, TX: VHA. Online at https://www.vha.com/research/public/research_beyondbricksandmortar_meth.asp.

7 Organizational challenges facing the European academic health center

Tom Smith

Introduction

In Britain, the interface between the health system and universities was once described as "the place where the present meets the future in health care" (Dainton, 1981). It is difficult to reconcile this grand portrayal with the picture that organizational partners face now, more than 20 years later. Research and clinical communities are more fragmented than in the past. New policy in both health and university sectors has unwittingly created incentives for partner organizations to point strategies in different directions. Universities are more focused on the future – with only a minority of medical research directly concerned with clinical problems. And university hospitals are more concerned than ever with present service demands. The capacity to relate ideas and research with practice is said to have diminished within European health care settings.

This situation has serious implications. The strength of collaboration between the clinical and research domains determines to a large degree the capacity to transfer knowledge to practice, to focus research on critical clinical issues, to develop new services, and to prepare professionals for interdisciplinary and reflexive practice.

Local or central health authorities fund hospitals and manage their performance. Separate central ministries fund and manage the performance of universities. European AHCs, as the collaborations between faculties and university hospitals might be labeled, have been weakened by a gradual untangling of policy strands between education, service, and research. With the exception of the Netherlands, which has three or four integrated models, organizational partners in other European countries

Tom Smith is Senior Policy Analyst in the Health Policy and Economic Research Unit at the British Medical Association.

are finding it difficult to relate across different sectors and institutional boundaries.

This chapter sets out the key organizational challenges facing the European AHCs. In particular, it explores the implications of organizational fragmentation and discusses ways in which this fragmentation might be overcome. The chapter is divided into two parts. The first explores the managerial perspective, outlining strategic and organizational fragmentation between health and university partners. The second part introduces a case study from Sweden and adds the voice of clinicians and researchers to the discussion of overcoming fragmentation. It adds an understanding of cultural fragmentation and the need to develop more engaging relations between preclinical and clinical groups. Neither policy makers nor organizational leaders have paid as much attention to cultural issues as they have to structural issues between sectors. The cultural analysis provided by people within departments offers some practical insights into ways in which fragmentation can be directly addressed.

This chapter draws on two main sources. The first source is the summary of an Organization for Economic Coordination and Development (OECD) seminar held in November 2002. The meeting brought together pairs of CEOs and deans from cities in 15 countries. Quotations from a survey of participants appear throughout the report (Smith and Davies, 2003). The second source of quotations is from a project to enhance the capacity for clinical research between the University of Lund and university hospitals based in Malmö and Lund, 40 km apart in the Skåne region of Sweden (Smith, 2003).

Both sources take an organizational perspective and are concerned with ways to improve joint working, but have slightly different emphases. The OECD meeting was concerned with a macro perspective. The Skåne project focused on a departmental or micro level with discussion on human factors, group relationships, and the culture of working. Both perspectives help us to understand the nature of fragmentation in many European AHCs. They also provide some insight into tensions between bottom-up and top-down approaches to overcoming fragmentation.

Global trends in partnership

Although it is common to consider difficulties between university and hospital partners as local problems, a number of global trends are apparent that have contributed to the slow separation between partners. Many of the organizational problems faced are international concerns.

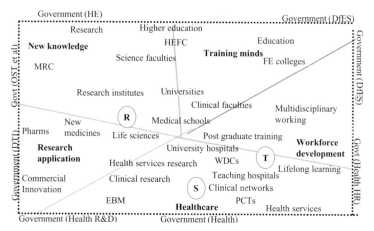

Figure 7.1   Strategic fragmentation (UK Example). DfES – Department for Education & Skills; EBM – Evidence-based medicine; FE – Further education; HEFC – Higher Education Funding Council; MRC – Medical Research Council; OST – Office for Science & Technology; PCTs – Primary Care Trusts; R&D – Research and development; WDCs – Workforce Development Confederations. The encircled R, S, and T stand for research, science, and teaching, respectively

Efforts to contain the cost of health care have resulted in tighter performance management and delivery targets. University hospitals have not been immune to the drive to contain costs in health care or any other health sector reform, far from it. They are often the chief targets of such initiatives designed to change the behavior of institutions, sometimes seen as black holes for resources and resistant to change. Leaders of university hospitals have been focused almost entirely on service issues.

At the same time, within universities, deans have been focused more on research, facing incentives to maximize scholarly over clinical impact. In education, the trend for students to be trained in a wider variety of clinical settings has complicated relations between universities and the health sector. Universities relate to a larger number of health providers and have a wider range of relationships to manage. To illustrate the scale of the problem, University College London has students placed with over 100 different health service providers.

Strategic fragmentation

Figure 7.1 illustrates the strategic fragmentation that exists in Britain (Moss and Smith, 2002). The same tensions are visible in many countries, though they take a different form. Around the border of the strategic picture are different agencies and departments with different interests, which are not necessarily aligned. The demands of different agencies pull strands apart, making it difficult for senior management to hold them together in institutions at the center of the picture.

A key problem is that policy in both sectors is formulated independently. Although university hospitals and faculties must pool resources and plan jointly to meet targets in research, education, and health care, targets for each are set externally and performance managed independently. There is no central overview of the integrated mission (relating research, service, and education). While policy is created categorically it is implemented in the thick of cross-cutting priorities, making it difficult to manage.

Structural fragmentation

A dean attending the OECD meeting summed up the views of many others in explaining their motivation for exploring organizational problems at the interface:

Creating strategic approaches whereby both the organizations work jointly together rather than existing side by side would be the single most important development that we could achieve (United Kingdom).

As the dean of medicine from the university of Belgrade explained, one of the consequences in Europe of introducing tighter budgetary management in the public sector has been that "all business affairs were separated and subordinated to the jurisdiction of different ministries." This has made it very difficult for organizational leaders to relate priorities from different sectors.

The details of the management difficulties faced in working across university and clinical boundaries are complex and, to be blunt, can be boring – which is one of the main reasons the problems are not well understood outside the confines in which they are experienced. Perhaps they are better presented through a dramatic metaphor.

Imagine a group of playwrights (policy-makers) scripting acts to be performed by separate companies of actors (university and clinical partners). Companies are independent of each other and performances are judged differently. But they are also interdependent. They share the same stage as well as the actors needed to put on a good performance. Although many think a joint production would improve performance, directors have found it difficult to persuade playwrights (who are also financial backers) to write more integrated scripts that would make it easier for the acts to work together. Each shows more passion for his own direction than for the picture as a whole.

Different scripts are played out on a complex stage where stage directors try to piece different lines (of accountability) into coherent scripts and choreograph the limited number of actors to fill all parts. It is difficult to manage without either requirement or incentives for a joint production and without the notable will and effort from actors who perform multiple roles. In such difficult circumstances, creative differences inevitably emerge between groups.

Models of partnership

In Britain, there have been numerous reports from government agencies that describe problems of managing at the interface in technical ways. One suggested partners should "combine as if a single entity in order to discharge their shared mission" (Steering Group on Undergraduate Medical and Dental Education and Research, 1994). But there has been a reticence to take this idea forward or experiment with different organizational models. There is a good deal of political caution about treating some organizations differently to others (i.e., teaching hospitals and nonteaching hospitals).

Although organizational heads have considered different organizational models, with the traditional US AHC model attractive to many, without political blessing organizational leaders have not felt able to marry. The most notable examples of institutionalized partnership in Europe are in the Netherlands, where Government has been supportive of the change.

The Amsterdam model is illustrated in Figures 7.2, 7.3, and 7.4. The hospital reorganized itself into ten new clinical departments and the university into three educational and seven research institutes. After a year, the two organizations came together into a single entity to form a matrix organization (as shown in Figure 7.4) where everyone, including academics, is based in a clinical department. The approach has not been formally evaluated as far as we are aware, but people within the organization consider great progress to have been made.

Why aren't new organizational models emerging in other places?

The kind of analysis outlined above has led to increasing support for the idea of creating University Clinical Centers (UCC), a concept introduced by the

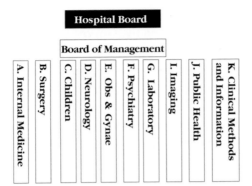

Figure 7.2   Matrix model from Amsterdam AMC. First the hospital reorganized

Figure 7.3   Then the university organized itself into research and educational institutes

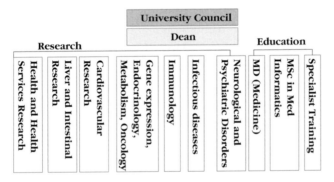

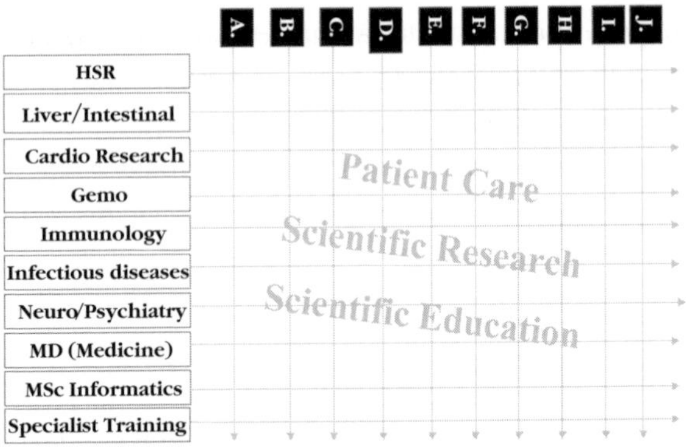

Figure 7.4   After a year the new structures came together in a matrix structure

Nuffield Trust in London (Smith, 2001) and inspired by the AHC model. It is an organizational concept that seeks to establish a vehicle for university and clinical partners to jointly manage activities.

Prior to the OECD conference, attendants were asked to contribute issues for discussion in advance. A chairman of a UK teaching hospital asked, "Why is progress not being made when the need for University Clinical Centres is so obvious?" But unfortunately, the case for University Clinical Centers is not obvious outside research-intensive institutions.

Talk of closer interaction raises cries of elitism. People ask why university hospitals should be treated any differently than any other hospital. They point out that medical students are trained in many settings, there is nothing particularly distinctive about the role of university hospitals in medical education. They argue that research needs to be patient based and only a minority of patients are in university hospitals and then for a very short length of stay.

While policy-makers are coming around to the view that there should be greater collaboration between university and health sectors, others think that this should happen everywhere. Again, why should there be special arrangements for university hospitals even if they are closely located and in many cases embedded in universities?

The limits of institutional thinking

There are valid points within these criticisms, but also an underestimation of what is required to better relate knowledge and practice. Academic health centers make little sense unless embedded within the health system to which they relate. There has been too much discussion of relations between university faculties and university hospitals to the exclusion of considering wider relations. One of the factors holding up organizational development has been the search for the perfect organizational model, which has acted as a bit of a red herring because there are limits to institutional thinking.

The clearest message from the OECD meeting of leaders was that a systemic view is required across local health systems. Partnership is needed not only with hospitals, but also with other nonmedical academic institutions that are sometimes located in different universities than medical faculties.

Achieving effective collaboration between health and university sectors requires networks to be developed across health economies that relate to service, research, and education. With this approach, partnership can be more effectively pursued across disciplinary and institutional boundaries, permitting closer relations among a wider number of academic and clinical partners. However, this broader concept of system-wide university clinical partnership does not negate the view that organizations should develop closer institutional relationships. In addition to broadening the network between health and education sectors, greater depth is also needed to underpin effective partnership. Academic health centers need to facilitate more intense collaborations among different communities. We know, for example, that the challenge of translating research into practice will not occur simply through the dissemination of research findings.

Leaders at the OECD meeting articulated a notion of collaboration that will introduce new academic disciplines into the knowledge base, aiming to understand more about relationship between knowledge and practice. But before coming back to ways in which partnership might develop, it is important to consider another perspective on the nature of fragmentation and ways to overcome it.

What happened to clinical research in Skåne, Sweden?

The need for greater depth in collaborations between service and research communities is supported by the experience of a project in Sweden to explore ways to develop capacity for clinical research. The project began from a concern that clinical research was declining and that this was symptomatic of a contraction in strategic liaison between two university hospitals and medical school. Research activity is dominated by basic science and service by politically established targets, such as waiting lists.

An appreciation of the structural separation that has occurred between university and health sectors is crucial to understanding the decline of clinical research in Skåne. But while discussion so far has detailed strategic and management perspectives, a third dimension is needed to fully understand the problem of fragmentation between the sectors. When talking to researchers and clinicians it is obvious that what preoccupies them is not structures linking academic and clinical departments, it is the cultural fragmentation that has arisen between clinical and preclinical spheres. This is not to say that people are not aware of structural fragmentation, far from it. The two are closely related, but dealing with cultural manifestations is more pressing in the minds of many.

The current climate

People we spoke to in Skåne see an institutional bias to basic science. Funding structures do not encourage clinical research and over time this has had a tremendous cultural impact. Universities are funded to maximize research activities that lead to scholarly rather than clinical impact. As one observer noted, "The money goes to preclinical research, but the results come from clinical research." The value of research qualifications in hospitals has dwindled and clinical research does nothing to advance either the academic or clinical career. Basic science is a greater source of academic credibility for researchers, and clinical careers are built leading services. Fewer and fewer people pursue clinical research.

University hospitals have a more distinct service identity than in the past. Fewer people teach, see patients, and undertake research – working across the so-called tripartite mission. Current structures do not allow people to bridge activities across what are increasingly separate domains. One young clinician determined to undertake research essentially does two jobs. After seven hours in the clinic, she goes to the laboratory and works for three or four more.

The health system is thought to have limited and diminishing capacity for the research activities. Winning research grants has become more competitive and people say they do not have time to write research proposals. Clinicians interested in research tend to work in very small groups, or alone, at a time when applications from large multidisciplinary groups are favored.

There are too few links between clinics and research groups. Many research groups are thought to be distant from clinics. Fewer researchers have clinical backgrounds than in the past. The number of medically qualified PhD students is diminishing. Consequently, there is said to be a lack of understanding of clinical problems and issues among researchers.

Individuals with an interest in research find it difficult to compete for funding, and applications from established research groups tend to be more successful, so research groups do not have strong links to clinics. There are concerns that research is moving away from service when "clinical research needs to happen in clinics with patients." People fear the "clinic" has been taken out of clinical research.

There is little daily contact between clinicians and researchers. The problem everyone highlighted was the limited capacity for learning between clinicians and researchers. There are few opportunities to meet and talk. There are not uniformly strong links between preclinical and clinical departments. There is misunderstanding between groups. Although there is a great will to work more closely, some academics say clinicians are not interested in research and clinicians say academics are uninterested in clinical problems.

There are different views on research. Over time, preclinical and clinical communities have become more distinct. In discussions, it was not clear that different people mean the same thing when talking about clinical research. While the university wants to develop "good" clinical research and spell out the findings for the health system to put in practice, the hospital sector is keener on research that can influence and raise service quality more directly. There is a view that ALF money, which is paid by the Swedish state to support research in hospitals, is not funding the kind of research needed to develop clinical services and improve patient care. Evaluation and follow-up projects are not regarded as "good science." Many activities that might benefit the clinic lie in "gray" areas.

Strengthening collaboration

In interviews in Skåne, despite there being overwhelming support for formalizing closer working, a good deal of caution is expressed about structural, top-down approaches. With too few opportunities to learn and work across disciplinary and organizational boundaries, people say management needs to concentrate on creating an environment that is conducive to effective collaboration rather than uniformly prescribe the form interaction should take.

For many people, the starting point in resolving problems faced at the interface is to focus on clinical issues faced by patients.

There is limited capacity for clinical research and a fear that current trends will lead to narrow research and the loss of any capacity to apply new knowledge to clinical practice or to explore clinical problems. The decline of patient-centered work can only be reversed through a bottom-up focus on clinical problems and ways to explore them.

Within departments there is some concern that structural solutions might constrain the kind of working that is required. They do not want what they see as essentially an administrative solution to a cultural problem. The point of organization from their perspective is to encourage as much interaction as possible between different groups. In one group discussion, someone drew a series of chaotic inter-crossing lines on a piece of paper and said, "That's the kind of organizational structure we need."

One of the key insights from researchers and clinicians based in Malmö and Lund is that, from their perspective, organization is temporary whereas the mission of relating research and service is permanent. The way this mission is pursued will inevitably change over time. Although today there is concern about relations between academic and clinical departments, it may be that over time the boundaries of researchers and clinicians will change.

The development of clinical research and development may contribute to the process of changing traditional boundaries. To develop clinical research, one group asks:

Have we got the right kind of local organization in place, the right teams? Today departments are administrative structures rather than scientific homes and in that sense are becoming increasingly obsolete.

The chief problem is seen as the lack of engagement between research and service communities. As one forthright person explains, there are two main problems.

First, they do not meet. Second, some preclinical researchers seem to have a lot of prejudice towards clinicians, whom they do not count as "real" scientists. They might not like to collaborate with "simple" doctors. I also suspect the two groups may have difficulties understanding each other: the lab researchers may have no or little clinical experience, whereas the doctors are unfamiliar with lab work. Solution: make them meet. This will increase respect and understanding between the two groups and could generate ideas about common projects.

Through exploring people's aspirations for clinical research and views of how it might develop, the project in Skåne has laid the foundations to evolve a unified framework for closer working. It will follow three principles: (1) necessitate links between clinical and preclinical groups and perspectives; (2) create an environment that is conducive to greater interaction between people; and (3) build bridges between different research islands, providing incentives for work between them.

The views of clinicians and researchers in Skåne help to make sense of the organizational reality involved in developing partnership.

Developing organizations to sustain partnerships

Prior to the OECD meeting in November 2002, several heads of research and service institutions highlighted questions in advance they hoped discussion would explore. Two questions from Nordic countries were:

- What is a university hospital, what makes it distinctive? (Finland)
- What will the university hospital look like in 2010? (Sweden)

Most often, answers to the first question are institutionally defined rather than related to purpose. While university hospitals have distinctive service profiles in certain clinical areas, it is not true that service profiles are hugely different from a large general hospital. The presence of teaching is not unique either. A wider number of clinical providers are involved in undergraduate education.

The scale of research activity is one genuine difference. But the extent to which this is related to service, as an integrated environment would wish, is questionable. As we have seen, significant bridge building activity is required to develop the interface at a number of levels. Organizational development is required to build up muscle between research and clinical communities.

It is impossible to say what the university hospital will look like in 2010. We can say a bit about the kind of organization leaders would like to create, drawing on submissions prior to the OECD conference. There is a lot of overlap with the kind of organization clinicians and researchers want to work in.

What kind of organizations do leaders want to create?

Leaders want to work in closer collaboration with partners. They would like to work as a joint entity explicitly charged with creating a dynamic across research, service, and education. There is a view that the giants of research and service eclipse the education mission within institutions. European heads want to see a greater emphasis on teaching and learning, and stronger links between research and service communities. An organizational entity that enables more interorganizational cooperation is thought necessary to cope with the organizational pressures that a more disjointed structure cannot. This is not suggesting a merger between organizations, but a formal partnership engaged in a joint venture. The shape of collaborations is likely to change over time.

More faculties would be brought into the partnership, including non-biomedical disciplines, such as operations research, humanities, and other disciplines that might enhance our understanding of behavior. Academic health centers should seek to establish an interdisciplinary understanding of the relationships between theory and practice, developing organization capacity to translate clinical and health services research into practical and service improvements. Academic health centres need to develop much stronger links to primary care and nonuniversity hospitals. Networks need to be developed for research, service, and education to link up different organizations and enhance system-wide capacity for knowledge sharing and collaboration in research.

What kind of organization do clinicians and researchers want to work in?

In answer to the question, "What kind of organization do you want to see?" someone countered, "I'd like to know, what kind of organization are we?" People want a clear recognition of the mission they are engaged in, as do leaders. People want to work in an organization with a "questioning mentality" in which research and learning activities are considered core to service. Rather than structures, management should think more about relationships and aim to create an environment that is conducive to working across institutional and disciplinary boundaries. They need "to concentrate on people because the social interaction of groups matters." Researchers and clinicians want organizations to create an environment that is conducive to learning.

The aspirations of people within AHCs are similar. They each hope to overcome fragmentation between sectors, organizations, departments, and groups. They hope to develop more engaging relationships between people with different perspectives in order to develop clinical practice and health services.

How will this vision of a less fragmented collaboration be realized?

Bridges between partners are needed at a number of levels. The problems are structural, relating to misaligned incentives and organizational structures that fail to bridge departments. But they are also cultural, inextricably related to diminished capacity for engagement between different perspectives. Perhaps unsurprisingly, managers and department heads are concerned more with structures while those in departments suggest the main problems are cultural.

It is interesting that "a bridge" was the most commonly used metaphor in discussions. Structural links are needed to enable organizations to develop coherent strategies. Cultural bridges are needed to create the milieu for relating the different worlds of research, education, and practice. European AHCs have to build bridges at a variety of levels.

In the past, leaders in countries such as Britain and Sweden have rightly identified the dislocation in performance management and structures as major problems. But even if structures were aligned, the cultural tensions will not be resolved. Experience in Britain supports this view. Although limited funds have recently been available to support clinical research projects, high-quality applications are not always forthcoming. Making clinical research a mainstream activity will require significant development. The kind of collaborations required between twenty-first century research and service communities are different than in the past. More complex interactions are required to bridge all the steps from the laboratory bench to the patient, wherever they are located.

So how are these initiatives likely to emerge? Organizations want to develop relationships, but are aware of the structural limits to what can be done. It is likely that the fragmentation between health and university sectors will take time to erode. In any case, organizational partners cannot wait for blessing to begin to strengthen organizational partnerships.

There are things they can do. The cultural perspective from Skåne offers some suggestions. Partners can introduce initiatives to engage projects between research and clinical communities. They can face research and clinical work toward each other. They can encourage the growth of networks for research and service.

The need for local development

The complexity contained with the kind of collaboration people hope to see emerge will require fundamentally different relationships among learning, research, and clinical communities. The capacity to work across boundaries is critical to fulfilling the social missions of relating scientific knowledge to practice. But the process of translating research into practice is often characterized as linear and more straightforward in practice than it actually is. Understanding links between different research activities (e.g., basic science, technology evaluation, the testing of procedures, and audit of clinical practice) and their development will require greater engagement between groups. The problem is there are significant cultural barriers between people and insufficient opportunities for cross-boundary interaction. Because of the different perspectives of groups and individuals, what is needed are ways of ensuring a kind of "multicultural" communication between different perspectives.

The need for systemic development

Organizations can also help to develop links across the health system to better relate research, service, and educational communities. A group in Skåne suggested research and clinical groups should "promote regional networks for clinical research." Stronger links could be gained through "greater use of honorary academic titles." These kinds of approaches could help stimulate clinical research groups. Groups can play an important role in the development of research networks. They will provide a focus for clinicians with research questions, and academics with clinical concern.

People could be kept in touch with clinical research and development initiatives through regular conferences, and by email, which would support the dissemination of information across institutional boundaries and contribute to professional development across Skåne.

People need to be aware of conferences and about opportunities to join research activities. Researchers who are remote from clinical environments need to join these to ensure they are aware of clinical problems.

Activities like this are part of the necessary process to relate clinical and research perspectives. Some networks may need dedicated network coordinators to support development.

Conclusion

This chapter has outlined the challenges faced by European AHCs. A slow and gradual fragmenting of organizational priorities has weakened collaborations. There is great will to overcome this and an appreciation that bridges need to be built at several levels. Creating structural links between organizations will ease some pressures on management but will not alone guarantee that in 2010 AHCs in Europe will live up to the aspirations that senior management, clinicians, and researchers have for them. Academic health centers need urgently to address cultural fragmentation between clinical and preclinical perspectives. The cultural perspective from people in departments may help build new foundations for university clinical partnership.

REFERENCES

Dainton, F. (1981). *Reflections on the Universities and the NHS*. London: Nuffield Provincial Hospitals Trust.

Moss, F. and Smith, T. (2002). *Challenges to Academic Medicine: a UK Perspective*. London: UK University Hospitals Forum. Online at http://www.uhf.nhs.uk/publications/.

Smith, T. (2001). *University Clinical Partnership: a New Framework for NHS/University Relations*. London: The Stationary Office.

 (2003). *Developing Organizational Capacity for Clinical Research: Creating a Framework for University Clinical Partnerships in Skåne*. Report presented to Medical Faculty, Lund University Sweden.

Smith, T. and Davies, S. (2003). *Managing University Clinical Partnership: Key Organisational Issues in Relating Health Services, Teaching and Research*. Paris: Institute for Management in Higher Education.

Steering Group on Undergraduate Medical and Dental Education and Research (1994). *Report of the Steering Group on Undergraduate Medical and Dental Education and Research*. London: Department of Health. Online at http://www.info.doh.gov.uk/doh/coin4.nsf/page/ HSG-(96)21?OpenDocument.

Commentary

Haile T. Debas, M.D.

This chapter provides a graphic description of the strategic, management, and cultural fragmentation confronting the European AHC. The challenges facing European AHCs are not dissimilar to those experienced by their American counterparts with some significant differences. However, such comparisons and generalizations should be made with awareness that AHCs in the United States, as is probably also true in Europe, are different from each other.

In the United States, AHCs are made up of a medical school, a teaching hospital(s), which may or may not be owned by the university, and one or more allied professional schools (nursing, pharmacy, dentistry). Day-to-day governmental or political regulatory interferences are significantly less in the United States than in Europe because no national health system exists in the United States. Instead, managed care and market-driven payment mechanisms have provided the greatest challenge to American AHCs. Academic health centers in the United States have a cost structure typically 20 to 30 percent higher than community hospitals where education and research are not core missions.

Failure of the Clinton Health Plan and the institution of a market-driven health care payment system provided a serious threat to the existence of AHCs in the past decade, causing much structural fragmentation. In response, AHCs lowered their cost structure as much as they could and demanded higher clinical productivity of their faculty. Clinical faculty's time for teaching, research, and other scholarly activities became compromised. The number of NIH research grants awarded to medical schools in areas of the country with the highest managed care penetration declined, presumably because faculty had less time to write proposals.

However, a far greater dislocation of academic medicine occurred as a result of the survival strategies AHCs themselves chose to implement. Such

Haile T. Debas is Executive Director for Global Health Sciences and Chancellor and Dean Emeritus at the University of California San Francisco.

strategies included buying primary care networks and feeder community hospitals, merging with each other wholly or partly, or selling the university hospital to for-profit corporations such as Tenet and Columbia. Acquisition of primary care networks and hospitals largely proved to be an economic failure. Full mergers such as University of California San Francisco-Stanford, Pennsylvania State and Geisingher failed. Partial mergers such as Partners between the Massachusetts General and Brigham and Women's Hospital and between Columbia Presbyterian and New York Hospital have been more successful, but they are little more than holding companies. During the turmoil caused by managed care, AHCs in America saw a transformation of the job description of their department chairs and deans who, in addition to providing academic leadership, had to become financial managers of multimillion-dollar clinical enterprises.

Mr Smith describes management fragmentation in the European AHC. Management fragmentation exists in the American AHC for a different reason. In an attempt to become more business competitive, several prominent university-owned AHCs created a reporting structure in which the dean and the chief operation officer (CEO) were placed in potential rivalry, with the CEO reporting either directly to the university president or to a separate private board. This structural fragmentation proved untenable in several universities (Johns Hopkins, Chicago, UCLA, for example). They corrected the problem by making the dean vice president for clinical affairs, with the CEO reporting to the vice president. This restructuring realigned the academic and clinical enterprise missions of the hospitals and has served to show that management in academic centers is profoundly different from that in industry.

Mr Smith also describes the cultural fragmentation seen in European AHCs. Cultural differences between the basic science and clinical communities also exist in the United States and in all countries and are an important deterrent to the transfer of scientific advances from the bench to the bedside and back again. Smith describes Skåne's imaginative approach: the promotion of "regional networks for clinical research" as an initiative to bridge the chasm between the research and clinical communities.

In the United States, we have recognized that several structural and traditional causes contribute to creating the chasm between our basic science and clinical communities. The departmental structure creates silos and does not promote broad collaboration across departments. A problem common in basic science departments is the "all-too-important" principal investigator with his/her fiefdom of postdoctoral fellows and graduate students. In the clinical departments, funds flow issues and the considerable clinical income generated by some departments serve to harden the silos. The strategy that is now being followed in many American AHCs is to break down these silos by developing multidisciplinary programs in cancer, cardiovascular disease, human genetics, neurosciences, gastrointestinal diseases, and immunology. Many AHCs have met success with this approach including the University of California San Francisco (UCSF).

Curricular reforms in medical school can be used as a powerful method to bring together faculty from the basic science and clinical departments. The new UCSF curriculum integrates a significant part of the teaching in the first two years so that it is done as small group teaching by both clinicians and scientists. Similarly, basic sciences topics have been introduced in the third and fourth years again with the goal of not only providing an integrated curriculum, but also bringing together teachers from the basic science and clinical departments.

Some 18 years ago, the basic science departments organized themselves into the Program in Biological Sciences (PIBS), which is run as an executive committee of the basic science departments. All graduate student and faculty recruitment and the development of new programs are done through PIBS. The departments are still important in controlling space and faculty positions, but have ceded important responsibilities to PIBS in order to break departmental barriers. Our clinical departments have clinician scientists performing basic biomedical research. To create a bridge between them and the basic scientists in PIBS, a program in biomedical sciences (BMS) was created with membership from both groups. Both PIBS and BMS are grounded in graduate education.

Developing multidisciplinary programs in the clinical departments has been harder. The UCSF Comprehensive Cancer Center, the AIDS Research Institute, and the Wheeler Center for the Neurobiology of Addiction have been particularly successful in providing the environmental and core resources to integrate basic and clinical scientists, clinicians interested in population research and outcome studies, and clinicians and nurses interested in community outreach. Similarly, multidisciplinary centers and institutes in social and behavioral sciences and public health have been successful: The Center for Health and Community (CHC), The Institute for Health Policy Studies (IHPS) and The Institute for Global Health (IGH). A move towards this type of multidisciplinary organization is seen in many US AHCs.

In the United States, a misalignment exists between the organization of clinical service delivery and the needs and demand of an increasingly sophisticated public. Clinical delivery in AHCs has traditionally been physician centered and based on fragmented departmental services. The public wants a coordinated, "one stop" service. It is likely that in the twenty-first century, clinical care given by AHCs has to be patient and disease centered rather than discipline based. The challenge to AHCs is how to create these comprehensive care centers given the reluctance of major clinical departments with large clinical revenues. The one area AHCs have been successful in doing this is in the treatment of neoplastic disease in their Cancer Centers. An important reason for the success of Cancer Centers is federal funding through the National Cancer Institute.

Finally, US AHCs seek to differentiate themselves from their clinical competitors in community hospitals by providing complex tertiary and quaternary care. They see translational research as a growth area. The impact of being providers of complex care is the need to send students and residents far afield to obtain experience in primary and secondary care. This leads to strategic fragmentation in the United States not dissimilar to that drawn by Tom Smith in Figure 7.1.

In summary, although the causes and potential solutions of fragmentation may be different in the European and American AHCs, the problems and challenges are similar. Academic health centers must provide the environment for education, patient care and discovery in a collaborative fashion. As we seek the same goal, European and American AHCs have much to learn from each other.

Index

Note: page numbers in *italics* refer to figures and tables; those with suffix 'n' refer to footnotes.